Download Yo[ur]
Ebook With Supplemen[t]

MW01152487

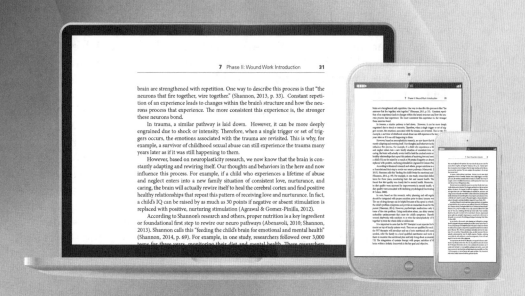

Your print purchase of *Advanced Public and Community Health Nursing Practice Population Assessment, Program Planning, and Evaluation,* Second Edition, **includes an ebook download** to the device of your choice— increasing accessibility, portability, and searchability!

Download your ebook today at: http://spubonline.com/communhealth and enter the access code below:

1P734HE7B

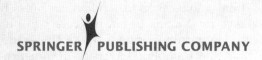

SPRINGER / PUBLISHING COMPANY

SPC

springerpub.com

Naomi E. Ervin, PhD, RN, PHCNS-BC, FNAP, FAAN, is board certified as a public health clinical nurse specialist. She earned her bachelor's degree in nursing, master's degree in public health, and PhD in education from the University of Michigan. She is a fellow in the National Academies of Practice and the American Academy of Nursing. Previously she served as president of the Association of Community Health Nursing Educators and of the Chicago Nurses Association. She is a recipient of the Ruth B. Freeman Distinguished Career Award for contributions to public health nursing presented by the Public Health Nursing Section of the American Public Health Association and the Pearl McIver Public Health Nurse Award presented by the American Nurses Association. Dr. Ervin had the opportunity to chair the task force that developed the first certification examination for the clinical specialist in public health nursing and to revise *Nursing's Social Policy Statement* in 2002–2003. As chair and a member of the Quad Council of Public Health Nursing Organizations, she was involved in revising the public health nursing standards and core competencies of public health nursing. Dr. Ervin's career in public and community health nursing spans from staff public health nurse to director of public health nursing of a large city health department. In her academic career, Dr. Ervin has held positions from assistant professor to endowed chair and professor. Her academic administrative positions include department head to director of a school of nursing. Throughout her career, she has been involved in research about the quality of public health nursing care and the use of evidence in public health nursing practice. Her work can be found in over 70 publications. She most recently held adjunct professor positions at two colleges of nursing.

Pamela A. Kulbok, DNSc, RN, PHNA-BC, FAAN, is the Theresa A. Thomas Professor of Primary Care Nursing and professor of public health sciences at the University of Virginia (UVA). She holds a bachelor's degree in nursing and a master's degree in community health nursing from Boston College. She earned her DNSc from Boston University and completed postdoctoral work in psychiatric epidemiology at Washington University. She is a fellow in the American Academy of Nursing. Dr. Kulbok received the 2016 Ruth B. Freeman Distinguished Career Award from the American Public Health Association, Public Health Nursing (PHN) Section. Previously, Dr. Kulbok served as chair of the Environmental and Public Health Expert Panel of the American Academy of Nursing, as a member of the Congress on Nursing Practice and Economics of the American Nurses Association (ANA), as president of the Association of Community Health Nursing Educators, and as chair of the Quad Council of PHN Organizations. In addition, she was a member of the ANA workgroup to revise the *Nursing Social Policy Statement* (2010) and was a member and chair of the ANA workgroups to revise *Public Health Nursing: Scope and Standards of Practice* (2007, 2013). She coordinated the public health nursing leadership track of the master of science in nursing (MSN) program at UVA from 1994 to 2017 and codirected two advanced education nursing training grants at UVA to prepare leaders in public health nursing and rural health nursing. Her funded research includes examination of adult and adolescent health behavior patterns and predictors, youth tobacco prevention, and community-based participatory research to design a substance use prevention program for rural youth. Her current research is focused on sustainable wellness and health behavior transitions from adolescence to adulthood. Her scholarly work includes more than 80 publications. Dr. Kulbok began her career in public health nursing as a visiting nurse. She held PHN faculty positions at the University of Illinois at Chicago, St. Louis University, and the Catholic University of America in Washington, DC.

Advanced Public and Community Health Nursing Practice

Population Assessment, Program Planning, and Evaluation

Second Edition

Naomi E. Ervin, PhD, RN, PHCNS-BC, FNAP, FAAN

Pamela A. Kulbok, DNSc, RN, PHNA-BC, FAAN

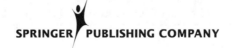

SPRINGER PUBLISHING COMPANY

Springer Publishing Company, LLC
11 West 42nd Street
New York, NY 10036
www.springerpub.com

Acquisitions Editor: Elizabeth Nieginski
Compositor: Graphic World

ISBN: 978-0-8261-3843-9
ebook ISBN: 978-0-8261-3844-6
Supplementary Material ISBN: 978-0-8261-2577-4

Supplementary Exemplars are available at springerpub.com/ervinkulbok2e

18 19 20 21 22 / 5 4 3 2 1

The author and the publisher of this Work have made every effort to use sources believed to be reliable to provide information that is accurate and compatible with the standards generally accepted at the time of publication. Because medical science is continually advancing, our knowledge base continues to expand. Therefore, as new information becomes available, changes in procedures become necessary. We recommend that the reader always consult current research and specific institutional policies before performing any clinical procedure. The author and publisher shall not be liable for any special, consequential, or exemplary damages resulting, in whole or in part, from the readers' use of, or reliance on, the information contained in this book. The publisher has no responsibility for the persistence or accuracy of URLs for external or third-party Internet websites referred to in this publication and does not guarantee that any content on such websites is, or will remain, accurate or appropriate.

Library of Congress Cataloging-in-Publication Data

Names: Ervin, Naomi E., author. | Kulbok, Pamela A., author.
Title: Advanced public and community health nursing practice: population
   assessment, program planning, and evaluation / Naomi E. Ervin, Pamela Kulbok.
Other titles: Advanced community health nursing practice
Description: Second edition. | New York, NY: Springer Publishing Company,
   LLC, [2018] | Preceded by Advanced community health nursing practice /
   Naomi E. Ervin. c2002. | Includes bibliographical references and index.
Identifiers: LCCN 2017052270 | ISBN 9780826138439 (hardcover : alk. paper) |
   ISBN 9780826138446 (e-book) | ISBN 9780826125774 (Instructor's material)
Subjects: | MESH: Community Health Nursing | Public Health Nursing |
   Community Health Services | Needs Assessment | Health Services Needs
   and Demand | Program Evaluation
Classification: LCC RT98 | NLM WY 106 | DDC 610.73/43—dc23
LC record available at https://lccn.loc.gov/2017052270

Contact us to receive discount rates on bulk purchases.
We can also customize our books to meet your needs.
For more information please contact: sales@springerpub.com

Printed in the United States of America.

To public health nurses everywhere who work to maintain and promote health

Contents

Contributors

Sue Ellen Bell, PhD, RN, PHN, APRN, CNS
Professor
School of Nursing
Minnesota State University, Mankato
Mankato, Minnesota

Julia Muennich Cowell, PhD, RN, PHNA-BC, FAAN
Executive Editor, *The Journal of School Nursing*
Professor Emerita
College of Nursing
Rush University
Chicago, Illinois

Joan E. Kub, PhD, MA, PHCNS-BC, FAAN
Adjunct Professor
Department of Nursing
Suzanne Dworak-Peck School of Social Work
University of Southern California
Los Angeles, California

Paul L. Kuehnert, DNP, RN, FAAN
Assistant Vice President
Robert Wood Johnson Foundation
Princeton, New Jersey

Pamela F. Levin, PhD, PHNA-BC
Professor
Community, Systems, Mental Health Nursing
College of Nursing
Rush University
Chicago, Illinois

Diane B. McNaughton, PhD, PHNA-BC
Associate Professor
College of Nursing
Rush University
Chicago, Illinois

Preface

Since the first edition of *Advanced Public and Community Health Nursing Practice* was published, it has been a challenge for nurses to keep up with the tremendous amount of information and data generated every day. Healthcare delivery system reforms initiated by the Patient Protection and Affordable Care Act emphasized the health of populations and social determinants of health; these areas are central to public/community health nursing practice. Throughout these reforms, public/community health nursing has retained focus on the core foundations of practice: social justice, interdisciplinary practice, community involvement, disease prevention, and health promotion. The core processes of community assessment, program planning, implementation, and evaluation remain relevant to advanced public/community health nursing practice. These processes are also useful for advanced practice nursing roles in many community settings. Incorporating these foundations into the second edition, *Advanced Public and Community Health Nursing Practice* will assist graduate students in public/community health nursing and other nursing specialties who focus on population health to become competent advanced practice nurses.

Content of this book is organized into six sections. The chapters in Section I provide the learner with an introduction to public/community health nursing specialty practice and foundations for this advanced level of practice. Section II provides the depth of knowledge needed by the advanced practice nurse to competently conduct community assessments. In Section III, the five chapters take the learner through the steps needed to develop coherent and high-quality program plans. Section IV provides the learner with the necessary information to implement program plans at the individual, group, or community level. The five chapters of Section V address program evaluation in depth, providing detailed content on how to develop an evaluation plan and revise programs. The one chapter in Section VI directs the learner's attention to graduate preparation in public/community health nursing as well as to the leadership role in creating a professional practice environment.

Updated content is provided throughout the text. Suggested clinical or practicum activities that assist the learner to apply the content in a variety of ways and settings are new to this edition. Throughout the text, there are examples of actual programs or projects conducted by advanced public/community health nurses.

We sincerely hope that this textbook helps you, the learner, gain knowledge and skills needed for advanced public/community health nursing practice in the evolving healthcare system. Please let us know what you think. **Open access through Springer's website allows readers to view exemplars based on essential content in various book chapters that contain discussion questions related to the textbook. Go to springerpub.com/ ervinkulbok2e.**

Naomi E. Ervin
Pamela A. Kulbok

SECTION I

Public/Community Health Nursing
at the Specialty Advanced Level

CHAPTER 1

Introduction to Advanced Public and Community Health Nursing Practice

■ STUDY EXERCISES

1. Define and describe the key components of advanced practice.
2. How are the key components of advanced practice incorporated into advanced public/community health nursing practice?
3. How does the focus of advanced public/community health nursing practice relate to health?
4. How are the core processes of advanced public/community health nursing practice related to the health of the public?
5. What are the models of advanced public/community health nursing practice? Describe one model.
6. How does the advanced practice public/community health nurse incorporate elements of interdisciplinary practice into practice?
7. Why are leadership skills important to advanced practice?

The terms *community health nursing* and *public health nursing* are often used interchangeably to indicate the specialty of nursing that has the community or population as the focus of practice. In this textbook, public/community health nursing is used for both terms. The term *public health nursing* has become more widely used since the first edition of this book was published and is often used to refer to nursing practiced in official public health agencies. The term community health nursing remains in wide use, whereas the term *population health nursing* is being seen more frequently in the titles of courses and graduate programs and advocated by some authors as the new name for public health nursing (Canales & Drevdahl, 2014).

This book contains required content for the preparation of specialists in public/community health nursing and builds on knowledge acquired at the undergraduate level. Incorporating content from biostatistics, epidemiology, and other public health sciences as well as nursing, advanced practice public/community health nurses seek to apply a synthesis of nursing and public health knowledge and skills to maintain and improve the health of communities. Thus, this book provides major parts of the core content for advanced public/community health nursing practice that focus on the community or populations, prevention of disease and injury, health promotion, and comprehensive care for maintaining and/or improving a community's health. This book is also a resource for graduate-level degree programs, such as master of science in nursing (MSN or MS) and doctor of nursing practice (DNP), that prepare nurse practitioners or clinical nurse specialists with an emphasis on community or population assessment, program planning, and program evaluation.

■ DEFINING ADVANCED PUBLIC/COMMUNITY HEALTH NURSING AS A SPECIALTY

Advanced public/community health nursing is a nursing specialty and is classified as advanced through graduate-level preparation in the field (APRN Consensus Work Group, 2008). Advanced practice within public/community health nursing is specifically related to the essential areas of graduate study (Levin et al., 2008) listed in Box 1.1. Advancement, which includes both specialization and expansion, is accomplished through formal course work; clinical practicums in public/community health nursing areas with qualified preceptors; and the completion of a scholarly project, thesis, or major paper in the specialty.

In addition, specialization in public/community health nursing involves course content and clinical practice in public/community health nursing administration, organizational theory, management theory, and fiscal operations. Grant writing and administration skills are needed for most positions that have a population or community focus.

■ DEFINING ADVANCED PUBLIC/COMMUNITY HEALTH NURSING PRACTICE

Throughout the past few decades, four professional organizations have defined and shaped the structure of public/community health nursing practice through publication of definitions, standards, white papers, resolutions, and other documents: the American

---

BOX 1.1 CRITICAL CONTENT AREAS FOR ADVANCED PRACTICE PUBLIC HEALTH NURSING

- Advanced nursing practice
- Population-centered nursing theory and practice
- Interdisciplinary practice
- Leadership
- Systems thinking
- Biostatistics
- Epidemiology
- Environmental health sciences
- Health policy and management
- Social and behavioral sciences
- Public health informatics
- Genomics
- Health communication
- Cultural competence
- Community-based participatory research
- Global health
- Policy and law
- Public health ethics

Source: Levin, P., Cary, A., Kulbok, P., Leffers, J., Molle, M., & Polivka, B. (2008). Graduate education in public health nursing: At the crossroads. *Public Health Nursing, 25*(2), 176–193. Used with permission John Wiley & Sons, Inc.

Nurses Association (ANA), the Public Health Nursing Section of the American Public Health Association (APHA), the Association of Community Health Nursing Educators (ACHNE), and the National League for Nursing. The Public Health Nursing Section of the APHA has been prominent among the organizations in providing leadership to bring order to the confusion of defining the specialty of public/community health nursing. Thus, the latest definition of public health nursing from this organization is presented.

Advanced public/community health nursing practice requires the synthesis of public health sciences and nursing science in order to promote the health of the community (APHA, 2013). Although the advanced practice public/community health nurse may be responsible for only a specific subcomponent of the community, such as enrollees in a health maintenance organization or mothers and children enrolled in a local health department program, the focus of the nurse's practice is to promote and protect the health of the entire community or population.

The following definition applies to advanced public/community health nursing practice as used in this book. The Public Health Nursing Section of the APHA developed the following definition in 1996 (APHA, 1996), and affirmed it in 2013: "Public health nursing is the practice of promoting and protecting the health of populations using knowledge from nursing, social, and public health sciences" (APHA, 2013, p. 2).

This definition of public/community health nursing does not explicitly indicate the level of practice, generalist or advanced, or the education required to practice within the scope of these definitions. However, this book takes the view that this statement defines a specialty level of practice that requires a master's or doctoral degree.

In public/community health nursing, the application of theory, principles, skills, and resources is on a continuum from the individual to the population. All nurses within the field of practice are held to the same standards according to their level, that is, generalist or specialist, or type of practice, such as public health, home healthcare, or school health.

The nurse prepared at the graduate level in public/community health nursing is designated as a specialist. Practice aimed at care of the community is advanced practice in public/community health nursing. In generalist practice, the nurse has knowledge and skills to care for individuals, families, and groups and beginning skills for some aspects of aggregate care. The minimum educational preparation for this practice is a baccalaureate degree in nursing. Figure 1.1 demonstrates the differences in division of practice between the generalist and the specialist (Kuehnert, 1995), with the specialist-level positions of

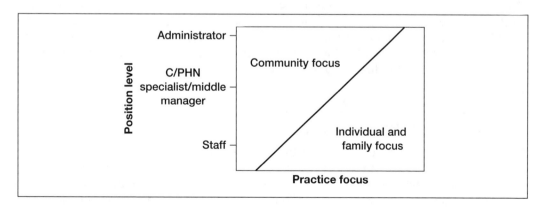

FIGURE 1.1 Focus of practice.

Source: Adapted from Kuehnert, P. L. (1995). The interactive and organizational model of community as client: A model for public health nursing. *Public Health Nursing, 12*(1), 11. Used with permission John Wiley & Sons, Inc.

clinical specialist, supervisor, and administrator having increasing focus of practice on the community as a whole. If a specialist is responsible for community-level programs, the practice would incorporate more focus on the community than indicated in Figure 1.1.

The Quad Council of Public Health Nursing Organizations competencies for public health nursing reflect the differences in generalist and specialist in three tiers of practice. Tier 1 competencies apply to generalist practice, whereas tiers 2 and 3 apply to practice at specialist levels (Swider, Krothe, Reyes, & Cravetz, 2013).

The definition of public/community health nursing has two key components: (a) promoting and preserving the health of populations, and (b) synthesis of knowledge from nursing and public health. These skills are acquired through graduate education and clinical experience.

Promoting and preserving the health of populations implies that the nurse will use knowledge about health promotion and prevention of disease and injury. Educational preparation for advanced practice provides the nurse with knowledge and skills to develop and evaluate population-level programs and services. The process of graduate education also provides nurses with educational experiences to synthesize knowledge from nursing and public health. Putting the two areas of knowledge together, however, requires clinical experience.

This depiction of practice is not to indicate that the specialist never takes care of an individual or a family. On the contrary, because the specialist is qualified to practice across the spectrum from individual to population, this nurse's practice may contain aspects of all client groups. For example, the nurse who is a family nurse practitioner often has a caseload of individuals and families seen for primary care. A second aspect of the practice may be a group of elderly individuals living in a housing unit. A third part of practice may be planning programs for a community health center's service area. Another component of advanced practice is working with others to achieve goals for a healthy community, which requires a wide span of knowledge and skills in areas such as human behavior, management, leadership, and communications. Successfully combining these aspects of a role is a challenge for advanced practice public/community health nurses.

Related Practice Areas

The practice areas of home healthcare, occupational health nursing, and school nursing also use the core knowledge and skills at the advanced level to focus on populations, subpopulations, communities, or aggregates. The roles of family nurse practitioner, community health nurse practitioner, school nurse practitioner, and occupational health nurse practitioner are included in public/community health nursing practice because of the belief by experts that primary care must be provided within the context of the community (Marion, 1996). More recent, the integration of primary care and public health has been promoted (Institute of Medicine [IOM], 2012).

Settings and Positions for Advanced Practice Public/Community Health Nurses

Settings for practice and positions held by advanced practice public/community health nurses are numerous and diverse. Titles vary a great deal. For example, in public health units, advanced practice public/community health nurses may have titles such as director of patient services, assistant commissioner of health, public health consultant, public health clinical nurse specialist, or public health nursing supervisor. In some states, nurses hold the top positions in local and state health departments with titles such as commissioner of health or director of public health.

As mentioned earlier, nurses who are prepared as nurse practitioners in school health, occupational health, community primary care, and family primary care often hold positions that require skills in community assessment, program planning, and program evaluation. These positions may have nurse practitioner titles with added responsibilities for program-level activities.

In managed care settings, the title may be director of patient services, vice president for patient services, director of community services, or director of community outreach. Case management is currently prevalent in many settings, including managed care, inpatient units, and home care, so titles dealing with case management are common. Usually, the advanced practice public/community health nurse is not a case manager but the director of a case management unit or a home care coordination unit.

In home healthcare agencies, advanced practice public/community health nurses may direct the operations of an agency and have titles such as chief executive officer, president, or chief operating officer. Other positions may be middle management, such as coordinator, supervisor, or director of specific programs. Another area for advanced practice skills is in quality assessment and improvement in any setting in public health and community health.

Nonprofit organizations provide opportunities for advanced practice public/community health nurses to use their skills in working with populations and communities. Positions may be available with titles such as program director, program coordinator, executive director, program specialist, or president.

Advanced practice public/community health nurses are also entrepreneurs who develop their own healthcare businesses. Consulting firms, community nursing centers, private practice, and home healthcare agencies are some businesses operated by public/community health nurses.

■ MODELS OF ADVANCED PUBLIC/COMMUNITY HEALTH NURSING PRACTICE

As mentioned earlier, the definition of public/community health nursing and public health nursing does not specifically state that the practice level is advanced. Likewise, most models of public/community health nursing practice do not specify the level of practice. In keeping with current professional standards that advanced practice requires graduate-level preparation, the models of practice in this section are introduced as those for the advanced practice public/community health nurse. The baccalaureate-prepared nurse may undertake some of the responsibilities of advanced practice, especially if there are no master's- or doctoral-prepared nurses in the agency, but the total role of advanced practice as depicted in the models requires graduate preparation.

Three models of advanced public/community health nursing practice were selected because of their potential for guiding practice: Anderson and McFarlane's (2015) community-as-partner model, Helvie's (1998) energy theory, and the integrative model for holistic community health nursing (Laffrey & Kulbok, 1999). Nurses have different practice styles and practice settings differ, so one model may be preferred to the others.

Community-as-Partner Model

Anderson and McFarlane's (2015) practice model places the nurse in partnership with the community and encompasses the philosophy of primary healthcare. The community-as-partner model was developed to encompass the definition of public health nursing as the synthesis of public health and nursing. The model consists of two central features: a focus on the community, which is represented by the community assessment wheel, and the use of the nursing process (Figure 1.2).

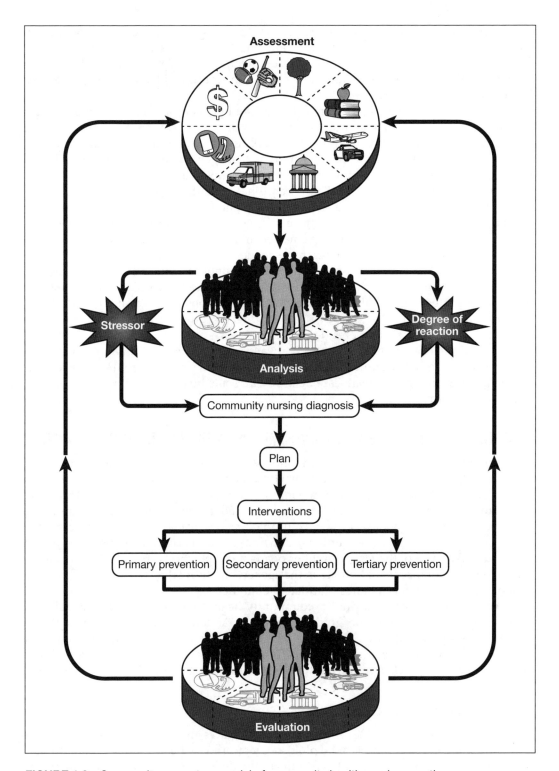

FIGURE 1.2 Community-as-partner model of community health nursing practice.

Source: Anderson, E. T., & McFarlane, J. (2015). Community assessment: Using a model for practice. In E. T. Anderson & J. McFarlane (Eds.), *Community as partner: Theory and practice in nursing* (7th ed., p. 168). Philadelphia, PA: Wolters Kluwer. Copyright © 2015 by Wolters Kluwer. Used with permission.

THE COMMUNITY-ASSESSMENT WHEEL

The community-assessment wheel provides a framework for organizing a community assessment. The wheel consists of two major parts: the core and eight subsystems. The core of the model represents the community residents who are described by demographics, values, beliefs, and history. The eight subsystems are physical environment, education, safety and transportation, politics and government, health and social services, communication, economics, and recreation. Community residents are affected by and influence the eight community subsystems.

A community is surrounded by its normal line of defense, which is the level of health obtained by the community members. Examples of the normal line of defense are characteristics such as low infant mortality or a high immunization rate among children. The flexible line of defense is "a 'buffer zone' representing a dynamic level of health resulting from a temporary response to stressors" (Anderson & McFarlane, 2015, p. 170). An example of an environmental stressor is flooding. How the community mobilizes to control damage is a temporary response to the flooding condition.

The eight subsystems are divided by broken lines to indicate that they both influence and are influenced by one another. There are the lines of resistance, or internal mechanisms within the community that defend against stressors. These strengths of the community are represented by lines of resistance throughout each subsystem.

In the community-as-partner model, stressors are tension-producing stimuli that may potentially cause disequilibrium in the system. Stressors, which may come from within or outside the community, penetrate the flexible and normal lines of defense, causing disruption of the community. The amount of disruption or disequilibrium is known as the *degree of reaction*. Using the community-assessment wheel is addressed in Chapters 4, 7, and 8.

THE NURSING PROCESS IN THE COMMUNITY-AS-PARTNER MODEL

The components of the wheel are used as parameters for data collection for a community assessment. The nurse analyzes data with the community, which leads to the development of community health diagnoses. The advanced practice public/community health nurse derives goals for interventions from stressors by using the community health diagnoses. Interventions are planned to strengthen the lines of resistance or to alleviate the stressors.

Primary, secondary, or tertiary prevention interventions are designed to meet the specific assessed conditions of the community. Primary prevention interventions are used to strengthen the lines of defense so that stressors cannot penetrate them. Immunization of preschool-age children is an example of a primary prevention intervention. Secondary prevention interventions are used after a stressor has entered the community in order to support the lines of defense and resistance to minimize the degree of reaction to the stressor. An example of a secondary prevention intervention is an epidemiological investigation and implementing a disease control plan in a situation of an outbreak of a vaccine-preventable disease like measles. After the stressor has penetrated the lines of defense and a degree of reaction has taken place, tertiary prevention is applied. A quarantine of children with measles in a community is an example of application of a tertiary prevention intervention to prevent further spread of the disease.

Evaluation is the last step in the nursing process as part of the community-as-partner model of practice. Feedback from the community provides a major part of evaluation of the community health nurse's interventions. Parameters used for the assessment often provide criteria to use for the evaluation.

Helvie's Energy Theory

The energy theory developed by Carl O. Helvie (1998) is a systems theory that is used in conjunction with the nursing process to assess a community, plan nursing care, intervene for improving community health, and evaluate the results. This conceptualization is depicted in Figure 1.3. In this theory, the underlying concept of energy is defined as the capacity to do work. Energy is used to describe activity and capabilities of communities and individuals.

The theory incorporates the four major concepts of the nursing metaparadigm: humans, environment, health, and nursing. When using the theory for advanced practice, *humans* refer to the community population being given nursing care, *environment* means both the internal environment of the community (the subsystems) and the external environment (the suprasystem), *health* is that of the community population, and *nursing* is the work of

The client	The health focus	The goal
Aggregate or community	Balanced energies; deficit of energies	Maintain or regain balance of energies

The nursing process			
Assess	**Plan**	**Implement**	**Evaluate**
1. Community a. Balance b. Deficit (resulting from part energy exchanges) 2. Energy exchanges a. Balance b. Deficit c. Basis for exchange 3. Nursing diagnosis 4. Supported by a. Indicators of community performance b. Population statistics (effect of community performance) c. Population surveys d. Standards	1. Maintain or regain balanced energies 2. Objectives a. Aggregate or community b. Activity c. Time frame d. Standard 3. Planned activity	1. Community plan energies a. Maintain b. Increase c. Decrease	1. Goal met 2. Objectives met 3. Reassess energies 4. Terminate process

FIGURE 1.3 Nursing process and community energy theory.

Source: Helvie, C. O. (1998). *Advanced practice nursing in the community*. Thousand Oaks, CA: Sage. Used by permission of Sage Publications, Inc.

the advanced practice nurse who focuses on the total community or aggregates to improve its health.

The theory encompasses "community subsystems such as health, education, and economics as energy subsystems because of the work expended by both the provider and the recipient of services" (Helvie, 1998, p. 24). The community population, or human system, is viewed as a changing energy field that both affects and is affected through exchanges with the other energies in the environment. The exchanges may be internal, as with air, water, food, or services, or external, as exchanges with state and national resources. Past and present exchanges, and the balance achieved by the exchanges, influence the health of the population and determine the placement of the populations on an energy or health continuum. The continuum may range from high energy (high-level wellness) to low energy (poor health).

In using the energy theory, the nurse assesses and compares past and present balances with those of other energy systems (e.g., a state or the nation). Placement on the continuum is determined by an assessment that uses health statistics and information about subsystems. Nursing diagnoses that result from the community assessment are written in energy terms; this approach is explained in Chapter 7.

The Integrative Model for Holistic Community Health Nursing

The integrative model was developed by Laffrey and Kulbok (1999) to expand holistic nursing to the community as client. The model allows nursing care to focus on any level, individual, family, aggregate, and community, "with the awareness that each is part of the unified whole" (Laffrey & Kulbok, 1999, p. 88). The model is based on two interrelated and continuous dimensions: focus of care and client system. The three foci of care are health promotion; illness, disease, or disability prevention; and illness care. Health promotion is the central focus of the model, indicating that all interventions are aimed at optimizing health (Figure 1.4). "The community health nurse's primary concern is promotion of optimal health as it is defined with and by the client" (Laffrey & Kulbok, 1999, p. 92). Health promotion encompasses both prevention and illness care. With this approach to care, the nurse is contributing to health promotion even when care is aimed at alleviating or preventing illness or injury. For example, when the nurse provides relief from pain through teaching meditation or relaxation techniques, the client has gained skills for promoting health in general.

In the integrative model, it is important to view the levels of clients as parts of the whole rather than viewing the specific part with which one is concerned as the whole system. The client system is continuous from the individual-as-client to the community-as-client. Thus, when working with an individual, the context or environment of care includes the family, aggregate, and community. "The mutual human/environment interaction affects the planning of care for the client either directly or indirectly by intervening on the client's behalf with one or more aspects of the environment" (Laffrey & Kulbok, 1999, p. 93).

This model of advanced public/community health nursing practice provides a framework to facilitate and organize care at multiple levels—individual, family, aggregate, and community—with various foci of care. Participation of the client is a key basis of practice with this model. One nurse cannot provide care to all levels, so a team approach is essential to meet the needs of the total community.

■ MAINTAINING THE FOCUS OF PRACTICE

Making the community or population the focus of practice requires the nurse to synthesize knowledge from both the general and specific areas of graduate nursing study. The advanced practice public/community health nurse is charged with providing care to an

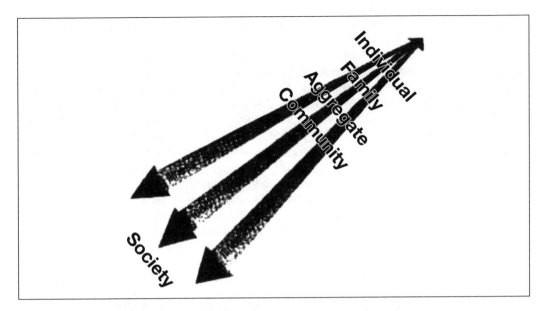

FIGURE 1.4 The integrative model for holistic community health nursing.

Source: Laffrey, S. C., & Kulbok, P. A. (1999). An integrative model for holistic community health nursing. *Journal of Holistic Nursing, 17*(1), 92. Copyright © 1999 by SAGE Publications. Reprinted by permission of SAGE Publications. doi:10.1177/ 089801019901700107

entire population, which may seem overwhelming unless you recall that it is the conceptual ideas that drive the practice, not the ability for one person to give care to an entire population. In fact, the advanced practice public/community health nurse is often part of a team that is responsible for the health of an entire community or population.

In practice, a population focus means that the advanced practice public/community health nurse considers the health of the entire group (community, subpopulation, or aggregate) when developing programs and interventions to solve or prevent health problems. Programs and services are designed and provided for all people in the population, which is usually defined by geographic boundaries, not just those who choose to come for care or for those who can afford a specific type of care. Although the focus of a specific program may be a subgroup of the population, the program contributes to the goal of a healthy community.

In order to maintain the focus of practice at the community level, the advanced practice public/community health nurse must acquire key knowledge and skills in the areas of community assessment, program planning, program implementation, and program evaluation. Brief descriptions of these processes are presented next.

■ UNDERSTANDING THE CORE PROCESSES OF ADVANCED PRACTICE

The four processes that form the core of advanced public/community health nursing practice are community assessment, program planning, program implementation, and program evaluation. These processes are the same as described in the practice models earlier. The challenge for the advanced practice public/community health nurse is to make the shift from applying the processes to care of the individual to care of the community.

The advanced practice public/community health nurse often undertakes the four processes with collaboration and cooperation from the community and appropriate teams. Team membership will vary depending on many factors, including the sources of funding, mission of the organization, level of community ability, and available resources. A brief description of each process is presented next to provide you with a conceptual map for navigating the concepts of advanced public/community health nursing practice. Box 1.2 summarizes the basic differences in the specialist and generalist roles with regard to focus of practice, processes used in practice, and practice models. The core processes of advanced public/community health nursing practice are discussed in depth in the chapters that follow.

Community Assessment

The community assessment process is composed of data collection, data analysis, synthesis of data, and community diagnosis. Section II of this book contains details about the four components of the community assessment process. *Data collection* is the gathering of pertinent quantitative and qualitative information, statistics, data, and facts about the status of a population or community. Although the description implies that this is an ongoing activity, usually the advanced practice nurse works with others to complete or update an assessment at regular intervals, perhaps once a year or every 2 to 3 years. For example, with the implementation of the Patient Protection and Affordable Care Act (ACA, 2010), nonprofit hospitals must meet new community benefit requirements to retain their nonprofit status (James, 2016). Nonprofit hospitals are mandated to complete a community health needs assessment (CHNA) every 3 years. The advanced practice public/community health nurse may be part of a community team responsible for updating the community assessment. However, just as care of an individual involves continuous updating of the assessment database, the care of a community requires that the public/community health nurse remain current about community changes. The second component of the community assessment process is analysis of data. *Data analysis* is the cognitive process of ordering data to allow for the higher level function of synthesis. *Data synthesis*, the third component, is the process of combining elements from several data sources to create a coherent whole or a new, complete picture of what is known or unknown (Grove, Burns, & Gray, 2012).

BOX 1.2 BASIC DIFFERENCES IN SPECIALIST AND GENERALIST ROLES		
Component of Practice	**Specialist**	**Generalist**
Focus of practice	Communities and populations	Individuals and families
Practice models	Advanced practice models	Comprehensive care of individuals and families
Processes	Community assessment, program planning, program implementation, and program evaluation	Assessing, diagnosing, planning, intervening, and evaluating

Data and information need to be examined while applying the knowledge of the public health sciences and the research, theories, and models from nursing. Effective analysis and synthesis are based on the skills of the nurse, but involvement of other team members and community residents is essential in order to obtain a broad perspective and to avoid the domination of the process by professionals.

Community diagnoses, or statements of the conclusions from data analysis and synthesis, are the fourth component of the community assessment process. Community diagnoses are problems, strengths, trends, and situations about communities that may or may not require intervention. If community diagnoses are done thoroughly and objectively, their statements provide a picture of a community.

Program Planning

In program planning, the advanced practice public/community health nurse addresses one or more of the situations identified in the community assessment process. Program planning is covered extensively in Section III. The process of developing programs is usually an interdisciplinary or interprofessional endeavor that involves community members who provide guidance needed to tailor a program for them. Effectiveness of programs is increased when the specifics of interventions are culturally accurate, gender and age specific, and based on research. The ACA provides another relevant example related to the need for program planning and the role of the advanced public/community health nurse. Nonprofit hospitals must also complete a community health improvement plan (CHIP) to address health and social problems that were identified in the community. Nonprofit hospitals must plan for a community benefit that goes beyond their basic provision of services to the community. The advanced practice nurse with preparation in public/community health nursing has the requisite program planning knowledge and skills to lead and collaborate with interprofessional teams in the creation of meaningful health improvement plans for their local community.

Program Implementation

In the third core process of practice, program implementation, the results of the assessment and program plan are put in place. Section IV addresses major aspects of program implementation. An implementation plan and careful monitoring of the process can help to ensure that the program is implemented accurately. Usually, staff must be recruited, oriented, and supervised in order to develop the skills required in the new program. If the program plan is not detailed enough to allow for smooth implementation, adjustments will be needed as the program is put in place.

Program Evaluation

Program evaluation is the process of examining the effectiveness of a program. Section V focuses on program evaluation and how to conduct a program evaluation. The results of program evaluation are used to make revisions in the program, if they are indicated, or to make adjustments for better performance. The advanced practice public/community health nurse is interested in the health of a community or population, so program evaluation includes aggregate- or community-level measures of effectiveness.

The processes of community assessment, program planning, implementation, and evaluation are cyclical and ongoing. A comprehensive community assessment conducted by an advanced public/community health nurse in partnership with community-based organizations and local citizens is vital. The assessment focuses on multiple determinants of health that are addressed in later chapters. These determinants, or indicators, are useful in the subsequent steps of developing program objectives and establishing program evaluation procedures.

■ UNDERSTANDING THE CORE PUBLIC HEALTH FUNCTIONS

In 1986, a study was undertaken at the Institute of Medicine by the Committee for the Study of the Future of Public Health to address a growing perception that "this nation has lost sight of its public health goals and has allowed the system of public health activities to fall into disarray" (IOM, 1988, p. 1). The results of that study were published in 1988 in the report, *The Future of Public Health*. One recommendation in the report was that all public health agencies should carry out three core functions: assessment, policy development, and assurance. These three core functions were affirmed in the 2003 IOM update on the 1988 report in a publication titled *The Future of the Public's Health in the 21st Century* (IOM, 2003).

Many public health units throughout the country implemented the recommendations given in this report. Over past decades, these core public health functions have become a part of the advanced practice role for public/community health nurses, especially in official public health agencies. Changes in the public health system affect other segments of the healthcare system, so it is important that nurses understand the core functions as well as the implications these have for advanced practice. All advanced practice public/community health nurses need to become familiar with these functions of public health because all healthcare agencies collaborate with public health to fulfill the core functions.

Assessment

One of *The Future of Public Health* report recommendations was that every public health agency regularly and systematically collect, assemble, analyze, and make available information about the health of the community.

The recommendation at the federal public health level specifically includes support of knowledge development and dissemination through data collection, research, and information sharing. State public health responsibilities include assessment of health needs in the state on the basis of statewide data collection. Local public health agencies are given the responsibility to assess, monitor, and conduct surveillance of local health problems and needs as well as the resources for addressing them.

Advanced practice public/community health nurses may perform assessment functions as part of their roles or work with others to carry out the core public health function of assessment. Nurses may hold positions at the local, state, and federal levels that require them to have the knowledge and skills to perform assessments. In addition, many health agencies work with public health agencies to develop a broad understanding of the health of communities.

Policy Development

The Committee for the Study of the Future of Public Health recommended that every public health agency should exercise responsibility "in the development of comprehensive public health policies by promoting use of the scientific knowledge base in decision-making about public health and by leading in developing public health policy" (IOM, 1988, p. 8). The 2003 IOM report went a step further to recommend that research be funded "to guide policy decisions that shape public health practice" (IOM, 2003, p. 9).

For the federal level of public health, these policy development responsibilities included the establishment of national health objectives and priorities and the encouragement of debate on interstate and national public health issues. It was recommended that states assure an adequate statutory base for health activities in the state as well as establishment of overall state health objectives. Local public health units were given the responsibility to lead and foster local involvement and a sense of ownership in policy development.

Advanced practice public/community health nurses have numerous opportunities to be involved in policy development. Some of this role is discussed in Chapter 21. Nurses may hold policy positions or influence policy development and change at all three levels of the healthcare system. Being aware of how to become involved and becoming active in policy development are key parts of the advanced practice role.

Assurance

The core public health function of assurance involves making certain that necessary services are provided to reach the agreed-upon goals by encouraging private sector action, requiring private sector action, or directly providing services.

For the federal level of action, recommendations from *The Future of Public Health* report included providing technical assistance and funds to states and local units so that they can strengthen their capacities for services. The federal level is also responsible for assuring actions and services that are in the public interest of the entire nation, such as control of communicable diseases.

States are recommended to assure appropriate organized statewide efforts to develop and maintain essential personal, educational, and environmental health services; provide access to necessary services; and solve problems antithetical to health. The state public health units are also charged with guaranteeing a minimum set of essential health services and supporting local service capacity.

The Committee on the Future of Public Health recommended that local public health units ensure the availability and accessibility of high-quality services for the protection of public health of all people in the community. Furthermore, local units are responsible for seeing that the community receives appropriate consideration in the allocation of federal, state, and local resources for public health. Informing the community about how to obtain services and how to comply with public health requirements also falls within the assurance core function at the local level.

Advanced practice public/community health nurses are involved in many assurance activities, from assisting with planning-needed services to evaluating services provided by various agencies. The quality assessment and improvement activities of many healthcare agencies are also part of the assurance core function of public health.

■ UNDERSTANDING THE INTERDISCIPLINARY NATURE OF ADVANCED PRACTICE

The field of public health has evolved into a mix of workers, including nurses, physicians, dentists, health educators, sanitarians, epidemiologists, attorneys, economists, political scientists, social workers, engineers, and many others. Much of public health practice is carried out in teamwork. The specific healthcare team varies greatly depending on the setting, the client focus, and the type of agency. Thus, the advanced practice public/community health nurse should expect to interact with numerous individuals, both lay and professionally trained.

Interdisciplinary practice refers to different professions working together in a coordinated manner to address various aspects of patient care or community care. Studies have demonstrated the benefits of interdisciplinary care for some types of patients, for example, geriatric and infant patients, including greater patient satisfaction, decreased cost, fewer hospitalizations, and lower infant mortality rates (Baldwin, 1996). In contrast to interdisciplinary practice, multidisciplinary practice refers to aspects of patient or community care addressed independently by appropriate providers from different professions. The care is not integrated, but the problems are divided and handled in parallel with providers responsible for their own areas of expertise (Walker et al., 1998).

Interprofessional practice is sometimes used instead of interdisciplinary practice. The World Health Organization has defined *interprofessional collaborative practice* as multiple health workers from different professional backgrounds providing "comprehensive services by working with patients, their families, carers and communities to deliver the highest quality of care across settings" (Hopkins, 2010, p. 13). In some settings in which public/ community health nurses practice, staff may consist of both professionals and nonprofessionals such as community health workers or lay community members. In these instances, the term *multidisciplinary* may be used as a more accurate term. For the purposes of this text, the terms will be used interchangeably or as the context implies.

Acquiring the Knowledge and Skills for Interdisciplinary Practice

Interdisciplinary work requires that the members of each discipline know its strengths and limitations. Often, conflict arises when two disciplines have overlapping practice boundaries, for example, family practice physicians and family nurse practitioners or social workers and public health nurses. Competent skills in collaboration or the ability to work jointly will assist the advanced practice nurse to develop and maintain the relationships needed to care for the community. In addition to being able to work with other professionals, it is important that advanced practice public/community health nurses are able to work with community members.

In addition to knowing one's own discipline, effective interdisciplinary practice requires knowledge of other disciplines. This knowledge may be acquired in practice, by reading or group work, but preferably through formal education in interdisciplinary or interprofessional courses. Being familiar with the content of other disciplines is a manifestation of courtesy and respect for others' professions.

The nurse must be competent in interpersonal relations and have good communication skills in order for her or him to be effective in interdisciplinary practice. Interpersonal competence is recognition of the skill and distinctiveness of all individuals involved. "It encompasses and includes a flexible, nonhierarchical stance with open communication both verbally and nonverbally." Competence in communication is part of interpersonal skill and encompasses "a fine-tuned and responsive communication style" (Walker et al., 1998, p. 48).

Interdisciplinary or interprofessional examples are presented throughout the text for continued emphasis on this important component of advanced practice. In addition, nurses are encouraged to seek experiences of working with other disciplines during graduate study. Learning to work together will greatly enhance a nurse's skills and abilities to practice in an interdisciplinary manner.

■ ACQUIRING LEADERSHIP SKILLS FOR ADVANCED PRACTICE

Leadership, or the ability to influence the action of others, is needed in all aspects of advanced practice. Leadership style is a pattern of consistent behavior that leaders use when working with others and perceived by others (Hersey & Blanchard, 1988). Graduate preparation provides opportunities for the student to obtain theoretical and practical knowledge. All leadership activities and roles call upon both kinds of knowledge.

Leadership Styles

Leadership exercised by nurses takes on various approaches depending on each nurse's background, philosophy of leading, and experience in being led. Two major approaches to leadership are situational leadership and participatory leadership.

SITUATIONAL LEADERSHIP

Situational leadership theory is based on two key outcomes of research: There is no one successful leadership style, and communication between leader and follower is the most important variable in leadership (Hersey & Duldt, 1989).

The situational leadership model consists of two leader behaviors: task behavior and relationship behavior. In the former component, the leader's communications are primarily one way and are about the structure of the job or task. The leader informs the followers about what is expected of them. For example, the advanced practice public/community health nurse would tell the interdisciplinary team members what tasks to accomplish each day. Relationship behavior involves primarily two-way communications by the leader, who facilitates interactions among people and provides support and encouragement. For example, in contrast to telling the team members what tasks to accomplish, the advanced practice public/community health nurse would regularly hold team meetings to discuss progress on a project and encourage discussion about assignments and improving performance.

In the model, *readiness* refers to the follower and how well the individual is able to do a task and whether the individual is willing to do the task when asked. Readiness thus consists of two elements: ability and willingness. The follower's ability can be viewed on a continuum from a great deal to little, indicating the degree of knowledge and skill possessed by an individual. Likewise, willingness occurs on a continuum from usually willing to seldom willing, indicating the degree of confidence and commitment possessed by an individual.

The leader's function is to set goals and develop guidelines to show how the work can be completed. Goals must be set that are moderately difficult yet potentially achievable with some risk. Goals set too low will be too easy and uninteresting for followers. For example, nurses may be asked to implement a complex intervention but would not likely be able to competently design a complex intervention based on research.

The situational leadership model contains four leadership communication styles: telling, selling, participating, and delegating. Each of these four communication styles is combined with the leadership behaviors of task and relationship for an appropriate leadership style for each of the four levels of follower readiness—low, moderate, moderate to high, and high.

A telling style of leadership is appropriate for people who are unable and unwilling (low readiness) to take responsibility to do something. Clear, specific directions and supervision will most likely be successful with people at this readiness level.

The selling style of leadership is needed with people who are unable to take responsibility but willing to take responsibility (moderate readiness). The selling style provides not only direction and help as well as support to reinforce the willingness of the followers. High task behavior and high relationship behavior are involved in the selling style of leadership.

Working with individuals who are able but unwilling (moderate to high readiness) to take responsibility calls for the participatory style of leadership. In this style, the leader and follower share decision making but the leader is primarily responsible for facilitation and communication. This style has high relationship behavior and low task behavior.

People at a high readiness level are both able and willing to take responsibility. The delegation style of leadership called for with these individuals involves providing little direction or support. Low relationship behavior and low task behavior characterize this style.

The advanced practice public/community health nurse needs to assess individuals' ability and willingness for each project because these characteristics of followers may vary with the type of tasks and content of a project. There is more likelihood of success in implementing projects, maintaining projects, and reaching the desired project outcomes with a careful matching of leadership style to the individual's style.

PARTICIPATORY LEADERSHIP

Even though participatory leadership is one type of leadership covered in situational leadership theory, special attention is given to the participatory type of leadership because of its importance in advanced practice for working with a variety of people in various social and political situations. Often seen as outsiders, nurses need to be able to work with people rather than give direction to complete tasks. Participatory leadership skills assist the nurse to be able to effectively work with others rather than always being in charge.

Community Participation. Working with communities often requires the advanced practice nurse to take action to organize individuals and groups to prevent problems or to correct long-standing problems. The advanced practice nurse is not required to carry out all the activities needed to correct a problem but may need to monitor and provide resources until the problem is corrected.

Participation of the community is a keystone of advanced public/community health nursing practice. Little ownership of programs may occur without community participation. Lack of ownership may mean that a successful program fails for lack of community interest and support after outside funding has ended. Moreover, communities are often dependent on outside professionals to tell them what they need, to tell them how to get what they need, and to provide what they are told that they need (Minkler, 1997). This model has not always resulted in problems being solved or even prevention of the slide of a community toward deterioration.

Participation of the community has been described on five levels by Rifkin (1986). The first level is participation of people in a passive way as recipients of established programs. Second-level participation involves people actively supporting programs by contributing something, for example, money or labor. On the third level, people participate in implementing the program or managing it after it has been developed by planners. At the fourth level of participation, people participate in monitoring and evaluating programs. At the fifth and ideal level, people participate in planning activities. The fifth level of participation is rarely achieved, but one example is in the development of a nursing center (Glick, Hale, Kulbok, & Shettig, 1996), which is presented in Chapter 20. Rifkin suggested that the level of participation should be specified by the planners of each project.

Another area for application of participatory leadership skills is in forming coalitions or groups who are organized to address community-level problems. Community health problems are complex and multidimensional, so solutions frequently require collaborative work among several organizations. Advanced practice nurses may also be called on to provide consultation to coalitions.

As discussed in Chapter 3, the advanced practice public/community health nurse uses various approaches to working with communities. One of these approaches is to meet the community's request for assistance. This level of participation as described previously is not usual for most public/community health nurses.

Professional Participation. Active participation of professionals involved in community health work is also important if programs are to be effective in meeting goals and objectives. A leader with the attitude that the program activities are a result of everyone working together will probably find a richer outcome than a leader who believes in sole ownership.

Clinical direction provided in an organized nursing service contributes to the effectiveness of public/community health nursing care at the individual, family, aggregate, and community levels. Nursing has, for a long time, separated nursing administration and nursing practice, so the nursing manager, administrator, or supervisor is often a separate person from the expert nurse clinician. This book takes the position that the clinical specialist in public/community health nursing should be both the nurse manager and the expert clinician. In order to have effective clinical programs, an integration of the clinical and program management processes is desirable. The advanced practice public/community health nurse should be the product of a formal educational program that facilitates the realization of this philosophy.

Often, the advanced practice public/community health nurse is also a manager who is responsible for directing the work of others. The leadership called for in supervision includes helping others to develop their skills through teaching and coaching employees in areas of performance (Ervin, 2005) that contribute to improved effectiveness of the total unit.

Developing Leadership Skills

Developing skills for leadership is one of the most important tasks for the advanced practice public/community health nurse. A first step in this process is to examine your leadership style. This can be accomplished by taking an assessment test or by rating yourself on an instrument designed for that purpose. Assessment tools are located in books and articles on leadership style.

If the self-assessment shows a high level of one type of leadership style, you may want to consider the development of skills in other types of leadership. If your experience has been primarily in leadership of work groups, you should seek out experiences in leading community groups or community efforts. Interdisciplinary experiences should also be included as part of your development in leadership competence.

▪ SUMMARY

The description of advanced public/community health nursing practice is presented in this chapter as a foundation for the remainder of this book. The terms *community health nursing* and *public health nursing* have the same meaning in this text; thus, the term public/community health nursing is used throughout. The specialty practice is focused on protection of the health of a community or population.

Advancement in nursing encompasses both specialization and expansion. The nurse specializes in public/community health nursing and expands skills in care of the community through course work in epidemiology; biostatistics; community organization; community development; and the core community health nursing processes of community assessment, program planning, program implementation, and program evaluation. Expansion of skills includes clinical experience involving the use of the processes of advanced public/community health nursing practice.

The interdisciplinary nature of advanced public/community health nursing practice requires knowledge and skills in working with other disciplines as well as with community members. Leadership for interdisciplinary practice and community participation is best visualized as that described in the theory of situational leadership. Success in reaching work goals is more likely if the leader uses a leadership style that matches the readiness level of the followers.

The next chapter focuses on the foundations and context of advanced public/community health nursing practice. These areas provide guidance for the advanced practice nurse in formulating a philosophy and practice style for working with communities and organizations.

■ SUGGESTED CLINICAL OR PRACTICUM ACTIVITIES

1. Meet with an advanced public/community health nurse at a local health department to discuss how she or he uses the core processes of advanced practice. How does she or he work with members of other disciplines?
2. Set up an observational field experience with an environmental health (EH) professional at a local health department. What is the job description of the EH professional? What educational preparation and experience are required for the specific position?
3. Observe an advanced public/community nurse leading a meeting or group session. What leadership skills did she or he use? How did she or he guide the group to make decisions, stay on topic, and have productive discussions? What decision-making processes were used?

REFERENCES

American Public Health Association Public Health Nursing Section. (1996). *The definition and role of public health nursing.* Washington, DC: Author.

American Public Health Association Public Health Nursing Section. (2013). *The definition and practice of public health nursing.* Retrieved from http://www.apha.org/~/media/files/pdf/membergroups/phn/nursingdefinition.ashx

Anderson, E. T., & McFarlane, J. (2015). Community assessment: Using a model for practice. In E. T. Anderson & J. McFarlane (Eds.), *Community as partner: Theory and practice in nursing* (7th ed., pp. 167–208). Philadelphia, PA: Wolters Kluwer.

Anderson, E. T., & McFarlane, J. (Eds.). (2015). *Community as partner: Theory and practice in nursing* (7th ed.). Philadelphia, PA: Wolters Kluwer.

APRN Consensus Work Group & the National Council of State Boards of Nursing APRN Advisory Committee. (2008). Consensus model for APRN regulation: Licensure, accreditation, certification & education. Retrieved from https://www.ncsbn.org/Consensus_Model_Report.pdf

Baldwin, D. C., Jr. (1996). Some historical notes on interdisciplinary and interprofessional education and practice in health care in the USA. *Journal of Interprofessional Care, 10,* 173–187.

Canales, M. K., & Drevdahl, D. J. (2014). Community/public health nursing: Is there a future for the specialty? *Nursing Outlook, 62*(6), 448–458.

Ervin, N. E. (2005). Clinical coaching: A strategy for enhancing evidence-based nursing practice. *Clinical Nurse Specialist, 19*(6), 296–301.

Glick, D. F., Hale, P. J., Kulbok, P. A., & Shettig, J. (1996). Community development theory: Planning a community nursing center. *Journal of Nursing Administration, 26*(7-8), 44–50.

Grove, S. K., Burns, N., & Gray, J. R. (2012). *The practice of nursing research: Appraisal, synthesis, and generation of evidence* (7th ed.). Philadelphia, PA: Elsevier.

Helvie, C. O. (1998). *Advanced practice nursing in the community*. Thousand Oaks, CA: Sage.

Hersey, P., & Blanchard, K. (1988). *Management of organizational behavior: Utilizing human resources* (5th ed.). Englewood Cliffs, NJ: Prentice Hall.

Hersey, P., & Duldt, B. W. (1989). *Situational leadership in nursing*. Norwalk, CT: Appleton & Lange.

Hopkins, D. (Ed.). (2010). *Framework for action on interprofessional education and collaborative practice*. Geneva, Switzerland: Author.

Institute of Medicine. (1988). *The future of public health*. Washington, DC: National Academies Press.

Institute of Medicine. (2003). *The future of the public's health in the 21st century*. Washington, DC: National Academies Press.

Institute of Medicine. (2012). *Primary care and public health: Exploring integration to improve population health*. Washington, DC: National Academies Press.

James, J. (2016). Nonprofit hospitals' community benefit requirements. *Health Affairs*. Retrieved from http://healthaffairs.org/healthpolicybriefs/brief_pdfs/healthpolicybrief_153.pdf

Kuehnert, P. L. (1995). The interactive and organizational model of community as client: A model for public health nursing practice. *Public Health Nursing, 12*, 9–17.

Laffrey, S. C., & Kulbok, P. A. (1999). An integrative model for holistic community health nursing. *Journal of Holistic Nursing, 17*(1), 88–103. doi:10.1177/089801019901700107

Levin, P., Cary, A., Kulbok, P., Leffers, J., Molle, M., & Polivka, B. (2008). Graduate education for advanced practice public health nursing: At the crossroads. *Public Health Nursing, 25*(2), 176–193.

Marion, L. M. (1996). *Nursing's vision for primary health care in the 21st century*. Washington, DC: American Nurses Publishing.

Minkler, M. (Ed.). (1997). *Community organizing and community building for health*. New Brunswick, NJ: Rutgers University Press.

Patient Protection and Affordable Care Act, Pub. L. No. 111-148. (2010). Retrieved from http://www.gpo.gov/fdsys/pkg/PLAW-111publ148/pdf/PLAW-111publ148.pdf

Rifkin, S. B. (1986). Lessons from community participation in health programmes. *Health Policy Planning, 1*, 240–249.

Swider, S. M., Krothe, J., Reyes, D., & Cravetz, M. (2013). The Quad Council practice competencies for public health nursing. *Public Health Nursing, 30*(6), 519–536.

Walker, P. H., Baldwin, D., Fitzpatrick, J. J., Ryan, S., Bulger, R., DeBasio, N., … Vanselow, N. (1998). Building community: Developing skills for interprofessional health professions education and relationship-centered care. *Journal of Gerontological Nursing, 24*(3), 45–49.

CHAPTER 2

Foundations and Context of Public/Community Health Nursing Specialty Practice

■ STUDY EXERCISES

1. How have historical factors shaped public/community health nursing practice?
2. What are the implications for practice of the philosophical and conceptual foundations of public/community health nursing?
3. How does the concept of health promotion relate to the philosophical orientation of social justice?
4. Explain how the standards of practice are applied in advanced public/community health nursing practice.
5. How are changes in the healthcare delivery system likely to affect the practice of public/community health nursing?
6. What are the strengths and weaknesses of public/community health nursing delivery organizations?

At the advanced level of practice, the public/community health nurse is required to make shifts in thinking. Two major components of the shifts are (a) from the individual and family to the community, population, or systems level; and (b) from treatment of disease to prevention of disease and injury and health promotion. Making these shifts in thinking is essential for competent practice, but not easy for many reasons.

Although the idea of community as the focus of practice has been in the literature since the early 20th century (Kub, Kulbok, & Glick, 2015), the concept has been slowly implemented. In a study of public health nurses in California, Grumbach, Miller, Mertz, and Finocchio (2004) reported that staff nurses were more likely to perform individual- or family-level interventions than interventions focused on the community or systems level. In fact, the most frequent intervention was case management, which was reported by 91% of staff public health nurses. Managers and directors responded similarly; they ranked interventions at the individual or family level as more important than interventions at the community or systems level.

Many community health programs are cited in the literature as having the purpose of prevention but are actually programs designed to detect diseases in their early stages, such as hypertension, breast cancer, cervical cancer, and diabetes. In addition, maternal and child health programs do not always focus on prevention except for childhood immunizations. In the past several years, maternal and child health programs have had a heavy focus on infants born with problems, but have few resources to prevent those problems.

With a scarcity of examples of prevention and health-promotion programs, public/community health nurses have more difficulty learning how to apply what they have learned. Often, nonnurses develop programs that are implemented by public/community health nurses and other team members. The nursing intervention, if there is one described in the program, is not always well developed or based on research.

An additional challenge for advanced practice public/community health nurses is that most nurses have been educated on a medical model. As noted by Fowler (2015), medicine is not nursing. Advanced practice nurses must not only reorient themselves but also make provision for the education of other nurses in an agency to shift their thinking. The medical model persists in most practice settings because medicine is the dominant controller of the practice environment, and physicians' decisions determine much of health expenditures. Some exceptions to a medically controlled practice environment are nursing centers, community nursing organizations, and some public health nursing divisions within health departments.

Using the foundations of practice and knowledge presented in this chapter, the advanced practice public/community health nurse now has the information necessary for developing a sound practice philosophy and for assisting staff to understand and apply standards of practice while implementing programs aimed at improving the health of the entire community. This chapter provides a foundation for practice that challenges the nurse to orient toward health, prevention, and nursing.

■ FOUNDATIONS OF PRACTICE

What constitutes public/community health nursing practice today is the result of over 100 years of organized practice that began as visiting nurse associations in the United States in the 1880s. These early voluntary societies were organized to care primarily for the poor sick at home and teach sanitary practices to families (Maxcy, 1956). The philosophical and value base of public/community health nursing practice today came from these early beginnings as well as the influence of the field of public health. A summary of the history of public health nursing may be found in other sources, such as Clemen-Stone, Eigsti, and McGuire (1998); Stanhope and Lancaster (2016); Spradley and Allender (1996); Sullivan (1984); and Kub et al. (2015).

The history of nursing care delivery organizations is truly the history of public health nursing in this country. Establishment of nursing in the community occurred in New York City in 1877. Visiting nurse associations were established in Buffalo in 1885, and in Boston and Philadelphia in 1886 (Brainard, 1985). The Henry Street Settlement was established in New York City by Lillian Wald and Mary Brewster in 1893, and is generally considered the first American community health agency (Silverstein, 1985). In addition, during the late 1800s, occupational health nursing and school nursing were established as offshoots of nursing in the community (Brainard, 1922/1985; Novak, 1988). Before the 1920s, most public health nurses were employed by voluntary agencies such as the Red Cross. During the 1920s, public health nursing services began to be absorbed by official agencies such as local health departments (Bigbee & Crowder, 1985).

These early beginnings were focused on care of the sick, but also had a major component of health teaching and health promotion. Changes throughout the 1900s resulted in more focus on primary care and care of the ill. However, advanced practice public/community health nurses have opportunities to direct change back to the origins of practice—prevention and health promotion.

The foundations of practice discussed in this section are categorized as philosophical, conceptual, and knowledge. Examples for applying these foundational precepts are brought out in the discussions. Nursing, of course, is the keystone of all advanced practice nursing.

Philosophical Foundations

The philosophy of a discipline defines its fundamental principles. At the fundamental level of public/community health nursing are nursing's contract with society and the principles of nursing that are basic for all nursing practice; for example, individualized care, respect for the individual, and involvement of the client and family in their care. *Nursing's Social Policy Statement* (American Nurses Association [ANA], 2010) focuses on the social contract between the nursing profession and society. The *Code of Ethics for Nurses* (ANA, 2015a) provides a guide to the moral obligations and duties for every nurse, including advanced practice public/community health nurses. In addition, social justice and self-determination are integral parts of the foundation of public health and public/community health nursing practice.

SOCIAL JUSTICE

Care of indigent individuals and families constituted the major focus of public health nursing during its early beginning in the United States. In the early 1900s, public health nursing services were extended to all residents of a community as it was recognized that prevention was an effective means to halt the spread of disease.

Women who were interested in helping others, who often had some financial means, started the early visiting nurse associations (Fulmer, 1902). Their early focus on service has been incorporated into many visiting nurse associations and community health nursing services today. The provision of services regardless of the ability to pay is part of the concept of social justice that has been incorporated into public health, with the goal of minimizing preventable death and disability.

In a society functioning under social justice, everyone is entitled equally to aspects of a healthy life such as health protection and a minimum standard of income. This ethical orientation requires that the total society addresses the challenge of protecting the public's health, as opposed to the idea that lifestyle is something that requires individual remediation (Beauchamp, 1976; Fry, 1985). For example, through research and demonstration projects, nursing and public health have attempted to discover interventions that work best with specific populations to improve their health status. Often, the interventions are aimed at changing individual behaviors of low-income people. Instead of changing behaviors, a social justice approach may focus on interventions to increase incomes above the poverty line so that individuals can buy what they need in order to be healthy, such as adequate nutritious food and shelter in a safe neighborhood. Public health nurses are often heard saying, "A mother who doesn't have enough food to feed her children does not have immunizations as a priority."

The approach to prevention of disease and injury by changing individuals' lifestyles has resulted in circumstances of blaming the victim—even though healthcare professionals are knowledgeable about the complexities of human behavior and the multiple societal influences on it. Beauchamp proclaimed, "The critical barrier to dramatic reductions in death and disability is a social ethic that unfairly protects the most numerous or the most powerful from the burdens of prevention" (1976, p. 3). This commentary remains true today.

Beauchamp proposed a new ethic to protect and preserve human life: "Controlling the hazards of this world, . . . to prevent death and disability . . . through organized collective action . . . shared equally by all except where unequal burdens result in increased protection of everyone's health and especially potential victims of death and disability" (Beauchamp, 1976, p. 7). This ethic is in opposition to market justice, which is the dominant model of justice in American life. According to market justice, people are entitled only to what they have earned by their own efforts, actions, or abilities. "Market-justice emphasizes individual responsibility, minimal collective action, and freedom from collective obligations except to respect other persons' fundamental rights" (Beauchamp, 1976, p. 4). Nurses in advanced public/community health nursing practice should be oriented toward practice that emphasizes social justice over market justice.

An extension of social justice that has become an important federal mandate is achieving environmental justice. The Environmental Protection Agency defined *environmental justice* as "the fair treatment and meaningful involvement of people regardless of race, ethnicity, income, national origin or educational level with respect to the development, implementation and enforcement of environmental laws, regulations, and policies. Fair treatment means that no population, due to policy or economic disempowerment, is forced to bear a disproportionate burden of the negative human health or environmental impacts of pollution or other environmental consequences resulting from industrial, municipal, and commercial operations or the execution of federal, state, local and tribal programs and policies" (Environmental Protection Agency, 1998, p. 2). There is evidence that minorities and lower income groups have higher levels of exposure to environmental hazards that are potential sources of risks to health (Bullard, 1996, 2005).

Practicing Within a Social Justice Context. Even though the concepts of social justice were delineated more than 40 years ago, the United States has not effectively dealt with the mechanisms needed to eliminate the disparities between the groups that have and the groups that do not have adequate income, access to healthcare, and other conditions necessary for health. Numerous publications have detailed the disparities in minority populations (Centers for Disease Control and Prevention, 2013; Institute of Medicine, 2003; Livingston, 1994). In addition, the role that racism plays in contributing to disparities in healthcare and in health continues to be documented (Williams & Mohammed, 2013; Williams, Priest, & Anderson, 2016; Williams & Purdie-Vaughns, 2016). Advanced practice public/community health nurses have unlimited opportunities to work with others to move toward the goal of social justice.

Providing access to healthcare for everyone, regardless of the ability to pay, is an obvious goal of social justice action in the United States. Working toward a universal healthcare system is a worthy goal for all advanced practice nurses. The ANA provided an early blueprint for such a system in the 1991 publication, *Nursing's Agenda for Health Care Reform* (ANA, 1991). According to this historic statement, the premises of an equitable healthcare system should include increased access and better healthcare for the population through primary care delivery and emphasis on disease prevention and health promotion. The Patient Protection and Affordable Care Act of 2010 has gone a long way in meeting the long-held goal of universal healthcare, but more effort is needed to continue toward that goal (Goldsteen, Goldsteen, & Goldsteen, 2017; Williams, McClellan, & Rivlin, 2010).

There are, however, many goals not as obvious as universal healthcare that require sustained effort. Nurses need to look within each organization for policies and practices that prevent equality from becoming a reality. For example, there are policies that require clients to adhere to very rigid behaviors in order to have access to care, for instance, arriving at

8 a.m. in order to get on a list to be seen by a provider that day. Often, clients are required to have payment in hand or have insurance before many providers will treat them. The realities of fiscal viability are that only limited care can be provided free, but healthcare institutions need to work together in order to provide care to everyone in a population.

Although assurance of the availability of healthcare is a core function of public health, the cooperation of all healthcare facilities is required to bring it to fruition. Advanced practice public/community health nurses may provide leadership to increase access to care for uninsured and underinsured people by developing programs. Examples of successful programs include health fairs to provide free preemployment physical examinations, a provider referral system for low-cost care, free dental clinics, and low-cost prenatal care.

Being active in policy development at the local, state, and national levels is another way for advanced practice public/community health nurses to actively engage in social justice implementation. With understanding of the philosophy of social justice, advanced practice nurses can work for development and implementation of legislation and policies that support families in an environment of equity. For example, social welfare policies can be formulated to assist families to become or remain independent of the system while still getting assistance to maintain the family structure. Health policies that allow families to care for an ill family member without having to declare bankruptcy or terminate employment are based on the concept of social justice.

Advanced practice public/community health nurses are role models for other nurses, staff, community members, and others. Practicing within the context of social justice allows the nurse to manifest in a small way what our society could be like if it were driven by social justice instead of market justice. Modeling social justice behavior is a key component of the role of the advanced practice public/community health nurse.

SELF-DETERMINATION

The right to self-determination for clients requires that they should be informed about their choices and be involved in planning their care. This ethical premise carries over to the total community in advanced public/community health nursing practice. A community has the right to self-determination and, therefore, should be involved in planning services and deciding what will be done in and to the community. The democratic structure of the United States is part of the basis of self-determination of the community.

Conflict over individual and community self-determination arises in many ways, not the least of which is in the meaning of the common good. What is good or desired for the individual is not always good for society (Fry, 1985). Alcohol and cigarettes are two examples that have deleterious effects on both individuals and society. Public health and safety are community interests that can take priority over individual, private interests. In the United States, legislatures determine these priorities when conflicts occur (Beauchamp, 1985; Shi, 2014).

The so-called police power of the state for public safety is another area of conflict between individual and community rights. In order to protect society in some instances, the rights of individuals must be curtailed (Goldsteen et al., 2017). For example, if an individual is spreading a communicable disease and refuses treatment, the person's activities may be restricted in some states.

Practicing Within a Context of Self-Determination. For the advanced practice public/community health nurse, learning to work with a community is an extension of working with individuals and families. Competent and ethical nursing practice requires that the nurse plan with clients for their care to the extent that they are able and choose to participate (ANA, 2015a). Communities also should be involved in all aspects of planning for their care or services (ANA, 2013). Examples of community involvement are presented and discussed throughout this textbook. Advanced practice public/community health nurses are encouraged to explore techniques and mechanisms to involve communities in all aspects of healthcare for improving the health of communities.

Conceptual Foundations

Guiding concepts for advanced public/community health nursing practice are numerous. Several are also basic to other specialties. The concepts that are central to advanced practice in public/community health nursing include nursing, public health, primary prevention, health promotion, population focus, community, autonomy, and interdisciplinary practice.

NURSING

Advanced public/community health nursing practice is the first and foremost nursing practice. The unique qualities of public/community health nursing as a specialty were introduced in Chapter 1 and continue here in Chapter 2. Much of what constitutes nursing as a discipline is contained in other courses at both the graduate and undergraduate levels. The content about nursing theory contained in this text is directed specifically to public/community health nursing but does not mean that other nursing theories are not useful. You are encouraged to explore the application of all appropriate nursing theories, even though they are not addressed in this book.

PUBLIC HEALTH

Public health was succinctly defined in the Institute of Medicine (IOM) study on public health as "what we, as a society, do collectively to assure the conditions in which people can be healthy" (IOM, 1988, p. 1). The mission of public health is to promote physical and mental health and to prevent disease, injury, and disability. Advanced public/community health nursing practice uses knowledge from nursing and public health (ANA, 2013; Kulbok & Ervin, 2012). In advanced practice, the nurse integrates these bodies of knowledge in ways that become the unique practice of public/community health nursing.

Often, public health is thought of as being practiced only in official public health agencies, such as state health departments and county health departments. The reality is that public health is practiced in a wide variety of organizations and agencies that have health, as well as other outcomes, as a goal. As funding for public health has decreased over the past two decades, some agencies have begun to deliver what were traditionally public health functions out of necessity. In addition, the trend to privatize public functions may be seen more in public health except for the functions that are not profitable such as disease control (Goldsteen et al., 2017).

PRIMARY PREVENTION

Another major foundation of public/community health nursing practice is prevention. The concept of levels of prevention (primary, secondary, and tertiary) is introduced in undergraduate study. For advanced public/community health nursing practice, the major focus is on primary prevention, which includes interventions aimed at keeping illness or injuries from occurring (Leavell & Clark, 1965), though secondary and tertiary prevention are part of the practice in most settings. Much attention has been directed to prevention in the past few years, but much more could be done in the way of effective prevention strategies (Wiley, 2016). One area of great interest to advanced practice public/community health nurses is health behavior. Nonnurse professionals have conducted much of the basic research, but application of the research results is an area ripe for developing and testing nursing interventions.

A focus on prevention in advanced practice requires that the public/community health nurse continue to read and learn about new approaches. Creativity and vision are key characteristics of the nurse who develops and implements preventive interventions. Often, the time to develop interventions is absent from the practice environment. Collaboration with university faculty is one approach for augmenting the talents of the nursing staff. Research-based interventions will more often be successful than those developed without a research base. Faculty can be very helpful in gaining access to the research literature as well as interpreting and critiquing the studies. Research-based examples are introduced later in this book.

HEALTH PROMOTION

There is confusion in the nursing profession about the concept of health promotion. *Health promotion*, defined as "healthcare directed toward high level wellness through processes that encourage alteration of personal habits or the environment in which people live" (Brubaker, 1983, p. 12) is not the same as primary prevention.

Nursing as a whole does not contribute a great deal of services in health promotion. Physicians who diagnose and treat illness control much of healthcare, so practice environments deal almost exclusively with these tasks related to illness. Thus, nurses are not free to develop and implement programs of health promotion. There are, however, some settings in which nurses have been more successful in health-promotion areas. One of these settings is occupational health. Evidence over the past three decades about workplace health-promotion programs that are well designed and founded on evidence-based principles has shown positive health and financial outcomes (Goetzel et al., 2014).

Numerous opportunities also exist in schools for health-promotion activities. Indeed, in years past, physical education classes and sports activities had a much greater emphasis on health promotion than on competition and winning. School nurse specialists have wonderful and frequent opportunities to develop health-promotion programs for children, school staff, and parents. In addition to promoting exercise through sports and physical education classes, health promotion in schools may encompass nutrition in the cafeteria, mental health through responsible decision making, and classes on healthy living, to list only a few examples.

Missing from much of the health-promotion movement is a focus on low-income and minority populations, which often have limited access to health-promotion activities and policy-making bodies. Interpreting environment broadly, the environment in low-income communities often lacks the control of hazards that result in death and disability much more often than in middle- and high-income communities. One example of this is a study done about billboard advertising. The number of cigarette advertisements per resident was 2.6 times greater in Black communities compared with White communities (Mayberry & Price, 1993). Other studies have found few or no grocery stores in inner cities, especially those providing fresh produce for the local community (Ghosh-Dastidar et al., 2014; Gordon et al., 2011).

POPULATION-FOCUSED PRACTICE

The concept of organized public health nursing grew out of the early epidemics, for example, cholera and typhoid fever, and the realization that illness could be prevented (Maxcy, 1956). Lillian Wald first used the title *public health nurse* in the first decade of the 20th century (Sullivan, 1984). Public health nurses were assigned to districts and thus were responsible for the total geographic area, and not just for the individuals who were ill or families that asked for help.

Thus, two key concepts in public/community health nursing are case finding and outreach. As nurses practice in the community, they find cases or encounter individuals and families with unmet needs for health or social services. The result of this discovery has always been to provide what is needed or to give information for families to obtain what is needed. This approach has been translated in advanced practice as conducting a community assessment in collaboration with community members and the eventual implementation of programs needed by communities to meet unmet needs. A **population focus** means that the community health nurse is interested in all people in a designated area even though they are not considered "clients" of the agency.

Care of a population may suggest an impersonal, anonymous approach to a large group of people with no faces. Although population-focused practice is meant to be an ideal of taking care of everyone within a given geographic area regardless of race, ethnicity, gender, age, religion, creed, beliefs, color, or sexual orientation, it does not need to be impersonal and distanced. Advanced practice public/community health nurses should guard against becoming the bureaucrat who stays at a distance from the "consumer."

Nursing was never meant to be a bureaucratic activity to deliver products to anonymous purchasers of health, so nurses must resist the trend to reduce healthcare to the industrial or business model. Healthcare is not building automobiles or selling financial products. A population focus must be implemented with the awareness that our actions have an effect on people.

The concept of community, as presented throughout this textbook, conveys the meaning of population-focused practice that is integral to advanced public/community health nursing practice. Advanced practice public/community health nurses should be interested in learning about the people, their interests, concerns, and ideas. It is the people of a community who are living with the situations at hand, not the nurse, so it is the people who must become involved in identifying and solving their problems. Thus, population-focused practice takes on a real-life form, not an anonymous focus on a mass of humanity.

FOCUS ON THE COMMUNITY

Focus on the community in public health practice has been present for many decades, and development of this focus of the specialty has continued in both academic and practice environments.

Community is an essential component of human experience (Hawe, 1994; Labonté, 1989; McKnight, 1987; McMillan & Chavis, 1986; Morris, 1996). Community as a part of everyday life is interrelated with the experiences of home, family, clan, or tribe. In different regions and cultures, the meaning and experience of community may be ascribed differently. Yet, as McKnight stated, "knowing community is not an abstract understanding. Rather, it is what we each know about all of us" (1987, p. 58).

Although it may be an everyday part of human experience, community is also a term used by professionals to describe an orientation to their practice. Public/community health nursing practice, by its professional focus, is closely tied to the concept of community (Maglacas, 1988; McKnight & Van Dover, 1994). Until now, there has been little literature exploring how different conceptualizations of community relate to nursing practice. At the same time, nursing has explicitly and implicitly relied on assumptions about the constituency of community. The language that is most prevalent in practice reflects a conceptualization of community as client.

In order to design and focus programs useful to a group of people, the concept of **community** is used in public/community health nursing to define the target group. The idea of community may be a physical place or groups composed of people who share institutions, values, culture, and life together. The idea of population-focused practice means that everyone is included in the program, whereas the idea of community means that the people have very definite rights to be involved in determining the direction of the program. Hence the two concepts, population focus and community, are combined to provide two important, yet compatible, strands in advanced public/community health nursing practice. Each of these concepts receives more attention throughout the book.

AUTONOMY

Public/community health nursing has had the unique position of developing for many decades free of the hospital environment, which has played a major role in shaping other current practice in the United States. The founder of public health nursing in the United States, Lillian Wald, thought nursing practice under the direction of physicians was inappropriate (Christy, 1970). Thus, one of the bases of practice is *autonomy*, though this has been somewhat diminished by the intrusion of reimbursement, especially Medicare, which often requires physicians' orders.

Public/community health nurses practice in many agencies without the requirement of physicians' orders for nursing interventions. Physicians or other healthcare professionals do not direct the advanced practice public/community health nurse in practice unless the tasks are dependent under a nurse practice act.

Often, advanced practice nurses go into new positions without previous experience in public/community health nursing, so they have not had the opportunity to observe autonomy in action or to practice it. Without this previous experience, the advanced practice nurse may be tempted to ask for direction from physicians in the agency. Often, this request for direction will be inappropriate, resulting in the physician's delegating medical tasks as opposed to nursing practice areas (of which a physician has little knowledge). The advanced practice nurse needs to enter practice with the knowledge and skills to undertake the new role with some assistance from other nurses, but not be dependent on others who have not had the appropriate preparation in nursing.

INTERDISCIPLINARY PRACTICE

Autonomy in practice must not exclude the ability to work with others in a team. Public health is all about teamwork used to accomplish goals that cannot be met by one discipline working alone. Interdisciplinary practice requires collaboration, which is a relationship of interdependence that necessitates the acknowledgment of complementary roles (Fagin, 1992; McCallin, 2001).

The team in public health may contain numerous disciplines and may change as the projects change. For example, in a food-poisoning outbreak, the environmental health personnel may take the lead, with nurses doing follow-up on people who are ill or recovering from the infection. In a voluntary agency, such as a community nursing center, the advanced practice public/community health nurse will be the lead person who seeks input from community professionals for specific projects. Working with the community also means that disciplines other than health disciplines are involved in projects. Lay members of the community may be involved in various ways, such as key informants and data collectors, and be considered part of a team. The advanced practice public/community health nurse can be more effective in meeting a community's needs with the ability to put a team together and guide the project.

Knowledge Foundations

Advancement in nursing practice encompasses both specialization and expansion, as discussed in Chapter 1. *Expansion* means acquiring new knowledge and skills. New knowledge and skills in nursing come from the core curriculum content for graduate study: nursing theory, research, health policy, organization of the healthcare system, ethics, professional role development, human diversity, and social issues. If the nursing role is preparation for care of the individual or family, advanced practice content should include health assessment, physiology, pathophysiology, and pharmacology. Depending on the role for which the advanced practice public/community health nurse is preparing, this latter content may not be part of the educational program. Although the inclusion of health promotion and disease prevention is recommended for all graduate nursing programs (American Association of Colleges of Nursing, 2011), this content is especially pertinent to the specialty of public/community health nursing.

In public/community health nursing, some new knowledge and skills come from the public health sciences, including biostatistics, epidemiology, and environmental health. Public health frameworks and theories, such as ecology, are important. In addition, knowledge of health-promotion and disease prevention theories is needed for program planning, which is part of the role of the advanced practice public/community health nurse (Levin et al., 2008). Graduate study should also include content in community assessment, program implementation, and program evaluation. A list of the essential areas of graduate study in advanced public/community health nursing practice is found in Chapter 1.

BIOSTATISTICS

Biostatistics provide knowledge about how to calculate and understand health statistics. The need to understand population changes in disease patterns in a statistical format is important knowledge for developing programs to prevent disease and to promote health in a population. Raw numbers are not useful for understanding disease patterns in a population, so rates, ratios, and proportions in a population become the equivalent of using physiological measures for the individual. Applications of biostatistics are made throughout the community-assessment process, program planning, and evaluation.

EPIDEMIOLOGY

Epidemiology is the study of the distribution of disease and injury, including examination of factors related to health and illness in a population, in order to prevent disease and injury (Friis & Sellers, 2014). The study of epidemiology at the advanced level in public/community health nursing, with a focus on the population, is parallel to the study of physiology and pathophysiology with a focus on the individual for a nurse practitioner role.

Although the investigation of disease and injury is the focus of epidemiology, the advanced practice public/community health nurse is interested in prevention of disease and injury. The study of epidemiology leads to knowledge about prevention because one can learn about how disease is spread, how injuries occur, and the surrounding circumstances. This knowledge can be used to develop evidence-based interventions for populations.

ENVIRONMENTAL HEALTH

Environmental health encompasses a broad range of content dealing with the quality of aspects of the environment, including water, air, and food. Health is inextricably tied to a healthy environment, so the advanced practice public/community health nurse is required to be knowledgeable about factors in the community that threaten the health of the population and how to address these factors. For example, the problem of lead poisoning in children has been recognized for many years. A major source of lead in the environment is house paint, which contained lead until the 1970s, when it was banned from use in most paint products. More recent, lead in the water supply and in soil has been explored (Hanna-Attish, LaChance, Sadler, & Champney Schnepp, 2016; Laidlaw et al., 2016).

■ STANDARDS AND ETHICS OF PRACTICE

Standards for professional nursing practice are statements that describe the duties that all registered nurses are expected to competently perform (ANA, 2015b). Building on the definition and scope of practice of the specialty of public/community health nursing, standards of practice were published by the ANA in 1973 and 1986 after wide review and suggestions from state nurses associations, individuals, and public health nursing and community health nursing organizations.

Until 1986, standards for the advanced practice community health nurse were not explicitly stated. At that time, the standards were separated into those for the generalist and the specialist; this book uses the specialist standards as the advanced practice public/community health nurse. In 1995, the ANA in collaboration with the Association of Community Health Nursing Educators, the Public Health Nursing Section of the American Public Health Association (APHA), and the Association of State and Territorial Directors of Nursing, began the process for revision of the community health nursing standards. In an effort to add clarity to the specialty practice, the resulting document was titled, *Scope and Standards of Public Health Nursing Practice* (Quad Council of Public Health Nursing Organizations [Quad Council], 1999). The latest scope and standards of practice were completed in 2013 (ANA, 2013).

Previous Standards

Standards published in 1973 and 1986 reflected practice laws, the healthcare system, and nursing science at those times. The 1973 standards of practice were basically the steps of the nursing process modified somewhat for community health nursing. For example, the 1973 standard V was "Nursing actions provide for consumer participation in health promotion, maintenance and restoration" (ANA, 1973, p. 3). Although there was some hint in this standard of the levels of prevention, it was so general that it could refer to many nursing specialties.

Each standard was accompanied by a rationale and assessment factors. Neither of these components of the standards document was oriented to what we now recognize as public/community health nursing. Indeed, there was very little reference to the community throughout the document. None of the eight standards contained the word *community*, though the term *consumer* was used in several standards.

One curious aspect about this lack of reference to community was that the definition of community health nursing that prefaced the standards had a clear population focus: "Community Health Nursing is a synthesis of nursing practice and public health practice applied to promoting and preserving the health of populations. The nature of this practice is general and comprehensive. It is not limited to a particular age or diagnostic group. It is continuing, not episodic. The dominant responsibility is to the population as a whole" (ANA, 1973, p. 1).

In contrast, the 1986 standards differentiated between the generalist, who concentrates on care of individuals and families, and the specialist, who is responsible for the care of the community or population. The definition of community health nursing offered in this document was: "Community health nursing practice promotes and preserves the health of populations by integrating the skills and knowledge relevant to both nursing and public health . . . . While community health nursing practice includes nursing directed to individuals, families, and groups, the dominant responsibility is to the population as a whole" (ANA, 1986, pp. 1–2).

Although the 1986 standards were also generic, the rationales and criteria were more specific to community health nursing. The criteria were divided into structure, process, and outcome statements. In addition, some of the process criteria were delineated into those for the generalist and the specialist, making role differentiation clear. This was one of the first documents that clarified the differences between the generalist and the specialist and identified a scope of practice for the field of community health nursing. Although this set of standards has been replaced by a new revision and was titled, *Scope and Standards of Public Health Nursing Practice* (Quad Council, 1999), it is an important document in the history of community health nursing practice.

The *Scope and Standards of Public Health Nursing Practice* (Quad Council, 1999) is also an important document that reinforced the 1996 definition of public health nursing proposed by the Public Health Nursing Section of the APHA: "Public health nursing is the practice of promoting and protecting the health of populations using knowledge from nursing, social, and public health sciences" (Quad Council, 1999, p. 2). In addition to this classic definition, the eight tenets of public health nursing (Quad Council, 1997), which advance the goals to promote and protect the health of the public, were reaffirmed. These tenets included population assessment, policy development, and assurance; partnering with community representatives; primary prevention; creating healthy environmental, social, and economic conditions; focusing on the whole population; concern for the greater good; resource allocation for maximum population health benefit; and multidisciplinary collaboration. These eight tenets or principles taken together distinguish public health nursing from other nursing specialties and were preserved in the current standards (ANA, 2013).

Current Standards

Specialty professional practice is constantly being shaped and refined by its own members. In 1995, the American Nurses Association Council of Community, Primary, and Long Term Care began the process of revising the standards of practice for community health nursing. Although some leaders desired to combine the standards for community health nursing and home health nursing, they did not come to an agreement on this. Although community health nursing had its beginning in home healthcare, the current trend in home healthcare has been away from the aggregate and community approach to that of caring for ill individuals. Reimbursement through Medicare was a major factor in creating this change of focus (Sullivan, 1984). As a result, the trend to separate community health nursing and home healthcare into two areas of practice continues, with each area having its own standards, certification examinations, and organizations.

After undergoing a lengthy development process, a statement about the scope of practice of community health nursing was written, and a draft scope-and-standards document was produced and sent to the state nurses associations for review and endorsement. Comments from the state nurses associations and by members of the Committee on Public Health Nursing Standards and Guidelines were used to make revisions in the draft document.

One major change in the latest standards is the name change to public health nursing, as noted earlier. The leaders of the Quad Council of Public Health Nursing Organizations (at that time composed of the American Nurses Association Council of Community, Primary, and Long Term Care; the APHA Section of Public Health Nursing; the Association of Community Health Nursing Educators; and the Association of State and Territorial Directors of Nursing) voted to change the title of the standards because the term *public health nursing* better reflects the specialty and differentiates it from community-based nursing.

The scope of practice outlined in the standards document includes practice at the public health nurse level and the advanced public health nurse level. The statements combine the nursing process with the core functions of public health: assessment, policy development, and assurance. The six standards of practice are components of the nursing process and address the areas of assessment, population diagnosis and priorities, outcomes identification, planning, implementation, and evaluation. Substandards in the area of implementation include coordination of care, health teaching and health promotion, consultation, and regulatory activities (ANA, 2013).

The second component of the public health nursing standards addresses standards of professional performance, including ethics, education, evidence-based practice and research, quality of practice, communication, leadership, collaboration, professional practice evaluation, resource utilization, and environmental health. Information about how the public health nursing standards may be used as a guide in evaluation is available in Chapter 16 (ANA, 2013).

In the second edition of the scope and standards document, public health nursing is defined as follows:

> Public health nursing practice focuses on population health through continuous surveillance and assessment of the multiple determinants of health with the intent to promote health and wellness; prevent disease, disability, and premature death; and improve neighborhood quality of life. These population health priorities are addressed through identification, implementation, and evaluation of universal and targeted evidence-based programs and services that provide primary, secondary, and tertiary preventive interventions. Public health nursing practice emphasizes primary prevention with the goal of achieving health equity. (ANA, 2013, pp. 2, 3)

■ CERTIFICATION

Certification is a process by which a profession recognizes a professional's expert level of knowledge and skill in a specific area of practice. The nursing profession certifies its members through a process similar to that of many professions. After a nurse has acquired the necessary formal educational credentials and meets the requisite practice requirements, the individual is eligible to apply to take a certification examination (ANA, 1996). The development of a certification examination is possible after the scope and standards of the specialty have been identified and endorsed by the appropriate organizations.

In 2013, the American Nurses Credentialing Center (ANCC) retired the certification examination for the specialist in public/community health nursing. The replacement for the examination is submission of a portfolio for the advanced public health nurse credential (PHNA-BC). "Certification through portfolio is a new assessment methodology to achieve ANCC board certification. No exam is required. Eligible applicants submit an online portfolio of evidence to document their specialized knowledge, skills, understanding, and application of professional nursing practice and theory" (ANCC, 2016). The Portfolio Content Outline found on the ANCC website contains details about the four domains of practice that must be included in the portfolio of applicants: professional development, professional and ethical nursing practice, teamwork and collaboration, and quality and safety. Certified public health nurses who renew by meeting the recertification requirements are allowed to retain the credential of public health clinical nurse specialist (PHCNS-BC) or change to advanced public health nurse (PHNA-BC).

A certified nurse has specific competencies that have been professionally normed, that is, the profession has determined which practice behaviors are necessary to achieve the recognition of certification. Thus, all certified nurses are expected to meet the standards of practice, maintain a minimum knowledge base, and be involved in professional activities. Becoming certified is one part of professional behavior that all advanced practice nurses will want to achieve.

Certification also serves the public by providing a known standard to guide the choice of a healthcare provider. Although certification alone is not sufficient to guarantee competence, it is one way for the nursing profession to fulfill part of its obligation to regulate itself and protect the public's safety.

■ THE CHANGING HEALTHCARE SYSTEM

In the late 20th century, the healthcare system continued to change greatly. The quest for cost control precipitated changes in the way that healthcare systems were organized and financed. Tremendous advances in technological and pharmacological research contributed to the increase in the cost of healthcare, while extending the lives of individuals who would have died in previous decades. In the 21st century, the focus on healthcare reform resulted in the Patient Protection and Affordable Care Act (PPACA), which was signed by President Barack Obama on March 23, 2010 (Mason et al., 2016).

The Patient Protection and Affordable Care Act

When the PPACA was signed, 49.9 million people were uninsured in the United States. In addition to providing healthcare coverage for uninsured individuals and families, the PPACA was amended by passage of the Healthcare and Education Reconciliation Act to include other provisions. The final law is titled the Affordable Care Act (ACA). Provisions of the ACA will be fully implemented tentatively by 2023.

The ACA contains nine titles that address various aspects of healthcare:

Title I: Quality, affordable health care for all Americans
Title II: The role of public programs
Title III: Improving the quality and efficiency of health care
Title IV: Prevention of chronic disease and improving public health
Title V: Health care workforce
Title VI: Transparency and program integrity
Title VII: Improving access to innovative medical therapies

Title VIII: Community living assistance services and supports
Title IX: Revenue provisions (Mason et al., 2016)

A 2014 web-based survey was conducted of 1,143 public health nurses to explore their practices under the ACA (Edmonds, Campbell, & Gilder, 2016). The investigators found that 45% of the respondents reported that their daily functions and tasks had changed a great deal or somewhat since the ACA enactment. Following were the leading activities reported by the public health nurses: 62% are involved in integration of primary care and public health, 60.3% in provision of clinical preventive services, 55.4% in care coordination, 55.3% in patient navigation, 55.3% establishment of private–public partnerships, 53.6% in population health strategies, 53.8% in population health data assessment and analysis, and 49% in community health assessments. Fewer proportions of respondents were involved in medical homes (37.8%), maternal and child health home visiting services (32.1%), and accountable care organizations (ACOs; 29.2%). Several nurses noted more involvement in community assessment because the ACA requires hospitals to engage in this activity every 3 years to maintain their nonprofit status.

Involvement of public health nurses in ACA activities was projected to continue by a majority of the survey respondents (Edmonds et al., 2016). Some nurses pointed out that leadership and knowledge were not always present in the public health nursing workforce.

Thus far in implementation of the ACA, research has shown a substantially decreased number of uninsured individuals with a decline of 43%, improvements in access to and affordability of healthcare, reduction in debts sent to collection (an estimated $600 to $1,000 per person with Medicaid coverage), and reforms in payment systems (French et al., 2016; Obama, 2016). Other outcomes are yet to be examined. In addition, legal and legislative challenges to the ACA continue to attempt to repeal and/or change some provisions of the law (Goldsteen et al., 2017).

Innovations in Healthcare Delivery

The ACA contains provisions for some new approaches to provide care and reducing cost. ACOs are one such innovation. These entities are composed of doctors, hospitals, and other healthcare providers who voluntarily come together to coordinate care for Medicare patients. Coordinated care, especially for chronically ill people, is aimed at providing high-quality care to avoid duplication of services and prevent medical errors. If a specified amount of cost savings is achieved, ACOs share in the savings (Centers for Medicare & Medicaid Services, 2016).

Another innovation in healthcare delivery is the patient-centered medical home (PCMH), also known as the *primary care medical home, advanced primary care,* and the *healthcare home* (Agency for Healthcare Research and Quality [AHRQ], n.d.-b). PCMH is a model of organization for primary care that delivers core functions of

1. Comprehensive care: PCMH is accountable for meeting the majority of patients' physical and mental healthcare needs.
2. Patient-centered: PCMHs are relationship based with a focus on the whole person.
3. Coordinated care: PCMHs coordinate care across the healthcare system.
4. Accessible services: PCMHs deliver services with access 24 hours a day via telephone or electronic means.
5. Quality and safety: PCMHs demonstrate commitment to quality by using evidence-based medicine, shared decision with patients and families, and practicing population health management (AHRQ, n.d.-a).

Focus on Prevention and the Community

The dual foci on prevention and the community have traditionally been the purview of the public health system. With passage of the ACA, some aspects of prevention have been incorporated into most health insurance plans. Hospitals are required to conduct community health assessments and to prepare community health improvement plans on the basis of assessment findings every 3 years, as mentioned earlier. These mandated changes have provided public health with greater access into the broader healthcare system. Partnerships have been encouraged for many decades, but the ACA has contained the first major thrust to impel the development of partnerships of healthcare entities with public health.

The ACA requires coverage for recommended preventive services that include 15 preventive services for adults; 22 services for women, including pregnant women; and 26 services for children. The services must be provided without copayment, coinsurance, and having to meet a deductible (U.S. Department of Health and Human Services, 2012). Although the services are categorized as preventative, most are screening for disease detection. The preventive services are primarily immunizations and some items of prophylaxis.

Although most health resources continue to be focused on acute care in hospitals, prevention has been featured in new initiatives to achieve a healthier population as well as to decrease the cost of illness care.

National Prevention Strategy

In 2011, the U.S. surgeon general issued a report titled *National Prevention Strategy* (National Prevention Council, 2011) as part of the ACA, which created the National Prevention Council, to focus attention on the need for prevention and health promotion to be part of the national agenda for health. The goal of the strategy is to move the healthcare system from that of illness care to a system based on wellness and prevention. The strategy contains directions and priorities about leading factors related to preventing disease, injury, and addressing the social determinants of health.

The four strategic directions are healthy and safe community environments, clinical and community preventive services, empowered people, and elimination of health disparities. The seven priorities of the strategy are tobacco-free living, preventing drug abuse and excessive alcohol use, healthy eating, active living, injury- and violence-free living, reproductive and sexual health, and mental and emotional well-being (National Prevention Council, 2011). With a focus on efforts that will have the greatest effect for the greatest number of people, the strategy offers evidence-based policy, program, and systems approaches to address each priority. This document provides the advanced public/community health nurse with an abundance of information to use in practicing at a high level of effectiveness.

Building a Culture of Health

Over a span of 18 months, the Robert Wood Johnson Foundation (RWJF) undertook the development of a document to contribute to the work of both governmental and voluntary organizations to create a healthier society (RWJF, 2015). Focusing on efforts to build a culture of health, the foundation proposed a framework containing four action areas within a context of equity: (a) making health a shared value, (b) fostering cross-sector collaboration to improve well-being, (c) creating healthier and equitable communities, and (d) strengthening integration of health services and systems. Citing statistics about the status of the U.S. population health, the foundation documented the need to create a movement for participation of all societal sectors to speed up the changes needed to reverse the trajectory of illness and injury.

The RWJF (2015) document provides a valuable source for advanced public/community health nurses of ideas that may work in specific communities and populations for inter-sectorial approaches to solve issues as well as prevent occurrences of others.

Healthier America Project

In 2007, the Trust for America's Health issued a report that emphasized the need to strengthen the nation's public health system. The report pointed out that the public health system must (a) provide people with information and resources to make healthier choices and live healthier lives and (b) protect people from health threats beyond the control of individuals, such as natural disasters, environmental risks, and infectious diseases (Trust for America's Health, 2007).

In order to accomplish the goal of a healthier America, the Trust for America's Health called for combined efforts of all levels of government plus partnerships with businesses, communities, and citizens. The focus on prevention to help avoid unnecessary costs and suffering was emphasized in the report. In addition, the Trust built on the premise that helping people to be healthier is important to improve the American economy as well as to help businesses be competitive in the global economy. The development of a national prevention strategy was proposed as one approach for highlighting prevention on a national health agenda. As of 2008, almost 150 organizations had signed on to support the vision for a healthier America (Trust for America's Health, n.d.).

Generation Public Health

At its 2015 annual meeting, the APHA launched Generation Public Health, a national movement to ensure that everyone has a right to good health. The vision of APHA is to create "the healthiest nation in one generation" (APHA, 2018). To achieve this vision, APHA is working with communities, organizations, and people, collaborating across public and private sectors to promote safety, education, economic mobility, health equity, healthy food, a healthy environment, healthcare for everyone, and a strong public health infrastructure.

The APHA website includes informational graphics that can be used by advanced public/community health nurses to educate the American public about the current poor state of our nation's health compared to the health of people in other developed countries and about social, environmental, and personal factors that affect the health-related choices and health status of the public (APHA, 2018).

■ NURSING CARE DELIVERY ORGANIZATIONS

With health departments concentrating on populations, public/community health nursing in community settings and voluntary organizations may be effective in reaching underserved segments of the population. Some examples follow.

Community Nursing Centers

Community nursing centers, nurse-managed health centers, nurse-led centers, or nursing centers have been around since the 1890s but were not called that until almost a century later. They often have the same purpose nowadays as they did 100 years ago: to serve low-income and underserved populations. Nursing centers are organizations administered by professional nurses and provide direct access to professional nurses who make services available at low or no cost as well as for reimbursement (National Nurse-Led Care Consortium, n.d.).

Studies have found that nursing centers are often affiliated with a school of nursing or other organization and serve a variety of clients. In a 1990 study, 56.2% of 80 centers reported that they were affiliated with a parent organization, whereas 43.8% described themselves as freestanding (Barger & Rosenfeld, 1995).

Edge Runner Models of Care

In 2006, the American Academy of Nursing began the Edge Runner program to recognize nurses who had "developed and implemented innovative models of care to promote health and manage illness across diverse and underserved populations" (Mason et al., 2015, p. 540). The American Academy of Nursing conducted a study of 39 nurse-designed models of healthcare designated as Edge Runner Models of Care. Some examples of nurse-developed and implemented models are as follows:

Centering Pregnancy and Healthcare. This program is a group healthcare delivery model that includes health assessment, education, and support. Results showed a 33% reduction in preterm birth, higher patient satisfaction, increased breast-feeding rates, and improved knowledge and readiness for birth and parenting. The model has been extended to parenting, diabetes, and other health areas. Significant cost reduction and cost-effectiveness have been demonstrated in two randomized clinical trials. Public health nurses delivered group care to pregnant women and partners in the 1960s, but we had no systematic data to demonstrate that this approach was efficacious and cost-effective.

Chicago Parent Program. This is a 12-session parenting program designed to reduce behavior problems in young children by strengthening parenting skills. The program was developed by working with "African American and Latino parents from different economic backgrounds to help parents tailor effective parenting strategies to their goals and values" (Mason et al., 2015, p. 541). Outcomes include a decrease in child behavior problems and parent reliance on corporal punishment. The program costs about $37/child/session with a potential return-on-investment (ROI) of over 900%.

Wise Health Decisions. This self-care management wellness program by RNs is built around the Wise Health Decisions Wellness Clinics. The aim is to identify employees with risks or at risk for chronic conditions. Individualized teaching/coaching services are given on the basis of screening results. Outcomes include reduction in insurance claims and lower health premium increases; reduction in risk levels across blood pressure, blood sugar, cholesterol, and weight measures that are sustained over time. ROI: for every $1 spent, $3 to $7 were saved in the first year.

Making Transitional Care More Effective and Efficient. This evidence-based model of hospital-to-home transitional care is led by advanced practice nurses working with the patient's healthcare team. Patients at risk for poor postdischarge outcomes are targeted. Outcomes demonstrated through the program include reductions in rates of rehospitalization, longer intervals before initial rehospitalization, shorter hospital stays, and better patient satisfaction. The average savings are about $5,000 per Medicare patient.

!Cuidate¡ This culturally specific program was designed to reduce rates of pregnancy and sexually transmitted diseases, including HIV, among Latina youth through abstinence and condom use. Outcomes include a decrease in reported sexual intercourse and being less likely to report multiple partners and more likely to consistently use condoms. A cost–benefit ratio of $2.50 saved for every $1 spent was observed.

These examples demonstrate the strengths of nursing for developing programs that reach populations that have historically been the focus of the work of public health nurses. Other examples can be found in the literature.

■ SUMMARY

Foundations of advanced public/community health nursing practice include nursing philosophy, nursing concepts, and nursing knowledge. Although it shares foundations of practice with all fields of nursing, public/community health nursing is especially concerned with equity and social justice issues of healthcare delivery. To this end, public/community health nursing has held to its history of caring for the total population.

With the changing healthcare system, public/community health nursing has an opportunity to return to its roots of a social justice model even though locating funding for such services is not easy. A focus on prevention and health promotion is easier to maintain in a practice environment controlled by nursing, such as in community nursing centers and other models of care delivery.

■ SUGGESTED CLINICAL OR PRACTICUM ACTIVITIES

1. After reading the complete set of standards for public/community health nursing practice, ask a public or community health nurse manger or administrator to provide job descriptions of advanced practice positions. Analyze how the standards of practice and philosophical and conceptual foundations of public/community health nursing are contained in the position descriptions.
2. Discuss with a public/community health advanced practice nurse how changes in the healthcare delivery system have affected or are likely to affect practice; especially, address the philosophical orientation of social justice in the changes.
3. Attend a variety of meetings of public/community health nursing staff to observe and analyze strengths and weaknesses of public/community health nursing delivery organizations. Discuss your observations and analyses with your preceptor.

REFERENCES

Agency for Healthcare Research and Quality. (n.d.-a). Defining the PCMH. Retrieved from https://pcmh.ahrq.gov/page/defining-pcmh

Agency for Healthcare Research and Quality. (n.d.-b). Transforming the organization and delivery of primary care. Retrieved from https://pcmh.ahrq.gov/#

American Association of Colleges of Nursing. (2011). The essentials of master's education in nursing. Retrieved from http://www.aacn.nche.edu/education-resources/MastersEssentials11.pdf

American Nurses Association. (1973). *Standards of community health nursing practice*. Kansas City, MO: Author.

American Nurses Association. (1986). *Standards of community health nursing practice*. Kansas City, MO: Author.

American Nurses Association. (1991). *Nursing's agenda for health care reform*. Washington, DC: Author.

American Nurses Association. (1996). *Scope and standards of advanced practice registered nursing*. Washington, DC: Author.

American Nurses Association. (2010). *Nursing's social policy statement: The essence of the profession*. Silver Spring, MD: Author.

American Nurses Association. (2013). *Public health nursing: Scope and standards of practice* (2nd ed.). Silver Spring, MD: Author.

American Nurses Association. (2015a). *Code of ethics for nurses with interpretive statements*. Silver Spring, MD: Author.

American Nurses Association. (2015b). *Nursing: Scope and standards of practice* (3rd ed.). Silver Spring, MD: Author.

American Nurses Credentialing Center. (2016). *Advanced public health nursing portfolio*. Retrieved from http://www.nursecredentialing.org/Certification/NurseSpecialties/AdvancedPublicHealth Nursing-Portfolio

American Public Health Association. (2018). *Generation public health*. Retrieved from https://www.apha .org/what-is-public-health/generation-public-health

Beauchamp, D. E. (1976). Public health as social justice. *Inquiry, 13*, 3–14.

Beauchamp, D. E. (1985). Community: The neglected tradition of public health. *Hastings Center Report, 15*(6), 28–36.

Barger, S., & Rosenfeld, P. (1995). Models in community health care: Findings from a national study of community nursing centers. *Nursing and Health Care, 14*, 426–431.

Bigbee, J. L., & Crowder, E. L. M. (1985). The Red Cross rural nursing service: An innovative model of public health delivery. *Public Health Nursing, 2*, 109–121.

Brainard, A. M. (1985). *The evolution of public health nursing*. New York, NY: Garland. (Original work published 1922).

Brubaker, B. H. (1983). Health promotion: A linguistic analysis. *Advances in Nursing Science, 5*(3), 1–14.

Bullard, R. D. (Ed.). (1996). *Unequal protection: Environmental justice and communities of color* (2nd ed.). San Francisco, CA: Sierra Club Books.

Bullard, R. D. (Ed.). (2005). *The quest for environmental justice: Human rights and the politics of pollution*. San Francisco, CA: Sierra Club Books.

Centers for Disease Control and Prevention. (2013). CDC health disparities and inequalities report— United States 2013. *Morbidity and Mortality Weekly Report, 62*(Suppl. 3). Retrieved from https://www .cdc.gov/mmwr/pdf/other/su6203.pdf

Centers for Medicare & Medicaid Services. (2016). Accountable care organizations (ACOs): General information. Retrieved from https://innovation.cms.gov/initiatives/aco/

Christy, T. (1970). Portrait of a leader: Lillian D. Wald. *Nursing Outlook, 18*, 50–54.

Clemen-Stone, S., Eigsti, D., & McGuire, S. (1998). Comprehensive community health nursing (5th ed.). St. Louis, MO: Mosby.

Edmonds, J. K., Campbell, L. A., & Gilder, R. E. (2016). Public health nursing practice in the Affordable Care Act era: A national survey. *Public Health Nursing, 34*(1), 50–58. doi:10.1111/phn.12286

Environmental Protection Agency, Office of Federal Activities. (1998). *Final guidance for incorporating environmental justice concerns in EPA's NEPA compliance analyses*. Washington, DC: U.S. Government Printing Office.

Fagin, C. M. (1992). Collaboration between nurses and physicians: No longer a choice. *Academic Medicine, 67*(5), 295–303.

Fowler, M. D. M. (2015). *Guide to nursing's social policy statement: Understanding the profession from social contract to social covenant*. Silver Spring, MD: American Nurses Association.

French, M. T., Homer, J., Gumus, G., & Hickling, L. (2016). Key provisions of the Patient Protection and Affordable Care Act (ACA): A systematic review and presentation of early research findings. *Health Services Research, 51*(5), 1735–1771. doi:10.1111/1475-6773.12511

Friis, R. H., & Sellers, T. A. (2014). *Epidemiology for public health practice* (5th ed.). Boston, MA: Jones & Bartlett.

Fry, S. T. (1985). Individual vs aggregate good: Ethical tension in nursing practice. *International Journal of Nursing Studies, 22*(4), 303–310.

Fulmer, H. (1902). History of visiting nurse work in America. *American Journal of Nursing, 2,* 411.

Ghosh-Dastidar, B., Cohen, D., Hunter, G., Zenk, S. N., Huang, C., Beckman, R., & Dubowitz, T. (2014). Distance to store, food prices, and obesity in urban food deserts. *American Journal of Preventive Medicine, 47*(5), 587–595. doi:10.1016/j.amerpre.2014.07.005

Goetzel, R. Z., Henke, R. M., Tabrizi, M., Pelletier, K. R., Loeppke, R., Ballard, D. W., … Metz, R. D. (2014). Do workplace health promotion (wellness) programs work? *Journal of Occupational and Environmental Medicine, 56*(9), 927–934. doi:10.1097/JOM.0000000000000276

Goldsteen, R. L, Goldsteen, K., & Goldsteen, B. Z. (2017). *Jonas' introduction to the U.S. health care system* (8th ed.). New York, NY: Springer Publishing.

Gordon, C., Purciel-Hill, M., Ghai, N. R., Kaufman, L., Graham, R., & Van Wye, G. (2011). Measuring food deserts in New York City's low-income neighborhoods. *Health & Place, 17*(2), 696–700. doi:10.1016/j.healthplace.2010.12.012

Grumbach, K., Miller, J., Mertz, E., & Finocchio, L. (2004). How much public health in public health nursing practice. *Public Health Nursing, 21*(3), 266–276.

Hanna-Attish, M., LaChance, J., Sadler, R. C., & Champney Schnepp, A. (2016). Elevated blood lead levels in children associated with the Flint drinking water crisis: A spatial analysis of risk and public health response. *American Journal of Public Health, 106*(2), 283–290. doi:10.2105/AJPH.2015.303003

Hawe, P. (1994). Capturing the meaning of "community" in community intervention evaluation: Some contributions from community psychology. *Health Promotion International, 9*(3), 199–210.

Institute of Medicine. (1988). *The future of public health.* Washington, DC: National Academies Press.

Institute of Medicine. (2003). *Unequal treatment: Confronting racial and ethnic disparities in health care.* Washington, DC: National Academies of Sciences.

Kub, J., Kulbok, P. A., & Glick, D. (2015). Cornerstone documents, milestones, and policies: Shaping the direction of public health nursing 1890-1950. *OJIN: The Online Journal of Issues in Nursing, 20*(2), Manuscript 3. doi:10.3912/OJIN.Vol20No02Man03

Kulbok, P. A., & Ervin, N. E. (2012). Nursing science and public health: Contributions to the discipline of nursing. *Nursing Science Quarterly, 25*(1), 37–43. doi:10.1177/0894318411429034

Labonté, R. (1989). Community empowerment: The need for political analysis. *Canadian Journal of Public Health, 80*(2), 87–88.

Laidlaw, M. A., Filippelli, G. M., Sadler, R. C., Gonzales, C. R., Ball, A. S., & Mielke, H. W. (2016). Children's blood lead seasonality in Flint, Michigan (USA), and soil-sourced lead hazard risks. *International Journal of Environmental Research and Public Health, 13*(4), 358. doi:10.3390/ijerph13040358

Leavell, H. R., & Clark, H. G. (1965). *Preventive medicine for the doctor in his community* (3rd ed.). New York, NY: McGraw-Hill.

Levin, P., Cary, A, Kulbok, P., Leffers, J., Molle, M., & Polivka, B. (2008). Graduate education in public health nursing: At the crossroads. *Public Health Nursing, 25*(2), 176–193.

Livingston, I. L. (Ed.). (1994). *Handbook of Black American health: The mosaic of conditions, issues, policies, and prospects.* Westport, CT: Greenwood Press.

Maglacas, A. M. (1988). Health for all: Nursing's role. *Nursing Outlook, 36*(2), 66–71.

Mason, D. J., Gardner, D. B., Hopkins Outlaw, F., & O'Grady, E. T. (Eds.). (2016). *Policy & politics in nursing and health care* (7th ed.). St. Louis, MO: Elsevier.

Mason, D. J., Jones, D. A., Roy, C., Sullivan, C. G., & Wood, L. J. (2015). Commonalities of nurse-designed models of health care. *Nursing Outlook, 63*(5), 540–553.

Maxcy, K. F. (1956). *Preventive medicine and public health* (8th ed.). New York, NY: Appleton-Century-Crofts.

Mayberry, R. M., & Price, P. A. (1993). Targeting blacks in cigarette billboard advertising: Results from down south. *Health Values, 17*(1), 28–35.

McCallin, A. (2001). Interdisciplinary practice—a matter of teamwork: An integrated literature review. *Journal of Clinical Nursing, 10*(4), 419–428.

McKnight, J. (1987). Regenerating community. *Social Policy, 17*(30), 54–58.

McKnight, J., & Van Dover, L. (1994). Community as client: A challenge for nursing education. *Public Health Nursing, 11*(1), 12–16.

McMillan, D. W., & Chavis, D. (1986). Sense of community: A definition and theory. *Journal of Community Psychology, 14*(1), 6–23.

Morris, E. (1996). Community in theory and practice: A framework for intellectual renewal. *Journal of Planning Literature, 11*(1), 127–150.

National Nurse-Led Care Consortium. (n.d.). About nurse-managed care. Retrieved from http://nurseledcare.org/about/nurse-led-care.html

National Prevention Council. (2011). *National prevention strategy*. Washington, DC: U.S. Department of Health and Human Services, Office of the Surgeon General. Retrieved from https:// www .surgeongeneral.gov/priorities/prevention/strategy/report.pdf

Novak, J. C. (1988). The social mandate and historical basis for nursing's role in health promotion. *Journal of Professional Nursing, 4*(2), 80–87.

Obama, B. (2016). United States health care reform: Progress to date and next steps. *Journal of the American Medical Association, 316*(5), 525–532. doi:10.1001/jama.2016.9797

Quad Council of Public Health Nursing Organizations. (1997). *The tenets of public health nursing*. Unpublished white paper.

Quad Council of Public Health Nursing Organizations. (1999). *Scope and standards of public health nursing practice*. Washington, DC: American Nurses Publishing.

Robert Wood Johnson Foundation. (2015). From vision to action: A framework and measures to mobilize a culture of health. Retrieved from http://www.rwjf.org/content/dam/COH/RWJ000_COH-Update_CoH_Report_1b.pdf

Shi, L. (2014). *Introduction to health policy*. Chicago, IL: Health Administration Press.

Silverstein, N. G. (1985). Lillian Wald at Henry Street, 1893–1895. *Advances in Nursing Science, 7*(2), 1–12.

Spradley, B. W., & Allender, J. A. (1996). *Community health nursing: Concepts and practice*. Philadelphia, PA: Lippincott.

Stanhope, M., & Lancaster, J. (2016). *Public health nursing: Population-centered health care in the community* (9th ed.). St. Louis, MO: Elsevier.

Sullivan, J. A. (Ed.). (1984). *Directions in community health nursing*. Boston, MA: Blackwell.

Trust for America's Health. (n.d.). Our vision for a healthier America. Retrieved from healthyamericans. org/healthier-america-project

Trust for America's Health. (2007). Vision for a healthier America. Retrieved from http://healthyamericans .org/assets/files/VisionHealthierAmerica.pdf

U.S. Department of Health and Human Services. (2012). Preventive services covered under the Affordable Care Act. Retrieved from www.hhs.gov/healthcare/facts-and-features/fact-sheet/preventive-services-covered-under-ace/index.html#CoveredPreventiveServices

Wiley, L. (2016). The struggle for the soul of public health. *Journal of Health Politics, Policy and Law, 41*(6), 1083–1096. doi:10.1215/03616878-3665967

Williams, D. R., McClellan, M. B., & Rivlin, A. M. (2010). Beyond the Affordable Care Act: Achieving real improvements in Americans' health. *Health Affairs, 29*(8), 1481–1488. doi:10.1377/hlthaff.2010.0071

Williams, D. R., & Mohammed, S. A. (2013). Racism and health I: Pathways and scientific evidence. *American Behavioral Scientist, 57*(8), 1152–1173. doi:10.1177/0002764213487340

Williams, D. R., Priest, N., & Anderson, N. B. (2016). Understanding associations among race, socioeconomic status, and health: Patterns and prospects. *Health Psychology, 35*(4), 407–411. doi:10.1037/hea0000242

Williams, D. R., & Purdie-Vaughns, V. (2016). Needed interventions to reduce racial/ethnic disparities in health. *Journal of Health Politics, Policy and Law, 41*(4), 627–651. doi:10.1215/03616878-3620857

SECTION II

Community Assessment Process

CHAPTER 3

Overview of Community and the Community Assessment Process

■ STUDY EXERCISES

1. Examine conceptualizations and definitions of community in the context of advanced public/community health nursing practice.
2. Discuss advantages and disadvantages of specific community-level outcome measures.
3. Why is it necessary to work with communities in the community assessment process?
4. Describe the major purposes of conducting community assessments.
5. Describe the components of the community assessment process.
6. How are community assessments applied in advanced public/community health nursing practice?
7. Discuss the differences and similarities between an interdisciplinary approach and an individual advanced public/community health nursing practice approach to community assessment.

Community as a unit of service is a cornerstone of advanced public/community health nursing practice. Indeed, the idea of conceptualizing community as a unit of care is historically rooted in the early public health movement (Kub, Kulbok, & Glick, 2015). Florence Nightingale's work in the Crimean War (Fee & Garofalo, 2010) illustrated using community as a unit of service in promoting health and well-being of wounded soldiers. Although the idea of community as a unit of service became accepted within the public health movement (Goodman, Bunnell, & Posner, 2014; Novick, 2005) and within public/community health nursing (Kulbok, Thatcher, Park, & Meszaros, 2012), less attention has been paid to the evolution of the concept of community itself.

Historically, the lived experience of community has evolved with changes brought about by evolving economic and family structures, cultural diversity, democratization, increased mobility, industrialization, integration, and urbanization. In public/community health nursing, there has been ongoing discussion of the relationship between the concept of community and practice, and how the concept of community influences practice. Yet, public/community health nurses use a wide range of conceptualizations, each having different influences on practice.

This chapter first focuses on conventional definitions of community and patterns of practice of advanced public/community health nurses within the context of community-as-client, community-as-relational-experience, and community-as-resource. Then, the focus shifts to the process of community assessment. Although community assessment is rarely conducted as a solo activity of an advanced practice public/community health nurse, in this chapter you will learn how a nurse conducts or directs most of these activities. The advanced practice public/community health nurse must have knowledge and skills of the community assessment process, irrespective of whether he or she is a member of a team. Moreover, the master's-prepared public/community health nurse may be the only member of an interdisciplinary team with formal educational preparation to plan and conduct a community assessment.

■ DEFINITIONS, TYPES, AND CONCEPTUALIZATIONS OF COMMUNITY

Definitions of *community* abound in the public/community health nursing literature. For many nurses, community is a setting of practice. However, as Laffrey and Craig (1995) stated, community as a setting of practice is an important definition but not "sufficient for community health nursing practice" (p. 127). Community, then, rather than simply being a setting in which practice occurs, is viewed as a focus of practice. In Blum's (1981) seminal article, he described several different types of communities, including face-to-face communities, neighborhood, community of identifiable need, community of problem ecology, community of concern, community of special interest, community of viability, community of action capability, community of political jurisdiction, resource community, and community of solution. Blum's types of communities infer both structural features of community, that is, a neighborhood within a defined region, and functional aspects of community, for example, a special interest group that crosses geopolitical boundaries.

Other theorists described specific characteristics of community. Higgs and Gustafson (1985) identified attributes of community that include size, population groups, culture, spatial characteristics or boundaries, organizations, laws, socioeconomic status, community history, occupations, schools, and community resources. Similarly, Anderson and McFarlane (2015) described community as encompassing eight components: physical environment, education, safety and transportation, politics and government, health and social services, communication, economic, and recreation.

The most common definitions of *community* that are useful for public/community health nursing practice encompass the ideas of an aggregate of *people*, in a *place* referring to geographic locality or time, and with specific *function* described as aim or activities (Shuster, 2014). Cassells (1993) described community as an aggregate of people, as a location in time and space, or as a social system. Anderson and McFarlane (1988) defined *community* as "a group, population, or cluster of people with at least one common characteristic (such as geographic location, occupation, ethnicity, or housing condition)" (p. 261). Shuster and Goeppinger (1996) described community as a "locality based entity, composed of systems of formal organizations reflecting societal institutions, informal groups and aggregates" (p. 290). In addition, they viewed the dimensions of community as interrelated, including personal, geographic, and functional components. More recent, in *Public Health Nursing: Scope and Standards of Practice*, the American Nurses Association defined *community* as "a set of people in interaction, who may or may not share a sense of place or belonging, and who act intentionally for a common purpose (e.g., live in a neighborhood; work at a given company; or share a common cultural or demographic characteristic, health condition, or threat to health)" (American Nurses Association [ANA], 2013, p. 3).

Definitions of community are both complex and variable. For advanced public/community health nursing practice, the definitions of *community* may have a dramatic influence on the nature and scope of practice. In order to examine this premise, three conceptualizations of community are considered next: community-as-client, community-as-relational-experience, and community-as-resource.

Conceptualizing Community-as-Client

Discourse on the conceptualization of community-as-client was dominant in the 1980s (Kulbok, Kub, & Glick, 2017). Within this conceptualization, *community* is defined as a group or aggregate of people within a geopolitical boundary and is the unit of practice. This conceptualization requires nurses to examine and focus their practice on the community as a whole and as the unit of service delivery. Mass screenings, immunization campaigns, public policy for the good of the community, and community education programs are common activities within a community-as-client framework.

Nurses work with the community to understand issues that permeate the community, to identify and assess health issues of the community as a whole, and to plan and implement services on a broad scale. Understanding the social determinants of health and the use of epidemiologic data are essential to identify patterns and trends of health, illness, and associated risk factors. In advanced public/community health nursing practice, the conceptualization of community-as-client emphasizes program planning on a mass scale, prevention and early-intervention programs for the population as a whole, and programs that are disease or injury specific. Notably, government statutes in relation to communicable disease control, child welfare, sanitation, and public health policy may guide advanced public/community health nursing practice.

Conceptualizing Community-as-Relational-Experience

A conceptualization of community that contrasts sharply with the community-as-client is community-as-relational-experience. Within this conceptualization, *community* is defined as the everyday experience of people "living" and "being" in community. Community is the experience of having "a shared culture, which entails having a mutual respect for every culture in a community. Through this collective experience, communities gain respect for their own and others' histories, resources, hopes, and dreams" (Creative City Network of Canada, 2007, p. 5). Although community pervades most people's lives, it is rarely talked about or put into words. When a nurse visits a subsidized housing complex, she must not rely solely on the social determinants of health or epidemiological data in her community assessment. The nurse also needs to consider community connections, relations, and experiences of the people of the community. The experiences of connection and power are inextricably interwoven. They determine the qualitative dimensions of the experience of community.

Within the conceptualization of community-as-relational-experience, advanced public/community health nursing practice requires nurses to engage in policy and community-development strategies. Nursing practice is participatory: working with people of the community for collective action and change. Although the basic impetus for the work is grounded in the relational experience, understanding sociopolitical–environmental factors that influence health is essential to understand the relational experience of power within the community.

Conceptualizing Community-as-Resource

Community-as-client and community-as-relational-experience have been examined as contrasting conceptualizations. Community-as-resource is the bridge that spans or brings together the previous two conceptualizations. Community-as-resource, as a bridge, reflects an emerging understanding and definitions of *health* and *health promotion* in its language. If *health* is defined as a resource for living and health promotion is designed to facilitate resourcefulness and capacity within the community (World Health Organization [WHO], 1986), then community becomes an alive and active agent in the health of its members.

In contrast to community-as-client and community-as-relational-experience, the emphasis of community-as-resource is on the vitality, capacity, and resourcefulness of the community members. With these three conceptualizations of community as a foundation, our discussion next turns to measuring outcomes of care at the community level and working with the community in advanced practice.

■ MEASURING OUTCOMES OF CARE AT THE COMMUNITY LEVEL

The choice of the most appropriate community-level outcome measures is guided by both program or project goals and the nurse's conceptualization or definition of *community*. For example, within the community-as-client perspective, if the program goals are to reduce the incidence and prevalence of disease, to reduce the incidence of injuries, and to increase health and longevity, then outcome measures must be congruent with these goals. A number of outcome measures may be appropriate. These outcome measures reflect the focus on epidemiologic data. Within the community-as-relational-experience perspective, it is important to choose outcome measures that (a) are relevant and meaningful to the community members and (b) capture the process as well as the potential outcomes of community development work and program goals. Moreover, the outcome-evaluation process must be completed in partnership with members of the community. Outcome measures for advanced public/community health nursing practice within the community-as-resource perspective need to address the multidimensional experience of practice. Evaluation may encompass the overall health status of the population as well as explicit health patterns or risk factors. In addition, documentation about community members' experiences, including meaning and relevance of particular health patterns for the community, is essential. Examples of outcome measures for the community-as-client, the community-as-relational-experience, and the community-as-resource perspectives and corresponding advanced public/community health nursing practice activities are given in Table 3.1.

■ WORKING WITH COMMUNITY IN ADVANCED PRACTICE

Advanced public/community health nursing practice involves working with communities as equal partners to achieve desired community-level health outcomes. In partnerships with community members, nurses often function in a shared leadership role and engage in a collaborative and participatory process with members of the community (Kulbok et al., 2012). In this participatory process, nurses facilitate, honor, and respect the self-initiated actions of community members and continuously encourage community members to voice their ideas and local knowledge of community assets and resources.

When advanced public/community health nurses work as equal partners with communities to implement community-wide programs, they strive to engage community members and trusted community leaders in all program activities, from problem identification to evaluation and dissemination. This type of participatory approach, similar to community-based participatory research (CBPR), is based on critical and social action theory (Israel, Eng, Schulz, & Parker, 2005). This approach creates partnerships with community members across socioeconomic status and seeks balance between community members and nurses through shared leadership, coteaching and colearning opportunities (Kulbok et al., 2012). Nurses achieve this balance as partners with community members through listening and

TABLE 3.1 Outcome Measures and Corresponding Examples of Nursing Activities

Outcome Measures for Community-as-Client	Examples of Nursing Activities
Morbidity and mortality of disease and injury patterns	Reviewing data about people who have a diagnosis of lung cancer and number of people who died from lung cancer to determine areas for priority interventions
Prevalence and incidence of disease and injury patterns	Analyzing the number of head injuries as a result of motor vehicle crashes (prevalence) or the number of people with head injuries within the population (incidence)
Rates of immunization and/or protection against disease	Analyzing records of immunizations to determine need for immunization clinics and/or working with healthcare partners to provide immunizations
Outcome Measures for Community-as-Relational-Experience	**Examples of Nursing Activities**
Overall health status of community related to the social determinants of health	Collecting statistics on socioeconomic status, local employment patterns, and people living below the poverty line
Outcomes identified by the community as being relevant and important	Documenting changes in access to transportation, costs of housing, numbers of people misusing substances
Community involvement and participation	Documenting town hall meetings, local support group meetings, emerging community activities
Outcome Measures for Community-as Resource	**Examples of Nursing Activities**
Measures of the resources available within the community	Evaluating the effectiveness of support groups by community members and education initiatives undertaken by the community
Health activities and patterns of a community of people	Documenting the results of broad health-focused surveys, identifying changes in measures of societal health (e.g., decreasing low-birth-weight infants), documenting the effectiveness of community-based events to support community health (e.g., health fair)
Connectedness within the community	Supporting the development of community coalitions, community support groups, the growth of community capacity, interdisciplinary and multidisciplinary initiatives

critical reflection. Listening provides nurses an opportunity to understand everyday life experiences of the people in their care. These life experiences exemplify both the meaning of community and the effect of power within and on the community members. People whose voices have been marginalized, or are not heard both by other members of the group or professionals, have the opportunity to come forth. Although many health professionals believe that they understand community members, listening and reflection often provide new insights, perspectives, and opportunities to understand the meaning and relevance of issues, and the emergence of priorities.

Advanced public/community health nursing practice occurs in partnership with community members with the overall intent of increasing the health of the community by engaging in community-based planning. The nurse views her or his role as a collaborative change agent and holds an explicit understanding that change occurs only through partnership with the community. Although the nurse brings expert knowledge about population factors, theoretical frameworks, change theories, risk factors, and etiology, community members are equally valued for "local knowledge" about their own experiences and individual and sociocultural meanings of health and community. The nurse as an expert brings professional knowledge of community assessment, planning, implementation, and evaluation. The nurse as a partner brings skills of listening, critical reflection, recognizing patterns, and facilitating community action by creating partnerships and coalitions with community members, such as clients, other practitioners, government agencies, and special interest groups.

Advanced public/community health nursing practice is complex and multilayered. Practice is characterized by the ability to bring together divergent sources of knowledge and a range of strategies to engage with community members in participatory processes of community assessment, planning, implementation, or evaluation. In daily practice, the nurse's work involves integration of both local knowledge and professional knowledge. The intricate balance between the nurse's responsiveness to community members and her or his professional knowledge and competencies fosters community collaboration and participation, which are critical for effective advanced public/community health nursing practice.

■ PURPOSES OF CONDUCTING A COMMUNITY ASSESSMENT

For the specialty of public/community health nursing, conducting community assessments assists nurses in fulfilling their social responsibility. Advanced practice public/community health nurses, as professionals concerned with the health of a total community or population, have the responsibility, along with others, to protect the health of the population. The community assessment is one of the autonomous components of advanced practice that should be part of all public/community health nursing positions (ANA, 2013; Quad Council of Public Health Nursing Organizations, 2011). Purposes of conducting a community assessment include learning about a community, addressing persistent problems, meeting requirements, prioritizing problems, and informing the decision-making process.

The activities of community assessment may not be written into a formal job description, though it is becoming a more common job component of many positions. The prepared public/community health nurse introduces the concept and activities of community assessment into a position as part of the autonomous functions of the registered nurse, who has independent and legal authority to provide nursing care. In the case of a community assessment, the nursing care is provided to a community, population, or groups in a community. An assessment is a necessary part of nursing practice whether the client is a family, a group, a community, or a population.

In recent years, the American Association of Colleges of Nursing (AACN, 2011) recommended that all master's degree programs should include content from public health science, including epidemiology, population health analysis, and program planning. Although community assessment (or population health analysis) has been one skill of the specialist in public/community health nursing for many decades, others have recently seen the need for a broader focus on the health of communities and populations as well as individuals who present with illness.

Many types of organizations, not just healthcare organizations, conduct community assessments. This discussion, however, focuses on community assessments done by advanced practice public/community health nurses. The reasons for conducting a community assessment may differ among organizations, but the process is essentially the same.

Learning About a Community

In general, a community assessment is conducted in order to learn about a community. Often groups, business leaders, or elected officials want to address health or social problems in their communities without a reasonable idea of where or how to begin (Maurer, 2002). They may not know how people feel about the problem or have local knowledge of trends or factors that may have shaped the community. Without a good base of information, funds and valuable resources may be used to start programs that are not acceptable to the community or that do not address the actual problem. A comprehensive community assessment corrects these deficiencies by bringing together data and information about specific community conditions and characteristics.

Addressing Persistent Problems

Persistent and emerging health and social problems, such as infectious diseases, the growing number of refugees and immigrants, and poverty, require new approaches and preventive techniques. Community assessments can assist nurses in looking at old situations in new ways. Although helpful, community assessments alone cannot provide answers to complex problems but can inform nurses about the factors that contribute to the complexity of specific problems and conditions in communities.

In addition to dealing with new diseases, the United States and other countries are experiencing a recurrence of vaccine-preventable diseases (Hinman, Orenstein, & Schuchat, 2011). Although medications and medical treatments are often seen as the panacea for such diseases, they alone will not control the spread of disease. There must be money to purchase drugs, then the individual must take the drugs, and finally the drugs must be effective against the organism. Poverty, nonadherence to drug regimens, illiteracy, adverse drug reactions, cultural admonitions against taking drugs, and a myriad of other factors compete with the medical model of diagnosis and treatment. Information and data collected in a community assessment can assist healthcare professionals to understand problems in more depth and with new insights.

Meeting Requirements

Community assessments are being conducted more often because the Internal Revenue Service (IRS) requires in the Affordable Care Act (ACA) that nonprofit hospitals conduct a community health needs assessment (CHNA) every 3 years (Stoto, 2013). Previously, public health professionals were the main advocates for assessing the health status of populations because of their responsibility to protect the population's health, and community assessment is a core function of public health. For years, local health departments have collaborated with other governmental departments to conduct assessments because they are needed for the development of municipal plans required by the city or county government. Often, foundations and governmental agencies require submission of a community assessment with a request for funding.

Nowadays, there is a move toward national accreditation of local health departments with a requirement that public health professionals participate in a collaborative community health assessment (CHA) process (Laymon, Shah, Leep, Elligers, & Kumar, 2015). Since 2011, when the national accreditation program was launched through the Public Health Accreditation Board (PHAB), 134 public health departments and one integrated local public health system have been accredited (PHAB, 2016). PHAB accreditation requires these health departments to collaborate with local partners to complete CHAs.

Prioritizing Problems

One impetus for conducting community assessments is a lack of sufficient resources to address all identified problems. A community assessment provides part of the information needed for prioritizing the multitude of competing problems that confront most communities every day. The community assessment provides a view of what the problems are, how many people are affected, strengths of the community to deal with the problems, and trends of current or potential problems. Often, busy personnel in healthcare do not think that they have time to pursue an extensive community or population health analysis, but if done, this is time well spent because a community assessment provides direction for program planning and for deletion of programs no longer needed.

Informing the Decision-Making Process

Other purposes for conducting community assessments include the need to verify some suspected change, such as a demographic population shift; need to obtain detailed information about a particular segment of a larger community, such as married housing units on a college campus; and need as part of a proposal for a new program or service, such as a childhood obesity prevention campaign.

Community assessments are usually undertaken every year or 2 by an agency. Updating an assessment is then a matter of gathering current data and obtaining the perspective of residents, business owners, leaders, and professionals regarding changing circumstances. A community assessment may also be continuously updated with ongoing data from usual sources, such as disease reports, population projections, and vital statistics. Continuous survey of many sources of data to maintain current information about the health and social status of a community or population is a part of the advanced practice public/community health nurse's job.

Irrespective of whether it is called a *community assessment, CHNA, CHA, population health assessment,* or another term, this increased emphasis on assessing the health of the entire community in the public and private healthcare sectors provides a leadership opportunity for advanced practice public/community health nurses.

■ COMPARING THE COMMUNITY ASSESSMENT PROCESS AND THE NURSING ASSESSMENT PROCESS

You have used the nursing assessment process as the basic approach to nursing care of individuals and families, so you may need time to adjust your thinking to the community assessment process. Although the community assessment process and the nursing assessment process are similar, the two differ in several important aspects.

Focus of the Processes

The nursing assessment process is used to assess the status of an individual. Even when the nursing assessment process is used to assess a family, the family is often not assessed as a whole but as individuals who are related. In the community assessment process, the public/community health nurse specialist is concerned with the entire community from the beginning rather than assessing individuals and then attempting to put together their data. For example, data about chronic disease levels in the community are the focus of data collection rather than data about care provided to individuals by a particular health agency.

Steps of the Processes

A second difference between the nursing assessment process and the community assessment process relates to the steps involved. The nursing process includes collecting data and diagnosing. The community assessment process consists of data collection, data analysis, data synthesis, and formulation of community diagnoses. Additional components of working with the community, program planning, program implementation, and program evaluation are presented as separate processes in this book.

Frequency of Conducting the Processes

A third area of difference between the nursing assessment process and the community assessment process is the frequency at which the processes are performed. The nurse may assess an ill individual every 15 minutes or an individual with a stable condition at home every week or perhaps once a month. In general, a community assessment may be completed once a year or less often. Communities do not change as quickly as individuals, so community assessments are useful for longer periods of time or may be updated in pertinent areas as new information is received or obtained by the advanced public/community health nurse or team members. However, if a community is perceived to be undergoing rapid change, an updated community assessment would be a logical activity before programs and services are altered.

Data Elements

A fourth area of difference relates to data elements. Although similar conceptual frameworks may be used in nursing and community assessments to guide data collection, the actual data elements differ. For example, an individual's circulatory and respiratory systems are very different from community systems for crime prevention and for recreation. Although the systems' frameworks may be similar for these examples, the details are very different.

Content of Processes

These two kinds of assessments differ in a fifth aspect. Although the nurse may address risk factors and potential health problems of the individual, the nurse's assessment efforts are usually centered on the immediate reason for the individual's visit or hospitalization. Community assessments should include problems, trends, strengths, potential problems, and community risk factors or multiple determinants of health and health-related factors, such as housing, crime, social isolation, and income levels.

■ USES OF COMMUNITY ASSESSMENTS IN SUBSPECIALTIES

Advanced practice nurses in all public/community health nursing subspecialties, including occupational health, primary care, home health and hospice care, faith-based care, and school health, use the community assessment process. The focus of a community assessment may be on a community specifically related to the nurse's practice, such as school children in a particular elementary school or the total school community, including children, their families, and school personnel. The community assessment process, being a general process, is applicable in all settings, for all communities, populations, or aggregates.

Occupational Health Nursing

Advanced practice occupational health nurses may have a variety of responsibilities within various position titles. Thus, conducting community assessments may differ from the general outline presented in this chapter. The advanced practice occupational health nurse in a management position may conduct an assessment of the physical plant where employees work instead of the physical community in which they live. In this instance, the plant or business is the community. Conducting an assessment of both the plant and the geographic community may be appropriate for some situations, as when the worksite is in a closed community, such as an oil field in an isolated part of the world or occupational health issues of Native Americans who live on or near reservations in a southwestern state.

Primary Care

The advanced practice nurse in primary care, either clinical specialist or nurse practitioner, may conduct an assessment of a specific community and not just the clients and families who come to the primary care site. This total community assessment provides knowledge to participate with other professionals in addressing community concerns. A population health focus for primary care is becoming the usual pattern as new models of patient-centered care evolve to achieve the "triple aim" of better quality, experience, and cost (National Committee for Quality Assurance [NCQA], 2015). Patient-centered medical homes (PCMHs) and accountable care organizations (ACOs) are becoming more common sources of coordinated primary care for selected patient populations or entire communities. In addition, the NCQA recognizes practices that meet rigorous standards for addressing patient needs through long-term partnerships and coordination of care and community resources.

Advanced practice public/community health nurses in primary care who have information about their clients' communities can be more effective. The community assessment gives the nurse practitioner and clinical specialist a comprehensive view of clients' backgrounds and contexts of life. In addition, the advanced practice nurse becomes knowledgeable about community resources to which clients may be referred. Knowledge of a total community is necessary for advanced practice public/community health nurses when participating in program planning, review of quality of patient care, and professional activities. For advanced practice nurses who develop and deliver primary care services in community nursing centers, knowledge of the community is crucial for successful development of the center (Ervin & Young, 1996).

Faith-Based Care

In faith-based care or parish nursing, the advanced public/community health nurse has many roles involving individuals, families, groups, or the entire faith or parish community, including health advocate, health counselor, health educator, and program developer. The nurse often relies on a community assessment to get to know the unique characteristics and health and social needs of the parish community. A congregational needs assessment provides the nurse with valuable information that can be used to design targeted health-promotion and disease prevention interventions. A novel community assessment survey with an interactive faith-based kiosk used by congregants in African American churches revealed that opportunities for targeted church-based health-promotion activities were enhanced by knowledge of congregants' characteristics and overall health status (Dulchavsky, Ruffin, Johnson, Cogan, & Joseph, 2014).

Home Healthcare and Hospice Care

In home healthcare and hospice care, the advanced practice public/community health nurse is often challenged to develop new programs in order to meet the service demands of a growing elderly population. One basis for program planning is a community assessment. Although the focus is generally on the elderly population, data about the total community are necessary because of the dependency of elderly individuals on others for some activities of daily living and the complexity of their needs, which require an interdisciplinary approach. A community assessment provides the nurse leader in home healthcare and hospice services with information to conduct in-service education for staff about the community, to educate physician providers about the elderly population, to mobilize resources, to coordinate care, and to provide a smooth transition from home to hospital.

Aggregate Focus

Community assessments in subspecialty practice are valuable tools for several other reasons. The advanced practice nurse may be part of a management team responsible for developing and implementing new programs and services that relate directly to aggregates within the target population, such as pregnant students in a high school or women of childbearing age in a chemical factory. The community assessment gives the advanced practice nurse a comprehensive picture of aggregates and the environment for program development through the data collected, analyzed, and synthesized in the community assessment process.

Community assessments also provide baseline data used for evaluating program outcomes. Often, the data needed in assessments of aggregates or subpopulations are not available from usual sources such as literature and government publications. Surveys and internal records often supply specialized data. Thoughtful planning for collecting data from various sources is required before any activities are begun. These aspects of conducting a community assessment are addressed in detail in Chapter 7.

■ INTERDISCIPLINARY APPROACH TO COMMUNITY ASSESSMENT

As described in Chapter 1, the terms *interdisciplinary* and *interprofessional* are used interchangeably throughout this book. Interdisciplinary practice involves a variety of disciplines from health and other fields that work together through collaboration on planning, decision making, and goal setting (AACN, 1997). An interdisciplinary team includes people from different disciplines who come together with a unified direction, common objectives, and a focus on an integrated outcome (Mariano, 1989). In conducting a community assessment, nurses work with other disciplines in their own agencies and other community agencies that agree to be involved in the assessment process.

An interdisciplinary approach to conducting a community assessment is desired because a community assessment deals with multiple facets of the community. The complexity of problems that our society faces calls for a melding of the knowledge bases from several disciplines. This is being done successfully in some research projects, but is not as common as many governmental and voluntary agencies would like. Several reports have been issued to identify the need for interdisciplinary education and practice (AACN, 1997; Advisory Committee on Interdisciplinary, Community-Based Linkages [ACICBL], 2013; Interprofessional Education Collaborative Expert Panel [IECEP], 2011). In addition, years of research have begun to accumulate evidence that cooperation among healthcare providers results in better client outcomes (ACICBL, 2013; IECEP, 2011). A team of various disciplines provides richness and expertise that nursing alone does not usually bring to the process, such as knowledge and experience in enforcing housing codes and evaluating environmental levels against quality standards.

Acquiring Interdisciplinary Experience

Public health, one of the bases of public/community health nursing practice, is an interdisciplinary enterprise. The original master's programs in public health nursing were often part of schools of public health where students from all disciplines interacted and learned to practice in teams. Nowadays, almost all public/community health nursing graduate programs are offered in schools of nursing, and interdisciplinary educational activities may be limited. Some students have opportunities to take courses with students from other disciplines, for example, medical students, but, by and large, graduate nursing education is conducted with only nurses in the classroom. Content about developing and working with teams may be included as part of the curriculum. In addition, practicum experiences provide opportunities to use the content about interdisciplinary teamwork.

Most nurses have not had opportunities to practice with an interdisciplinary team, so this aspect of the role is not always easy to grasp or achieve. Moreover, it is particularly difficult to implement a team approach because most practice settings do not contain team practice models. Although it is true that professionals come together to meet and discuss problems and issues, usually they return to their own disciplines and methods after the meeting. This is not to imply that professionals do not want to collaborate through teamwork; it is a matter of fact that most health professionals have not had formal preparation about working in a team (ACICBL, 2013; IECEP, 2011).

Interdisciplinary team practice means that the members identify with the team as much as with their own disciplines. A key to this identification is sharing a common knowledge base. Advanced practice public/community health nurses are fortunate to have preparation in biostatistics and epidemiology, both important public health science courses that are taken by and common to all public health professionals. These common areas of knowledge can facilitate effective communication between the advanced practice nurse and other team members. Other interprofessional collaborative practice competency domains (IECEP, 2011) are given in Box 3.1.

BOX 3.1 INTERPROFESSIONAL COLLABORATIVE PRACTICE COMPETENCY DOMAINS

Competency Domain 1: Values/Ethics for Interprofessional Practice

Competency Domain 2: Roles/Responsibilities

Competency Domain 3: Interprofessional Communication

Competency Domain 4: Teams and Teamwork

Source: Interprofessional Education Collaborative Expert Panel. (2011). *Core competencies for interprofessional collaborative practice: Report of an expert panel.* Washington, DC: Interprofessional Education Collaborative, p. 16. Used with permission.

An additional factor that binds a team together is sharing a common intended outcome or goal (Mariano, 1989). In public/community health nursing, as in public health, this common intended outcome is promotion, protection, and restoration of the health of the public or a community (Pickett & Hanlon, 1990). Although teams do not work together on all aspects of care, the skills to lead or to function as a team member need to be included in the public/community health nurse's practice.

Assessing a Community as a Team

The goal of a team is to complete a community assessment as efficiently as possible. Conducting a community assessment as an interdisciplinary team presents a challenge because each team member may have a different background from the others and function in a role different than that called for in the team effort. Furthermore, a community assessment may be conducted in addition to the regular work of team members. The advanced practice public/community health nurse may facilitate team functioning by providing an organizing focus, such as suggesting a format to follow, providing written materials, conducting an orientation to the process, and writing a suggested plan and timeline. Other team members, who should be encouraged to contribute to the team's efforts, may share these skills.

Building a Team

Effectiveness as an interdisciplinary team may be enhanced by activities to promote team building. In order for a team to benefit from these activities, all team members must be present. Attendance at meetings demonstrates a commitment to the successful functioning of the team. Building commitment to the team is one of the activities that foster effective functioning.

Efforts to encourage commitment to the team and thus improve interdisciplinary practice can come from activities such as team-building exercises, attending continuing-education programs as a team, holding social events as a team, attending classes together, and cooperatively initiating a project. Team members and the leader should be viewed as equally important in contributing to the team's functioning. Suggestions for activities and exercises to encourage team building are presented in Chapter 7.

Obstacles to Team Efforts

In leading teams, the advanced practice public/community health nurse may encounter individuals who are not interested in developing and working on teams. These individuals may be those who like to work independently and express that team members in other disciplines are not as qualified as they are. Other individuals may be the type characterized as not "team players." These are people who like to work alone and feel burdened if asked to work with others in any aspect of the job.

At times, team efforts may falter if uncooperative individuals remain on the team. One alternative is to ask the person to resign from the team and seek a replacement. A second approach is to ask the individual to take specific assignments that do not require team involvement. For example, during the community assessment process, one individual could collect all data from secondary data sources. The other team members would then be available to collaborate on other tasks that require team effort, such as conducting focus groups or using the nominal group process.

Leadership Skills

A true team effort will allow individuals to use their unique skills to accomplish the tasks and reach the objectives set forth through team agreement. Although each team member has skills to contribute, individuals should not be limited in their roles if they are interested in developing new skills. For example, all members should lead the group if they so desire. The experience of leading the group will help each person to develop skills in a comfortable situation and result in better team members because there is more understanding about what it takes to lead and organize the team's work. Workshops about developing leadership could be part of the team's continuing-education activities.

The skills required to lead a group in a participatory manner include communicating clearly, facilitating decision making, encouraging contributions from all members, organizing the agenda, keeping the meeting on the agenda, allowing time for free discussion without losing control, and keeping a record of decisions already made (Hersey & Duldt, 1989; Schmele, 1996). The interdisciplinary team offers a great opportunity to learn and apply participatory work skills that will allow everyone on the team to be part of the decision-making process and bring out the best ideas from everyone.

The development of an interdisciplinary team to conduct a community assessment is a valuable asset. The team may be used to continue work during program planning, program implementation, and program evaluation. All members will learn from the development efforts and be able to function better in other situations.

■ COMMUNITY ASSESSMENT PROCESS

A community assessment, within the practice of the advanced practice public/community health nurse, is a comprehensive examination of a community or population. This comprehensive examination includes the multiple factors that are related to health and a healthy community (Aday, 1993). The community assessment process is composed of four parts: data collection, data analysis, data synthesis, and community diagnosis formulation. Each part of the community assessment process is elaborated in Chapters 4 through 8.

Program planning, program implementation, and program evaluation are presented in this textbook as separate core processes of the advanced practice public/community health nursing role and are addressed in depth in later chapters. Separating the processes of community assessment, program planning, program implementation, and program evaluation allows nurses to understand the numerous ways in which they may be used together, separately, and in conjunction with other processes and in a variety of agencies and organizations.

Data Collection

Data collection involves the actual physical acquisition of facts, observations, opinions, statistics, and other types of information about the community. Sources of data and methods of data collection, which are covered in Chapters 5 and 6, vary somewhat with the specific purpose and focus of the assessment. The data-collection activities are begun after the community assessment is planned and the timeline determined. Data collection can consume a great deal of time, so the plan for the community assessment will provide guidance for data collection on the basis of available time, money, personnel, and purposes of the community assessment. Details about planning for the community assessment are presented in Chapter 7.

MULTIPLE DETERMINANTS OF HEALTH

Health and the lack of it have multiple determinants, so the task in a comprehensive community assessment is to examine not only health-related behavior but also the conditions of living, such as housing, eating, and working (Green & Kreuter, 2005; Commission to Build a Healthier America, 2008). Social, economic, and political conditions have been determined to play important parts in a society's health (U.S. Department of Health and Human Services [USDHHS], 2016). The relationship between a country's economic development and the population's health has been found to be strong (Anderson & McFarlane, 2015).

LIFESTYLE DATA

Lifestyle is part of the multiple determinants of health. Often, lifestyle is equated with personal choice, but a community focus takes a broader view. Green and Kreuter (1999, p. 13), leading authorities in health promotion, defined *lifestyle* as "a composite expression of the social and cultural circumstances that condition and constrain behavior, in addition to the personal decisions the individual might make in choosing one behavior over another."

This definition of *lifestyle* requires an understanding of the various factors that shape behavior and how a community (which is the context of behavior) both influences and is influenced by the individual. Data collection about the context of behavior is an important part of a community assessment.

COMPREHENSIVE DATA

Acquiring comprehensive data for a community assessment requires much time and effort but can be done over a period of time. If adequate time is available, data analysis can go on simultaneously with collection of additional data and information to fill in gaps in the data. With the intensified debate about healthcare reform in the United States during the past decades, professionals in healthcare are becoming more accepting of information that points to the need for a multipronged approach to improve the health of the population. This approach requires comprehensive data about numerous factors in the community.

The medical model of diagnosing, treating, and curing illness has dominated the healthcare system, especially since World War II (Green & Kreuter, 2005), so small amounts of resources and efforts have been put forth in the areas of prevention and health promotion. Despite the enactment of the ACA in 2010, recent policy debates have not emphasized serious expansion of prevention and wellness (Murray & Frenk, 2010). In fact, because of a continued medical model focus by third-party payers, data about health behaviors, disease prevention, and other useful information are not available as readily as illness statistics.

A narrow focus on only illness statistics and utilization of illness services, such as the number of hospitalizations, emergency room visits, diagnostic tests performed, or encounters at physicians' offices, provides very little insight into the actual health status of a community. Indeed, these data may be useful at some time and some place in a program-planning process but are not the content of a community assessment in the context of advanced public/community health nursing practice. A comprehensive approach to community assessment includes data about health behaviors, disease and injury prevention, and health promotion.

The first phase of the community assessment process, data collection, provides the necessary raw statistics and knowledge to begin data analysis.

Data Analysis

Analysis is a cognitive process of ordering data to allow for the higher level function of synthesis. Although analysis may occur throughout the community assessment process, this step is encouraged as a formal activity to allow the public/community health nurse to become better acquainted with the data and, thus, an opportunity to see patterns that may have been overlooked during the data-collection phase. Analyzing data is not a clearly delineated process and requires an ongoing commitment to seeking others' ideas and expertise during and after the formal phase of the community assessment process. An approach to data analysis is presented in Chapter 8.

An interdisciplinary or interprofessional team is a valuable asset during the data analysis phase of the community assessment. The team members comprise different areas of knowledge and viewpoints. The composition of a team should be based on the purpose of the community assessment, the agency conducting the assessment, and the community in which the assessment is conducted. There are often no right or wrong conclusions to be drawn, so varying perspectives allow for a healthy debate and convincing-each-other stage.

Data analysis is not an objective process. People's activities are likely to be influenced by their backgrounds, experiences, and knowledge. In addition, team members will have varying experience with the type of analysis used for community assessment. An analysis process that involves a number of the team members' disciplines provides some safeguard against biases. Chapter 8 includes content about analyzing data without bias.

A second important component is involvement of those who live in the community being assessed. As identified earlier, the community needs to be represented in as many ways as possible and as often as possible in the community assessment process. This is not an expedient way to accomplish the task, but a completed community assessment without community ideas represents only a professional viewpoint. Approaches to solving community problems require the whole community, not just professionals. Effective approaches for involving the community are presented throughout the book.

Data Synthesis

During synthesis of data, the advanced practice public/community health nurse combines data elements from several sources to create a coherent whole or a new, complete picture of what is known or not known (Grove, Burns, & Gray, 2013). In synthesizing data, the advanced practice public/community health nurse brings experience and knowledge of research, and community health in general, to bear on the analyzed data.

There are no rules to dictate right from wrong in the synthesis phase of the community assessment process, so the nurse must make use of literature, research findings, experts in specific fields, and other health professionals to come to conclusions that are as objective and unbiased as possible. Advanced practice public/community health nurses have an obligation to interpret data without a negative bias. In addition, data must be interpreted in the context of the specific beliefs, culture, history, and values of the community. Seeking ratification from a community of the community diagnoses is one way to obtain some verification about whether conclusions are valid. Community validation of conclusions can assist nurses in avoiding invalid negative conclusions (Anderson & McFarlane, 2015). In the future, there may be community diagnoses that have been tested for reliability and validity.

Just as with any new skill, data synthesis begins at an elementary level and becomes more advanced with experience and knowledge. Also, data synthesis is dependent on the level of knowledge of interdependent relationships in the community. For example, the discovery that lead in the environment results in poisoning led to more research to increase knowledge about sources of lead, behaviors related to lead ingestion, and prevention techniques (Green & Kreuter, 2005). Data synthesis is addressed in Chapter 8.

COMMUNITY DIAGNOSIS

The diagnosis phase of the community assessment process involves stating the conclusions drawn from synthesis of the data (Anderson & McFarlane, 2015; Shuster, 2014). Community diagnoses may be formulated about health issues (e.g., infant mortality), housing conditions (e.g., high lead content in interior paint), economic conditions (e.g., 30% of community residents below poverty level), strengths (e.g., three community coalitions formed to deal with potential environmental hazards), or trends (e.g., increasing employment opportunities). Chapter 8 presents and illustrates formats for stating community diagnoses.

■ SUMMARY

Purposes for conducting a community assessment vary with the organization, its functions, and requirements of external agencies. Determining the purpose of conducting a specific community assessment is one of the first steps in the total endeavor. The actual steps of the community assessment process include data collection, data analysis, data synthesis, and community diagnosis. These individual steps are elaborated in later chapters.

Within the field of public/community health nursing, subspecialties, such as faith-based care, home healthcare, occupational health, primary care, and school health, make use of community assessments to describe the targets of their services as well as to provide the basis for program planning and evaluation. At times, interdisciplinary or interprofessional teams are involved in conducting community assessments. The advanced practice public/community health nurse uses skills to develop, work with, and lead interdisciplinary teams.

The next chapter provides a variety of frameworks and models used in guiding a community assessment.

■ SUGGESTED CLINICAL OR PRACTICUM ACTIVITIES

1. Interview advanced public/community health nurses working in local or state public health agencies or different subspecialties about how they conceptualize the community. Compare and contrast different conceptualizations of the community, target populations, and the implications for advanced nursing practice.
2. Discuss with advanced practice public/community health nurses what outcome measures and nursing activities they most commonly use in their practice.
3. Identify a community coalition that is focused on a specific community health problem (e.g., childhood obesity, homelessness, opioid abuse). Attend meetings of the coalition and analyze interdisciplinary team roles of the coalition members. How might an advanced practice public/community health nurse facilitate the work of the coalition?

REFERENCES

Aday, L. A. (1993). *At risk in America.* San Francisco, CA: Jossey-Bass.

Advisory Committee on Interdisciplinary, Community-Based Linkages. (2013). *Redesigning health professions education and practice to prepare the interprofessional team to care for populations; Twelfth annual report to the Secretary of the United States Department of Health and Human Services and the Congress of the United States.* Rockville, MD: U.S. Department of Health and Human Services, Health Resources and Services Administration. Retrieved from http://www.hrsa.gov/advisorycommittees/bhpradvisory/acicbl/Reports/twelfthreport_.pdf

American Association of Colleges of Nursing. (1997). *Interdisciplinary education and practice.* Washington, DC: Author.

American Association of Colleges of Nursing. (2011). *The essentials of master's education in nursing.* Washington, DC: Author. Retrieved from http://www.aacnnursing.org/Portals/42/Publications/MastersEssentials11.pdf

American Nurses Association. (2013). *Public health nursing: Scope and standards of practice* (2nd ed.). Silver Spring, MD: nursesbooks.org.

Anderson, E. T., & McFarlane, J. (1988). *Community as client: Theory and practice in nursing.* New York, NY: Lippincott.

Anderson, E. T., & McFarlane, J. (2015). *Community as partner: Theory and practice in nursing* (7th ed.). Philadelphia, PA: Lippincott Williams & Wilkins.

Blum, H. L. (1981). *Planning for health: Genetics for the eighties* (2nd ed.). New York, NY: Human Sciences Press.

Cassells, H. (1993). Nursing process in the community. In J. M. Swanson & M. Albrecht (Eds.), *Community health nursing: Promoting the health of aggregates* (pp. 81–108). Philadelphia, PA: Saunders.

Commission to Build a Healthier America. (2008). *Where we live matters for our health: The links between housing and health* (Issue Brief 2). Washington, DC: Robert Wood Johnson Foundation. Retrieved from http://www.commissiononhealth.org/PDF/e6244e9e-f630-4285-9ad7-16016dd7e493/Issue%20Brief%202%20Sept%2008%20-%20Housing%20and%20Health.pdf

Creative City Network of Canada. (2007). *Creative city news, special edition 4.* Vancouver, BC, Canada: Author.

Dulchavsky, S. A., Ruffin, W. J., Johnson, D. A., Cogan, C., & Joseph, C. L. (2014). Use of an interactive, faith-based kiosk by congregants of four predominantly, African-American churches in a metropolitan area. *Frontiers in Public Health, 2*(106), 1–5. doi:10.3389/fpubh.2014.00106

Ervin, N. E., & Young, W. B. (1996). Model for a nursing center: Spanning boundaries. *Journal of Nursing Care Quality, 11*(2), 16–24.

Fee, E., & Garofalo, M. E. (2010). Florence Nightingale and the Crimean War. *American Journal of Public Health, 100*(9), 1591. doi:10.2105/AJPH.2009.188607

Goodman, R. A., Bunnell, R., & Posner, S. F. (2014). What is "community health"? Examining the meaning of an evolving field in public health. *Preventive Medicine, 67*(Suppl. 1), S58–S61.

Green, L. W., & Kreuter, M. W. (1999). *Health promotion planning: An educational and environmental approach* (3rd ed.). Mountain View, CA: Mayfield.

Green, L. W., & Kreuter, M. W. (2005). *Health program planning: An educational and environmental approach* (4th ed.). New York, NY: McGraw-Hill.

Grove, S. K., Burns, N., & Gray, J. (2013). *The practice of nursing research: Appraisal, synthesis and generation of evidence* (7th ed.). Philadelphia, PA: Saunders.

Hersey, P., & Duldt, B. W. (1989). *Situational leadership in nursing.* Norwalk, CT: Appleton & Lange.

Higgs, Z. R., & Gustafson, D. D. (1985). *Community as client: Assessment and diagnosis.* Philadelphia, PA: F. A. Davis.

Hinman, A. R., Orenstein, W. A., & Schuchat, A. (2011). Vaccine-preventable diseases, immunizations, and MMWR–1961–2011. *Morbidity and Mortality Weekly Report, 60*(Suppl. 4), 49–57. Retrieved from https://www.cdc.gov/mmwr/preview/mmwrhtml/su6004a9.htm

Interprofessional Education Collaborative Expert Panel. (2011). *Core competencies for interprofessional collaborative practice: Report of an expert panel.* Washington, DC: Interprofessional Education Collaborative.

Israel, B. A., Eng, E., Schulz, A. J., & Parker , E. A. (2005). *Methods in community-based participatory research for health.* San Francisco, CA: Jossey-Bass.

Kub, J., Kulbok, P., Glick, D., (2015). Cornerstone documents, milestones, and policies: Shaping the direction of public health nursing 1890-1950. *OJIN: The Online Journal of Issues in Nursing, 20*(2), Manuscript 3. doi: 10.3912/OJIN.Vol20No02Man03

Kulbok, P. A., Kub, J., & Glick, D. F. (2017). Cornerstone documents, milestones, and policies: The changing landscape of public health nursing 1950–2015. *Online Journal of Issues in Nursing, 22*(2). doi:10.3912/OJIN.Vol22No02PPT57

Kulbok, P. A., Thatcher, E., Park, E., & Meszaros, P. S. (2012). Evolving public health nursing roles: Focus on community participatory health promotion and prevention. *Online Journal of Issues in Nursing, 17*(2), Manuscript 1. doi:10.3912/OJIN.Vol17No02Man01

Laffrey, S. C., & Craig, D. M. (1995). Health promotion for communities and aggregates: An integrated model. In M. Stewart (Ed.), *Community nursing: Promoting Canadians' health* (pp. 125–145). Toronto, ON, Canada: Saunders.

Laymon, B., Shah, G., Leep, C. J., Elligers, J. J., & Kumar, V. (2015). The proof's in the partnerships: Are Affordable Care Act and local health department accreditation practices influencing collaborative partnerships in community health assessment and improvement planning? *Journal of Public Health Management and Practice, 21*(1), 12–17.

Mariano, C. (1989). The case for interdisciplinary collaboration. *Nursing Outlook, 37*(6), 285–288.

Maurer, R. (2002). Methods of community assessment. Retrieved from http://srdc.msstate.edu/trainings/presentations_archive/2002/2002_maurer.pdf

Murray, C. J. L., & Frenk, J. (2010). Ranking 37th—Measuring the performance of the U.S. health care system. *New England Journal of Medicine, 362*, 98–99. doi:10.1056/NEJMp0910064

National Committee for Quality Assurance. (2015). The future of patient-centered medical homes: Foundation for a better health care system. Retrieved from https://www.ncqa.org/Portals/0/Public%20Policy/2014%20PDFS/The_Future_of_PCMH.pdf

Novick, L. F. (2005). Defining public health: Historical and contemporary development. In L. F. Novick, G. P. Mays., & G. C. Benjamin (Eds.), *Public health administration: Principles for population-based management* (pp. 3–33). Sudbury, MA: Jones & Bartlett.

Pickett, G., & Hanlon, J. J. (1990). *Public health administration and practice* (9th ed.). St. Louis, MO: Times Mirror/Mosby College Publishing.

Public Health Accreditation Board. (2016). Accredited health departments. Retrieved from http://www.phaboard.org/news-room/accredited-health-departments

Quad Council of Public Health Nursing Organizations. (2011). Quad Council competencies for public health nurses. Retrieved from http://www.achne.org/files/quad%20council/quadcouncilcompetenciesforpublichealthnurses.pdf

Schmele, J. A. (1996). *Quality management in nursing and health care.* Albany, NY: Delmar.

Shuster, G. F. (2014). Community as client: Assessment and analysis. In M. Stanhope & J. Lancaster (Eds.), *Public health nursing: Population-centered health care in the community* (8th ed., pp. 392–426). St. Louis, MO: Mosby Elsevier.

Shuster, G. F., & Goeppinger, J. (1996). Community as client: Using the nursing process to promote health. In M. Stanhope & J. Lancaster (Eds.), *Community health nursing* (4th ed., pp. 289–314). Toronto, ON, Canada: Mosby.

Stoto, M. A. (2013). *Population health in the Affordable Care Act era.* Retrieved from http://www.academyhealth.org/files/publications/files/AH2013pophealth.pdf

U.S. Department of Health and Human Services. (2016). *Healthy people 2020 [Internet].* Washington, DC: Author, Office of Disease Prevention and Health Promotion. Retrieved from https://www.healthypeople.gov/2020/topics-objectives/topic/social-determinants-of-health

World Health Organization. (1986). *Ottawa charter for health promotion.* Ottawa, ON, Canada: Health and Welfare Canada. Retrieved from http://www.who.int/healthpromotion/conferences/previous/ottawa/en

CHAPTER 4

Exploring Frameworks and Models for Guiding a Community Assessment

■ STUDY EXERCISES

1. Why is a framework or model used as a guide to conduct a community assessment?
2. How is a framework or model used in conducting a community assessment?
3. Compare and contrast frameworks and models used for community assessments.
4. List some advantages and disadvantages of the various community assessment frameworks and models used for conducting a community assessment.
5. Which criteria could be used to select a community assessment framework or model?
6. Apply the criteria for selecting a community assessment framework or model, and then describe the community assessment framework or model you may want to use to guide an assessment of a specific community.

When an advanced practice public/community health nurse selects a framework or model to guide a community assessment, it reflects a commitment that goes beyond merely filling in the blanks on data-collection forms. The choice of framework or model can influence the types and methods of data collection and, in turn, the findings of the community assessment.

Framework is used in this book as a general term meaning a representation or view of reality. A framework provides a way of organizing data, variables, data-collection points, or data-analysis strategies. A model is a symbolic representation of reality that may be depicted in a schematic form, for example, diagram, picture, or word symbols. The purpose of a framework and a model is to communicate a perceived structure of reality (Morse, 2017). This chapter introduces some frameworks and models that can be used to guide a community assessment. Each approach has advantages and disadvantages, but you are provided with criteria to help you select an appropriate approach for conducting your own community assessment.

■ NURSING PRACTICE KNOWLEDGE

Knowledge for nursing practice is acquired from authority, borrowing, experience, intuition, reasoning, role modeling, traditions, trial and error, and research (Grove, Gray, & Burns, 2015). In keeping with one goal of this book, three levels of theory for advanced public/community health nursing practice are summarized to encourage nurses to base their practice on theory and research. The three levels of theory are grand theory, middle range theory, and situation-specific theory (Meleis, 2012).

Grand Nursing Theories

Grand nursing theories are "systematic constructions of the nature of nursing, the mission of nursing, and the goals of nursing care" (Meleis, 2012, p. 33). A synthesis of experiences, insights, observations, and research findings form the basis of grand theories. Grand theories are very broad in scope, highly abstract, and often include a large number of concepts or phenomena, so they are not directly testable (Meleis, 2012; Morse, 2017).

Although authors claim that the grand nursing theories or conceptual models of nursing are not knowledge that can be applied in practice (McKenna & Slevin, 2008), midrange theories based on the grand theories have been tested through research (Fawcett & Alligood, 2005). The grand theories have also been used to structure nursing services, to guide the development of interventions, and to serve as conceptual frameworks for nursing curricula (Meleis, 2012; Morse, 2017).

Hanchett (1988) made a valuable contribution to public/community health nursing with her book on application of nursing conceptual models, which were classified as grand theories (Walker & Avant, 2011), to community assessment. Even though the book was written before the concept of advanced practice became popular, you may find her applications useful.

Four nursing theorists were included in Hanchett's work: Dorothea E. Orem (1985), Callista Roy (1984), Imogene M. King (1983), and Martha E. Rogers (1983). Hanchett chose these four theorists because they shared a "common commitment to nursing as the study of persons and their environments and to increasing human health and well-being" (Hanchett, 1988, p. xv). As Hanchett pointed out, few nursing theories directly consider the community. Theories have been extended to be used with the family and, by greater extension, are applied to the community.

In applying the nursing theories to guide community assessments, Hanchett (1988) considered community to be an aggregate or a human–environmental field. The community, as an aggregate, is composed of individuals, population groups, or target groups, similar to the conceptualization of community-as-client (Chapter 3). Thus, epidemiologic studies and survey methods are consistent with an aggregate approach to community because they look at individual risk factors and individual responses (Hanchett, 1988).

The use of grand theories to guide a community assessment is not recommended because of the abstractness and absent or weak linkages between terms and indicators (Meleis, 2012; Morse, 2017). Other nursing theories are presented later in the chapter.

Middle Range Theory

Middle range theories are less abstract, narrower in scope, comprise fewer concepts, and more applicable to practice than grand theories (Peterson & Bredow, 2009). First proposed by Merton (1967) to guide empirical inquiry in sociology, middle range theory was introduced to nursing in 1974 (Jacox, 1974). Middle range nursing theories are currently being developed to provide more control for predicting outcomes of nursing interventions. Some examples of middle range nursing theories are the Interaction Model of Client Health Behavior (Cox, 1982; Cox et al., 2009), the theory of unpleasant symptoms (Lenz, Suppe, Gift, Pugh, & Milligan, 1995), and the Health Promotion Model (Pender, 1996). Although there are currently no middle range nursing theories specifically developed for guiding a community assessment, you will find the middle range nursing theories useful in other aspects of advanced practice, such as the Interaction Model of Client Health Behavior for interactions with individual clients (Ackerson, 2011; Cox, 1982).

Practice or Situation-Specific Theory

Nurse researchers have begun to develop a theory that is "less abstract, more specific, and narrower in scope than middle range theories" (Peterson & Bredow, 2009, p. 37). This level of theory is referred to as *practice theory* or *situation-specific theory*. Practice theory contains a desired nursing goal and prescriptions for action or actions to achieve the goal (Jacox, 1974; Walker & Avant, 2011). Situation-specific theory is theory developed from "other theories, from research findings, or from practice" (Meleis, 2012, p. 419).

Bigbee and Issel (2011) identified 12 models in a review of public health nursing conceptual models with most having limited evidence of application and/or testing. Two of these models, the community-as-partner model (Anderson & McFarlane, 2015) and Helvie's (1998) energy theory, may be categorized as practice models, but lack the specificity of prescriptive actions to achieve specific goals. Two other practice models, the intervention wheel (Keller, Strohschein, Lia-Hoagberg, & Schaffer, 1998) and the public health nursing practice model (Smith & Bazini-Barakat, 2003), provide more specific nursing actions. The intervention wheel has been incorporated into the Anderson and McFarlane and the public health nursing practice models (Bigbee & Issel, 2011).

Borrowed and Shared Knowledge

Advanced public/community health nursing practice requires the synthesis of nursing, public health, and social sciences (Levin et al., 2008). Many useful theories come from the public health sciences, such as epidemiology and environmental health, and from the social sciences, such as demography, ecology, and sociology. Knowledge from other fields is often referred to as *borrowed*. After theories have been adapted to nursing practice, the knowledge may be called *shared* knowledge (Meleis, 2012). Anderson and McFarlane's community-as-partner model (2015) and Helvie's (1998) energy theory are nursing theories based on borrowed knowledge.

■ FRAMEWORKS AND MODELS USED TO GUIDE THE COMMUNITY ASSESSMENT PROCESS

This section introduces frameworks and models useful to advanced practice public/community health nurses in conducting community assessments. The frameworks and models are grouped into three categories: nursing frameworks and models, epidemiologic frameworks and models, and equity frameworks. The last two groups of frameworks and models are classified as borrowed or shared knowledge.

In general, the concepts or components of a framework or model provide the categories for organizing the data collected for a community assessment. If the epidemiologic triangle framework is used, for example, the data will be organized by the categories of host, agent, and environment (Finnegan & Ervin, 1989). Proposed relationships among the concepts or components of the model or framework direct the assessor to examine these relationships among the data elements. Chapter 7 provides detailed information about using a framework or model for the community assessment.

Nursing Frameworks and Models

The two nursing frameworks presented in this section are community-as-partner (Anderson & McFarlane, 2000, 2015) and Helvie's energy theory (Helvie, 1981, 1998).

COMMUNITY-AS-PARTNER

Anderson and McFarlane (1996) renamed their community-as-client model (Anderson & McFarlane, 1988) as the community-as-partner model to focus on the philosophy of primary healthcare as defined by the World Health Organization (WHO, 1978). Primary healthcare is an essential healthcare and is discussed in Anderson and McFarlane (2015, pp. 13, 14) and later in this chapter. The two models are almost exactly the same, except for the important distinction found in the words *client* and *partner*.

A client is someone for whom professional services are rendered. A synonym for *client* is *customer*. Although nursing has used *client* to indicate a more equal and less dependent relationship than *patient* for recipients of nursing care, the term still carries with it an unequal connotation. Thus, Anderson and McFarlane chose to use the term *partner* to demonstrate equality in the nurse's relationship with the community. This focus has been further developed in the third through seventh editions of their book (Anderson & McFarlane, 2000, 2004, 2008, 2011, 2015).

Anderson and McFarlane (2015) based their model of community-as-partner on the model of a total -person approach to viewing patient problems developed by Betty Neuman (1972). Two major components comprise the community-as-partner model: the community assessment wheel and the nursing process. Only the community assessment wheel, which is used for conducting a community assessment, is discussed in this section (Anderson & McFarlane, 2015; Figure 4.1).

The community assessment wheel consists of two major parts: the core and eight surrounding subsystems. The core of the model represents the community residents who are described by demographics, values, beliefs, and history. The eight subsystems are physical environment, education, safety and transportation, politics and government, health and social services, communication, economics, and recreation. Community residents are affected by and influence the eight community subsystems.

Surrounding the community is its normal line of defense, which is the level of health obtained by the community. The solid line (circle) in Figure 4.1 represents this line of defense. Examples of the normal line of defense are characteristics such as a high immunization level among children. The broken line around the community in Figure 4.1 depicts the flexible line of defense, which is "a 'buffer zone' representing a dynamic level of health resulting from a temporary response to stressors" (Anderson & McFarlane, 2015, p. 170). An example of an environmental stressor is flooding. Mobilization by the community to control damage is a temporary response to the flooding condition.

Broken lines divide the eight subsystems to indicate that they both influence and are influenced by one another. There are the lines of resistance or internal mechanisms within the community, represented by circular broken lines in Figure 4.1, which defend against stressors. Lines of resistance throughout each subsystem represent the strengths of the community. In the community-as-partner model, stressors are tension-producing stimuli that may potentially cause disequilibrium in the system. Stressors, which may come from within or outside the community, penetrate the flexible and normal lines of defense causing disruption of the community. The amount of disruption or disequilibrium is known as *the degree of reaction* (Anderson & McFarlane, 2015).

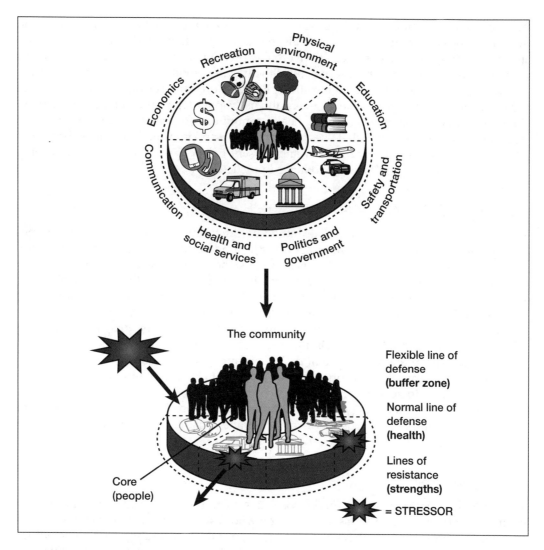

FIGURE 4.1 | Community assessment wheel.

Source: Anderson, E. T., & McFarlane, J. (2015). *Community as partner: Theory and practice in nursing* (7th ed.). Philadelphia, PA: Lippincott. Copyright © 2015 by Lippincott Williams & Wilkins, p. 171. Used with permission.

HELVIE'S ENERGY THEORY

Helvie's (1981, 1998) energy theory is based on systems theory and the underlying concept of energy as the capacity to do work. In addition to the capacity to do work, the word *energy* in Helvie's theory is used to mean the activity and capabilities of communities and individuals. The theory encompasses "community subsystems such as health, education, and economics as energy subsystems because of the work expended by both the provider and the recipient of services" (Helvie, 1998, p. 24).

In Helvie's energy theory, the community population or human system is viewed as a changing energy field that both affects and is affected through exchanges with the other energies in the environment. Energies in the human environment are composed of four categories: chemical, physical, biological, and psychological. Chemical energies include air pollutants, carcinogens, and pesticides; physical energies include health, light, and sound; biological energies include animals, bacteria, and plants; and psychological energies include feelings such as anger, nonverbal expressions, and sociocultural values. The exchanges of energies may be internal, as with air, water, food, or services, or external, as exchanges with state and national resources. Past and present exchanges, and the balance achieved by the exchanges, influence the health of the population and determine the placement of the population on an energy or health continuum. Placement on the continuum is determined by an assessment that uses health statistics and information about subsystems. The nurse assesses and compares past and present balances with those of other energy systems (e.g., state) as one basis for advanced practice.

Epidemiologic Frameworks

Epidemiology is the study of the distribution and determinants of diseases and injuries in populations (Gordis, 2014; Timmreck, 1998). In advanced public/community health nursing practice, epidemiology helps us to understand the intricacies of the multiple factors involved in injury and disease, both infectious and chronic. Although epidemiology is concerned with disease and injury, the major focus is maintenance of health through prevention. Epidemiologic methods are applied to infectious diseases and to many areas of health and prevention, such as injuries, chronic conditions, adverse drug reactions, drug addiction, and congenital defects. On the basis of the tenet that an ecological approach is necessary to explain the occurrence of disease in humans, epidemiology uses the framework of multiple causative factors: the requirement that more than one factor must be present for disease to develop or injury to occur (Gordis, 2014).

Two models of epidemiology are presented in this section. These models of epidemiology focus of multiple components of causation and include the epidemiologic triangle and web of causation.

EPIDEMIOLOGIC TRIANGLE

The epidemiologic triangle is a model consisting of three components: host, agent, and environment (Figure 4.2). The *host is* the person who is susceptible to a disease; the *agent* is the infectious organism; and the *environment* refers to both physical and social surroundings and biological conditions that are needed to result in disease in a person (Gordis, 2014).

In a broad interpretation of the agent and environment, one may look at the agent as a gene or a substance in a person's body; environment may include the factors that result

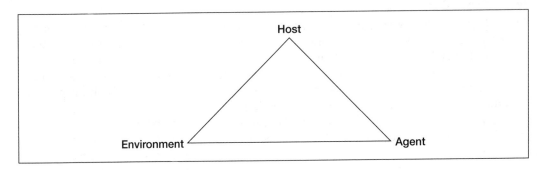

FIGURE 4.2 Epidemiologic triangle.

in disease or an injury, such as an automobile crash related to alcohol intake. This broad interpretation of the factors related to health has been useful in examining conditions, such as violence, farming injuries, and SIDS (sudden infant death syndrome), as well as newer diseases, such as AIDS.

In using the epidemiologic triangle, the nurse collects data related to its three elements of host, agent, and environment. For analysis and synthesis of data, the nurse is challenged to determine the relationships among the data items and relate them in ways that reflect the current epidemiologic knowledge, research, and practice bases. One example of the use of the epidemiologic triangle as a guide to conduct a community assessment is found in an article about the relationships of factors related to teenage pregnancy in a community. In the assessment of a community, the authors found a number of factors related to risk for teenage pregnancy, such as a high number of low-income single-parent families, high rates of school dropouts, and isolation of the community. The analysis and synthesis of the community data were facilitated by the use of literature on research about teenage pregnancy (Finnegan & Ervin, 1989).

THE WEB OF CAUSATION

The web of causation is a classic epidemiologic concept that posits that effects never depend on single isolated causes but result from chains of causation in which each link is the result of a complex mix of antecedents (Timmreck, 1998). The large number of antecedents and their complexity may be visualized as a web or an intricate design.

To use the web of causation, you may need to combine it with part of another framework because of the lack of categories within the web of causation to guide data collection. A useful framework may be the systems and subsystems of communities, such as those specified in the community-as-partner model (Anderson & McFarlane, 2015) and Helvie's energy model (Helvie, 1998).

Analysis and synthesis using the web of causation consist of using the research knowledge base to link the data elements to determine conclusions as community diagnoses. Although this framework does not provide as much concrete guidance as others, the concept of the complexity of antecedents helps the nurse to understand that problems or conditions are not the result of simplistic explanations. We are often tempted to dismiss behavior or situations as the result of one factor, such as the person's life choice, instead of searching for the real and more complex answer. Figure 4.3 depicts an examination of lead poisoning using the web-of-causation model.

Equity Models

Equity models contain a strong philosophy of community empowerment. The central theme of these models is that the professional is not in charge but provides information and assistance to the community upon request. Some equity models also support the philosophical foundation of social justice. A strong ethic of equality for all people may be seen in most equity models. The two models presented in this section are community capacity (McKnight & Kretzmann, 2012) and primary healthcare (WHO, 1978).

COMMUNITY CAPACITY

McKnight and Kretzmann's (2012) community-capacity approach views a community through a positive lens rather than a deficit scope. It is like seeing the glass as half full rather than half empty. Throughout the history of community assessment, communities,

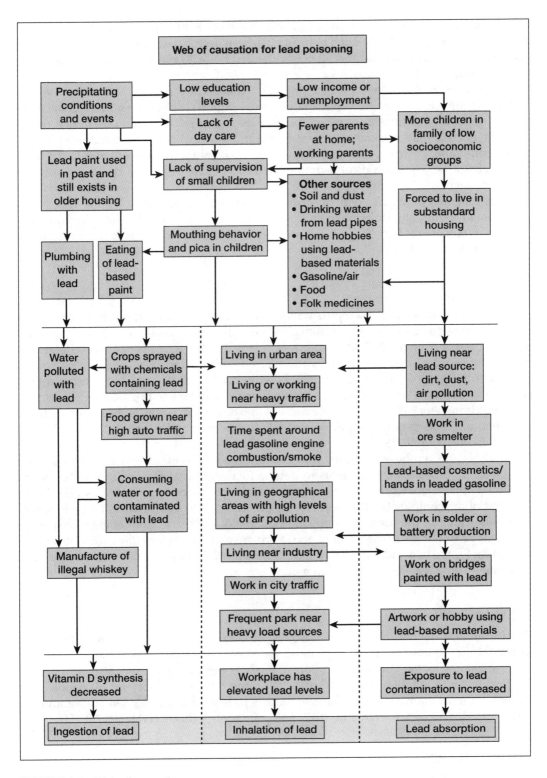

FIGURE 4.3 Web of causation.

Source: Timmreck, T. C. (2002.) *An introduction to epidemiology* (3rd ed.). Copyright © 2002 by Jones & Bartlett Publishers, Sudbury, MA, p. 350, www.jbpub.com. Reprinted with permission.

especially low-income communities, have been examined for problems, needs, or deficiencies. This approach is more compatible with helping communities to become stronger rather than concentrating on their weaknesses.

The information and data gathered for the community assessment using the community-capacity approach are used to create a map of assets and capacities. An example of a neighborhood assets map is shown in Figure 4.4. A beginning assets map is useful for developing more assets within the community, identifying processes to advance rebuilding the community, and building bridges to resources outside the community (McKnight & Kretzman, 2012).

To map community assets, one must assess the assets located in the community and controlled by those who live there (primary building blocks), assets located in the community but controlled elsewhere (secondary building blocks), and assets located and controlled outside the community (potential building blocks). These three categories of assets are the areas for data collection.

Primary building-block assets may be placed into two categories: individual and organizational. Individual assets include skills, talents, and experience of residents; individual businesses; home-based enterprises; personal income; and gifts of labeled people (such as elderly, disabled, retarded). When assessing organizational assets, the advanced practice public/community health nurse should include associations of businesses and citizens and organizations that address culture, communications, and religion.

To assess individual skills, talents, and experience, a data-collection instrument, Capacity Inventory, is available from John McKnight, Northwestern University, Evanston, Illinois. Information for the inventory is obtained by interviewing individuals. The interviews can take place in various locations within the community.

To assess a community's secondary building blocks, one would collect information about three community segments: private and nonprofit organizations, physical resources, and public institutions and services. Higher education institutions, hospitals, and social services agencies are included in private and nonprofit organizations. Physical resources are vacant land, commercial and industrial structures, housing that is sound but in need of repair, and energy and waste resources. Public schools, police, libraries, fire departments, and parks are the major categories of public institutions and services that almost all communities have and can be used for community-building purposes.

Potential building blocks include welfare expenditures, public capital improvement expenditures, and public information. Examples of public information are how much property in a community is off the tax rolls and what capital improvements the city or county plans for a community. One example of welfare expenditures comes from Cook County, Illinois, where "large, albeit shrinking funds are expended annually by government for low-income programs for people whose income falls below the official poverty line. This substantial investment is distributed so that on a per capita basis, poor people receive well over half of this money in the form of services rather than actual income" (McKnight & Kretzmann, 2012, p. 179). This creates more poverty in which poor families are dependent on services and creative community groups are developing approaches to invest welfare dollars in enterprise development and independence for families and communities (McKnight & Kretzmann, 2012). This kind of information can assist a community in developing approaches to neighborhood improvements.

In addition to the map of assets of the community, the community-capacity approach identifies potential strengths that can be called upon for building more community capacity. Policies and activities are based on the capacities, skills, and assets of residents and their communities.

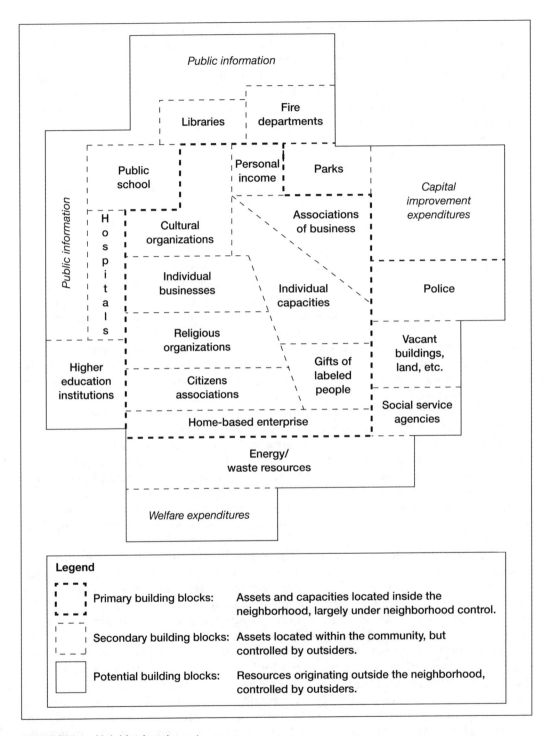

FIGURE 4.4 Neighborhood assets map.

Source: McKnight, J. L., & Kretzmann, J. P. (2012). Mapping community capacity. In M. Minkler (Ed.), *Community organizing and community building for health* (3rd ed., pp. 171–186). New Brunswick, NJ: Rutgers University Press. Used with permission.

PRIMARY HEALTHCARE

The concept of primary healthcare, not to be confused with primary care, originated at the 28th World Health Assembly of the WHO in 1975. The idea of primary healthcare culminated in a conference at Alma Ata, USSR, in 1978 with 134 nations committing to the achievement of health for all by the year 2000, through primary healthcare (Anderson & McFarlane, 2000).

WHO defines *primary healthcare* as "essential health care based on practical, scientifically sound and socially acceptable methods and technology universally accessible to individuals and families in the community through their full participation and at a cost that the community and country can afford to maintain at every stage of their development in the spirit of self-reliance and self-determination" (WHO, 1978, p. 3).

The eight essential elements of primary healthcare are promotion of food supply and proper nutrition; an adequate supply of safe water and basic sanitation; maternal and child care, including family planning; immunization against the major infectious diseases; prevention and control of locally endemic diseases; education about prevailing health problems and methods for preventing and controlling them; appropriate treatment for common diseases and injuries; and provision of essential drugs (WHO, 1978).

To use primary healthcare as a framework for conducting a community assessment, the advanced practice public/community health nurse would use the eight essential elements as the broad areas for data collection. The nurse would need to delineate the specific types of data to be included in each of the eight elements. For example, under the element of promotion of food supply and proper nutrition, several sources of data could be used about nutritional intake of the population. Also, statistics about food-related diseases, nutritional problems, and use of food pantries and soup kitchens are just a few of the areas that could be included.

Often in the literature, the terms *primary healthcare* and *primary care* are used interchangeably but have very different meanings (Muldoon, Hogg, & Levitt, 2006). The term *primary care*, in international use, essentially means personal health services; primarily, services provided by certain medical specialties, but some groups have included nurse practitioners and physician assistants as primary care providers. The term *primary healthcare* is broader and derives from core principles expressed by WHO. It is an approach to health policy and service provision that includes both primary care services delivered to individuals as well as population-level or public health services (Muldoon et al., 2006).

One way to conceptualize the differences between primary care and primary healthcare is to think of primary care as a component of primary healthcare. If the eight essential elements of primary healthcare are examined with this in mind, one can see that primary care or personal health services are part of several of the elements, such as maternal and child care and treatment for common diseases and injuries. Primary care is only one part of a comprehensive, accessible, acceptable, and affordable healthcare system.

Other Frameworks and Models

Several other frameworks and models to guide the community assessment process are found in the literature. Although not all are well developed or provide detail in guiding the assessment process, two are briefly described here for you to explore independently.

A COMMUNITY PARTICIPATION AND ETHNOGRAPHIC MODEL

The community participation and ethnographic model is primarily a qualitative approach to community assessment and evaluation that utilizes both qualitative and quantitative data collection and analysis. The model includes five community assessment domains: (a) community core and history, (b) physical environment, (c) idea systems, (d) social systems, and (e) behavioral systems. The community participation and ethnographic model facilitates gaining local knowledge of community members and allows public/community health nurses and their community partners to be sensitive to the ecological context and culture. It provides a useful framework for developing programs to promote healthy communities and health equality (Kulbok, Thatcher, Park, & Meszaros, 2012).

Strategies utilized in the community participation and ethnographic model include mapping, for example, geographic information systems (GIS), and picture-taking by community members and public health practitioners, for example, Photovoice. GIS is a tool that facilitates assessment and analysis of the ecological context of a population. Mapping enables community partners and practitioners to assess their community, target interventions, and identify geographic trends over time. Photovoice uses pictures taken by community members to facilitate sharing of beliefs, knowledge, and thoughts about the community. This form of engagement by the community often results in more balanced power, shared ownership, greater trust, and increased sensitivity to cultural preferences in the community assessment process (Kulbok et al., 2012).

WORKSITE ASSESSMENT GUIDE

Serafini (1976) provided a very useful assessment guide for advanced practice public/community health nurses in occupational health. This guide includes a description of the community in which the industry is located and continues to guide the assessor to gather data about aspects of the company, plant, working population, industrial process, and health program. The community assessment process is generally the same for any community or setting, but the items to be assessed differ as illustrated in the nursing assessment in industry. Box 4.1 is an example of an assessment guide for nursing in an occupational setting.

■ CRITERIA FOR SELECTING A COMMUNITY ASSESSMENT FRAMEWORK OR MODEL

As an advanced practice public/community health nurse, you have a variety of frameworks and models from which to choose, so how do you go about deciding which to use? Answering the questions in Box 4.2 will assist you in deciding which framework or model to use for a given situation. The following discussion elaborates the criteria indicated in the questions.

Compare Philosophical Foundations

The philosophical beliefs that form the foundation of how one relates to the world and, ultimately, how one practices nursing (Meleis, 2012) are part of a sound basis for choosing a framework. The foundations of public/community health nursing practice (delineated in Chapter 2) should be compatible with the beliefs one brings to practice. These foundations form the first level of criteria for review of any theory, framework, or model to be used in practice.

A framework provides a philosophical context in which community assessments are framed. Each framework is based on assumptions, values, beliefs, and, at times, ethical principles. Even though the philosophical context or underpinnings may not be explicit, you are encouraged to examine carefully a given framework on various levels.

BOX 4.1   EXAMPLE OF AN ASSESSMENT GUIDE FOR OCCUPATIONAL SETTINGS

I. Community in which the industry or business is located
   A. Description of the community
   B. Population: Demographic data
   C. Health information: Vital statistics, morbidity, mortality, health facilities, community resources
II. The company
   A. Historical development
   B. Organizational chart
   C. Policies
   D. Support services (benefits)
   E. Relations between workers and management
   F. Projections for the future of the company
III. The plant or business
   A. General physical setting
   B. The work area
   C. Nonwork areas
IV. The worker population
   A. General characteristics
   B. Type of employment offered
   C. Absenteeism
   D. Physically handicapped
   E. Personnel on medication
   F. Personnel with chronic illnesses
V. The industrial or business processes
   A. Equipment used
   B. Nature of the operations
   C. Exposure to toxic substances
   D. Faculties required throughout the industrial processes
VI. The health program
   A. Existing policies
   B. Existing facilities and resources
   C. Services rendered in the past year
   D. Unintentional injuries in the past year
   E. Reasons employees sought healthcare

Source: Adapted from Serafini, P. (1976). Nursing assessment in industry. *American Journal of Public Health, 66*(8), 755–760.

For example, one might choose to use the epidemiologic model, which is based on problem solving and an ecological understanding of health events. Epidemiology aims at a comprehensive view of disease, injury, and other conditions (Gordis, 2014), so one might view it as similar to nursing, which is concerned with a comprehensive approach to client care.

Another view of epidemiology is that it is based on a disease model that is not compatible with the health orientation of public/community health nursing (Hanchett & Clarke, 1988). Nurses may find that the epidemiologic models are not compatible with their beliefs because of the disease focus, which implicitly excludes the community as being involved

---

BOX 4.2 QUESTIONS FOR SELECTING A FRAMEWORK OR MODEL TO GUIDE A COMMUNITY ASSESSMENT

1. What are the philosophical foundations of the framework or model?
2. What are the ethical principles stated or implied in the framework or model?
3. How is the framework or model related to advanced public/community health nursing practice?
4. How does the framework or model fit with the culture, values, and beliefs of the community to be assessed?
5. How much structure is provided to guide the community assessment?
6. How feasible is it to use the framework or model within the available time and resources?

---

in the community assessment process. Fortunately, there are numerous other frameworks from which to choose. For example, in contrast to the epidemiologic models, the community-capacity model (McKnight & Kretzman, 2012), which is discussed in this chapter, encompasses a view of community empowerment with much involvement of community residents.

The ethical principles that form the basis of public/community health nursing practice may also be examined as part of the philosophical foundations of the specialty. The importance of the ethical orientation for practice is the compatibility with your orientation as well as that of the community to be assessed. Community assessment frameworks and models serve different purposes but also reflect different expressions of ethics. For example, some frameworks have a greater orientation toward including the community in the assessment process and, thus, have a stronger component of self-determination.

Identify Nurse's View of Practice

Although most advanced practice public/community health nurses hold similar views of practice, there are subtle nuances that make the selection of a framework an individual choice. Individual nurses may lean toward certain types of frameworks. For instance, some nurses view practice in terms of epidemiologic concepts, whereas others deal better with a nursing orientation such as those contained in nursing models. There are several frameworks with similar foundations, so the nurse will be able to choose among several frameworks for each community assessment.

Determine Compatibility With Community Values

Another criterion for choosing a framework is compatibility with the predominant community values, beliefs, and culture. Although a community usually has many different values and beliefs, communities may be characterized by a pervasive, if not dominant, way of viewing the world. For example, a framework to use with a community that values independence should have an orientation toward a great deal of community direction and involvement. Although you may not know the predominant community values before beginning the community assessment, you may be able to find out what community members identify as values by reading local publications and talking with people in informal settings.

Review the Structure Provided

In addition to using criteria related to philosophical orientation, practice components, and compatibility with the community, you should evaluate how much guidance the framework provides compared with the amount of structure desired. Some nurses feel comfortable with less structure and can perform the needed synthesis with a loosely developed framework. Others desire a structure that provides more guidance on data collection, analysis, and synthesis.

Using a framework or model to guide the community assessment process will not always be easy. When dealing with a large volume of data, the community assessor will be challenged to organize, analyze, and synthesize all available data. In addition, gaps in the data will become evident as the analysis and synthesis are being completed. The tendency is to continue to collect data and conduct interviews until the assessor feels comfortable that all bits and pieces of information are in hand. Large volumes of data are not useful unless they have been subjected to an orderly examination to detect patterns, trends, changes, and associations from the various parts of the framework or model. These activities are covered in Chapter 8 on community diagnosis.

Evaluate the Feasibility of Use

Another criterion for selecting a framework should be the ability to use the framework within the available resources. For example, some frameworks, such as community capacity (McKnight & Kretzmann, 2012), require extensive interviewing of individuals. If the work plan for a specific community assessment does not provide the resources in time or money to conduct extensive interviews, you should not select this framework.

Another consideration for feasibility of use of a specific framework is the knowledge and skills required to implement the components. For example, the epidemiologic frameworks require knowledge of epidemiology and some skills related to using epidemiologic techniques. The use of a team to conduct a community assessment will enhance the knowledge and skills available to use a variety of frameworks.

Box 4.3 contains a summary of the criteria for selecting a framework or model to guide the community assessment process.

BOX 4.3 CRITERIA FOR SELECTING A FRAMEWORK OR MODEL TO GUIDE THE COMMUNITY ASSESSMENT PROCESS

- Compare the philosophical foundations of various community assessment frameworks and models.
- Identify your view of advanced public/community health nursing practice.
- Determine the compatibility of the frameworks and models with the community's values, beliefs, and culture.
- Review the structure provided by the frameworks and models.
- Evaluate the feasibility of use in terms of resources and knowledge, skills, and abilities needed to use the framework or model.

■ APPLYING THE CRITERIA TO SELECT A FRAMEWORK

The criteria presented earlier are applied in this section to the frameworks and models introduced earlier in this chapter.

Nursing Frameworks and Models

The two nursing frameworks and models introduced earlier are community-as-partner (Anderson & McFarlane, 2000, 2015) and Helvie's energy theory (Helvie, 1981, 1998).

COMMUNITY-AS-PARTNER

Anderson and McFarlane's (2000, 2015) model exemplifies the following aspects of the criteria for selecting a framework to guide a community assessment.

Philosophical Foundations. The orientation of the community-as-partner model is primary healthcare, which is a philosophy of control by the community "in the spirit of self-reliance and self-determination" (WHO, 1978, p. 3). Primary healthcare is primarily a philosophy of approaching healthcare, so the community-as-partner model provides the nurse with clear direction to work with the community on every step of the community assessment. An ethical orientation that healthcare is a right fits well with the community-as-partner model.

Fit With the Nurse's View of Public/Community Health Nursing Practice. The community-as-partner model may fit within the conceptualization of practice of community-as-client or community-as-resource, as depicted in Chapter 3. The dominant conceptualization of community will depend on the readiness of the community to direct or be part of the assessment process. The community-as-resource conceptualization is more in keeping with the primary healthcare philosophy, but all communities may not be at a stage of development to seek assistance from the nurse and the healthcare system.

Compatibility With Community Values. The values reflected in the community-as-partner model are those of community control and involvement in the process of community assessment. A community that is active and involved is a good fit with the community-as-partner model.

Structure Provided. The community-as-partner model provides a well-developed structure for guiding the assessment of a community. The systems framework within the community assessment wheel gives concrete direction about what parameters to collect and how to organize the data into meaningful categories for later analysis and synthesis. The description of the dynamics among the factors in the model gives the advanced practice public/community health nurse assistance with the complexity of the eight subsystems contained in the wheel.

Feasibility of Use. Using the community-as-partner model is feasible for most nurses who are interested in gathering information about all aspects of a community. The model does not specify the sources of data and methods of data collection, so flexibility is a key attribute that lends to the feasibility of use of this model. In addition, much of the usable data for the model may be found in secondary data sources, thus making the model more economical in its use.

HELVIE'S ENERGY THEORY

Over several years, Helvie (1981, 1998) developed his energy theory to provide a comprehensive approach to organizing data collection and analysis of data.

Philosophical Foundations. Helvie's energy theory contains the four major concepts of nursing theories: humans, environment, health, and nursing. The energy theory is compatible with the community-as-relational-experience conceptualization of community as described in Chapter 3. The human energy system described in Helvie's theory is an open system that is characterized by exchanges both within the community and external to the community. Relationships are energy exchanges among the community population, which affect and are affected through these exchanges. Although no specific philosophical orientation is apparent in Helvie's energy theory, it appears to be compatible with the precepts of social justice and self-determination.

Fit With the Nurse's View of Public/Community Health Nursing Practice. The advanced practice public/community health nurse who uses Helvie's energy theory may view the community-as-relational experience as described in Chapter 3. This view of community implies a greater emphasis on process rather than community as place. The experience of everyday life is a key component of community-as-relational experience. Although it is not a perfect fit with the conceptualization of community-as-relational experience, Helvie's theory of energy offers a concrete approach to guiding a community assessment within a nurse's view of the community-as-relational experience.

Compatibility With Community Values. A community that values relationships more than the economy, for example, votes against gambling casinos because of the potential negative effects casinos may have on family life, may be a good fit with Helvie's energy theory. The emphasis in Helvie's theory on maintaining balance by adapting holistically to energy exchanges also lends itself to compatibility with a community that values a balance in community life. An open system implies that a community is open to new ideas and to input from within and outside the community while maintaining the community structure.

Structure Provided. Helvie's energy theory provides the structure to guide a community assessment in at least two areas: the use of subsystems and the direction for analysis. Although this discussion cannot provide great detail, descriptions of the theory provide adequate detail for use in conducting a community assessment.

Feasibility of Use. The decision about feasibility of use should take into consideration three factors: availability of data about the subsystems, the amount of time available to learn about the theory, and the nurse's comfort with the concept of energy as a theory of communities. Helvie's theory uses data that are readily obtainable and obtained by survey. Time to collect some of the needed data should be a factor in deciding to use this theory.

EPIDEMIOLOGIC FRAMEWORKS

This section addresses the two epidemiologic frameworks, the epidemiologic triangle and web of causation, based on multiple factors involved in diseases. The discussion of the criteria for use of these two models is consolidated because of their similarities.

Epidemiologic Triangle and Web of Causation. These epidemiologic frameworks reflect a philosophical foundation of equity because disease occurs in all people, and people and the environment may be examined for factors related to disease. Although many diseases are more prevalent in the presence of poverty and lack of education, epidemiology is judgment free on the surface. Conversely, epidemiology has no inherent values of social justice and equity. Epidemiologic frameworks offer unbiased approaches for all aggregates or subpopulations.

Fit With the Nurse's View of Public/Community Health Nursing Practice. The view of community that perhaps fits best with epidemiology concepts is that of community-as-client, described in Chapter 3. Viewing the community as a client focuses on the care of the community as a whole. Thus, an epidemiologic framework offers an approach to assess the total community and gain insights into the health status of the total community, especially as it relates to disease and the prevention of disease.

Compatibility With Community Values. The epidemiologic frameworks may fit with a wide variety of community values, cultures, and beliefs. A community that embraces diversity and the need for a total view of the community's health status, regardless of potential negative implications, is a good fit with an epidemiologic approach. Community values of helping the less fortunate and addressing problems or potential problems before they grow are also compatible with this approach.

Structure Provided. Although the epidemiologic frameworks provide structure for a community assessment, the structure is not as explanatory as some of the other frameworks. Each framework has categories that may be used for collecting and organizing data, as indicated in the descriptions. Details for each of the categories will need to be supplied by the nurse or team doing the assessment. The interaction among the various facets of data must be determined through knowledge of epidemiology as well as of research. Studies that have identified the relationships among various factors are found in the literature, so the nurse must be prepared to do more literature searches when analyzing the data.

Feasibility of Use. The additional time needed for literature searches is one factor to consider when determining the feasibility of use of an epidemiologic framework. The nurse's knowledge about epidemiology is a second factor for consideration. If the nurse is not knowledgeable about the use of epidemiology, the availability of others to assist in data analysis and synthesis may be a key factor in whether to use an epidemiologic framework. The fact that data about disease and injury are available for most geographic locations is a plus for using the epidemiologic frameworks.

Equity Models

The two equity models presented in this section are community capacity (McKnight & Kretzmann, 2012) and primary healthcare (WHO, 1978).

COMMUNITY CAPACITY

The community-capacity approach to community assessment is focused on building on a community's strengths.

Philosophical Foundations. Community capacity emphasizes the assets of a community for building more capacity. The identification of individual skills, talents, and experience exemplifies a social justice and self-determination approach to community assessment. Building the independence or interdependence of a community creates an environment of respect and empowerment for the community members.

Fit With the Nurse's View of Public/Community Health Nursing Practice. The advanced practice public/community health nurse who views practice as consultation to communities seeking professional knowledge will find a fit with the community-capacity approach to community assessment. The conceptualization of community-as-resource as described in Chapter 3 is closely related to the community-capacity approach.

Compatibility With Community Values. For the community with a strong value of self-determination, the community-capacity approach is a good fit. This approach to community assessment offers flexibility to accommodate the experiences of community members regardless of their values. A community that is not self-directed or lacks organizational components may not be a good fit with this approach.

Structure Provided. Structure for use of the community capacity model is provided in the neighborhood assets map, which is constructed according to the definitions provided in the written description. The Capacity Inventory provides guidance to assess individual skills, talents, and experience (McKnight & Kretzmann, 2012).

Feasibility of Use. A broad knowledge of community and community organizations is a prerequisite for use of the community-capacity approach to community assessment. Although it is time-consuming to collect information from many individuals, this model offers a thorough approach to knowing a community.

PRIMARY HEALTHCARE

The community assessment framework provided in the primary healthcare model emphasizes control of the process by the community.

Philosophical Foundations. More than any other framework, primary healthcare provides a social justice view of community assessment. Primary healthcare is primarily a philosophy of the community taking control of its own destiny, so the advanced practice public/community health nurse is called on when needed by the community. The actions of community intervention are initiated and controlled by the community. The original goal of primary healthcare was health for all by 2000 (WHO, 1978). Although this did not occur, the WHO will no doubt continue to seek ways to make health for all a reality in the true sense of equity for the world's population.

Fit With the Nurse's View of Public/Community Health Nursing Practice. A view of public/community health nursing practice as participatory and guided by the desires of community members fits well with the primary healthcare framework. The guidance of community members in conducting the community assessment would fit into this framework of grassroots activism.

Compatibility With Community Values. The expression of a variety of community values can be accommodated within the primary healthcare framework. The framework has been used extensively in other countries, so it may also be useful in communities of immigrants and refugees within the United States.

Structure Provided. The eight essential elements listed in the description of the primary healthcare model provide the basic structure for data collection and organization. Identifying the detail to be included in each of the eight elements would require time. In addition to these eight areas, data about the people and environment will make the data collection more complete. Analysis and synthesis of data using the framework present a challenge for the advanced practice public/community health nurse because no guidelines are provided. The use of other approaches, such as an examination of demographics by statistical methods, can assist with this.

Feasibility of Use. Data for the primary healthcare framework are available and should not usually be difficult to locate. If one's interest is in assessing a particular subgroup of the population, for example, immigrants from Mexico, specific data may be more difficult to obtain because most data are reported for larger segments of the population, such as cities, counties, and states.

■ SUMMARY

This chapter introduced you to several frameworks and models that can be used in conducting community assessments. These frameworks are organized into three categories: nursing models, epidemiologic frameworks, and equity frameworks. Criteria to use for choosing a framework include philosophical foundations, fit with the nurse's view of public/community health nursing practice, structure provided, compatibility with community values, and feasibility of use. The advanced practice public/community health nurse is encouraged to explore more than one framework or model in order to choose one that is suited to the purposes of the community assessment to be completed.

Conducting a community assessment is an interesting and exciting endeavor. Nurses often express how much they have learned about communities in which they have lived for years. When assigned to assess an unfamiliar community, nurses are often surprised to find how communities differ from each other. Being able to competently assess a community is equivalent to competently assessing an individual patient or family and is a necessary part of advanced practice in public/community health nursing. The next four chapters in this section will assist you in gaining the knowledge needed to conduct a community assessment.

■ SUGGESTED CLINICAL OR PRACTICUM ACTIVITIES

1. Go online to find community assessments conducted by nonprofit hospitals in your region. Were frameworks or models used for these assessments? What frameworks or models do you think would be most useful to conduct this type of community assessment? Provide a rationale for your response related to the criteria for selection of a framework.
2. Interview advanced practice public/community health nurses in a local health department and/or community-based agency. Describe the roles they have assumed related to community assessment and how the nurses' understanding of "knowledge for the sake of practice" influenced these roles.

REFERENCES

Ackerson, K. (2011). Interactive model of client health behavior and cervical cancer screening of African-American women. *Public Health Nursing, 28*(3), 271–280.

Anderson, E. T., & McFarlane, J. (1988). *Community as client: Theory and practice in nursing*. Philadelphia, PA: Lippincott.

Anderson, E. T., & McFarlane, J. (1996). *Community as partner: Theory and practice in nursing* (2nd ed.). Philadelphia, PA: Lippincott.

Anderson, E. T., & McFarlane, J. (2000). *Community as partner: Theory and practice in nursing* (3rd ed.). Philadelphia, PA: Lippincott.

Anderson, E. T., & McFarlane, J. (2004). *Community as partner: Theory and practice in nursing* (4th ed.). Philadelphia, PA: Lippincott Williams & Wilkins.

Anderson, E. T., & McFarlane, J. (2008). *Community as partner: Theory and practice in nursing* (5th ed.). Philadelphia, PA: Lippincott Williams & Wilkins.

Anderson, E. T., & McFarlane, J. (2011). *Community as partner: Theory and practice in nursing* (6th ed.). Philadelphia, PA: Lippincott Williams & Wilkins.

Anderson, E. T., & McFarlane, J. (2015). *Community as partner: Theory and practice in nursing* (7th ed.). Philadelphia, PA: Lippincott Williams Wilkins.

Bigbee, J. L., & Issel, L. M. (2011). Conceptual models for population-focused public health nursing interventions and outcomes: The state of the art. *Public Health Nursing, 29*(4), 370–379.

Cox, C. L. (1982). An interaction model of client health behavior: A theoretical prescription for nursing. *Advances in Nursing Science, 5*(1), 41–56.

Cox, C. L., Oeffinger, K. C., Montgomery, M., Hudson, M. M., Mertens, A. C., Whitton, J., & Robison, L. L. (2009). Determinants of mammography screening participation in adult childhood cancer survivors: Results from the childhood cancer survivor study. *Oncology Nursing Forum, 36*(3), 335–344.

Fawcett, J., & Alligood, M. R. (2005). Scholarly dialogue: Influences on advancement of nursing knowledge. *Nursing Science Quarterly, 18*(3), 227–232.

Finnegan, L., & Ervin, N. E. (1989). An epidemiological approach to community assessment. *Public Health Nursing, 6*(3), 147–151.

Gordis, L. (2014). *Epidemiology* (5th ed.). Baltimore, MD: Elsevier Saunders.

Grove, S. K., Gray, J. R., & Burns, N. (2015). *Understanding nursing research: Building an evidence-based practice*. St. Louis, MO: Elsevier Saunders.

Hanchett, E. S. (1988). *Nursing frameworks & community as client: Bridging the gap*. Norwalk, CT: Appleton & Lange.

Hanchett, E. S., & Clarke, P. N. (1988). Nursing theory and public health science: Is synthesis possible? *Public Health Nursing, 5*(1), 2–6.

Helvie, C. O. (1981). *The community as a system. Community health nursing: Theory and process* (pp. 87–109). Philadelphia, PA: Harper & Row.

Helvie, C. O. (1998). *Advanced practice nursing in the community*. Thousand Oaks, CA: Sage.

Jacox, A. (1974). Theory construction in nursing: An overview. *Nursing Research, 23*(1), 4–13.

Keller, L. O., Strohschein, S., Lia-Hoagberg, B., & Schaffer, M. A. (1998). Population-based public health interventions: A model from practice. *Public Health Nursing, 15*(3), 207–215.

King, I. M. (1983). King's theory of nursing. In I. Clements & F. B. Roberts (Eds.), *Family health: A theoretical approach to nursing care* (pp. 177–188). New York, NY: Wiley.

Kulbok, P. A., Thatcher, E., Park, E., & Meszaros, P. S. (2012). Evolving public health nursing roles: Focus on community participatory health promotion and prevention. *OJIN: The Online Journal of Issues in Nursing, 17*(2), Manuscript 1.

Lenz, E. R., Suppe, F., Gift, A. G., Pugh, L. C., & Milligan, R. A. (1995). Collaborative development of middle-range nursing theories: Toward a theory of unpleasant symptoms. *Advances in Nursing Science, 17*(3), 1–13.

Levin, P., Cary, A., Kulbok, P., Leffers, J., Molle, M., & Polivka, B. (2008). Graduate education for advanced practice public health nursing: At the crossroads. *Public Health Nursing, 25*(2), 176–193.

McKenna, H. P., & Slevin, O. D. (2008). *Nursing models, theories and practice*. Oxford, UK: Blackwell.

McKnight, J. L., & Kretzmann, J. P. (2012). Mapping community capacity. In M. Minkler (Ed.), *Community organizing and community building for health* (3rd ed., pp. 171–186). New Brunswick, NJ: Rutgers University Press.

Meleis, A. I. (2012). *Theoretical nursing development and progress* (5th ed.). Philadelphia, PA: Lippincott, Williams & Wilkins.

Merton, R. K. (1967). *On theoretical sociology*. New York, NY: Free Press.

Morse, J. M. (2017). *Analyzing and conceptualizing the theoretical foundations of nursing*. New York, NY: Springer Publishing.

Muldoon, L. K., Hogg, W. E., & Levitt, M. (2006). Primary care (PC) and primary health care (PHC). What is the difference? *Canadian Journal of Public Health, 97*(5), 409–411.

Neuman, B. N. (1972). A model for teaching total person approach to patient problems. *Nursing Research, 21*(3), 264–269.

Orem, D. E. (1985). *Nursing: Concepts of practice* (3rd ed.). New York, NY: McGraw-Hill.

Pender, N. J. (1996). *Health promotion in nursing practice* (3rd ed.). Stamford, CT: Appleton & Lange.

Peterson, S. J., & Bredow, T. S. (2009). *Middle range theories: Application to nursing research*. Philadelphia, PA: Wolters Kluwer.

Rogers, M. E. (1983). Science of unitary human beings: A paradigm for nursing. In I. W. Clements & F. B. Roberts (Eds.), *Family health: A theoretical approach to nursing care* (pp. 219–228). New York, NY: Wiley.

Roy, C. (1984). *An adaptation model*. Englewood Cliffs, NJ: Prentice Hall.

Serafini, P. (1976). Nursing assessment in industry. *American Journal of Public Health, 66*(8), 755–760.

Smith, K., & Bazini-Barakat, N. (2003). A public health nursing practice model: melding public health principles with the nursing process. *Public Health Nursing, 20*(1), 42–48.

Timmreck, T. C. (1998). *An introduction to epidemiology* (2nd ed.). Sudbury, MA: Jones & Bartlett.

Walker, L. O., & Avant, K. C. (2011). *Strategies for theory construction in nursing* (5th ed.). Upper Saddle River, NJ: Prentice Hall.

World Health Organization. (1978). *Primary health care: Report of the international conference on primary health care, Alma Ata, USSR 6–12 September 1978*. Geneva, Switzerland: Author.

CHAPTER 5

Locating Sources of Data

Pamela F. Levin and Joan E. Kub

■ STUDY EXERCISES

1. What are the strengths and weaknesses of the data provided in the census?
2. Where could you locate local vital statistics?
3. Why is it important to locate data using a variety of sources?
4. List some sources of information about culture in your community.
5. Which data source would give you information about the prevalence of smoking in your state?
6. If the nutritional status indicators you need for calcium intake and fat intake are not available at the local or state level, what national sources would you consult?

The usefulness of a community assessment in part depends on the accuracy, completeness, and reliability of the data collected. If the assessment is to realistically profile community strengths and weaknesses and precisely identify health problems and aggregates at risk, then the data used must be appropriate, provide adequate detail, and be of the highest quality possible. This chapter discusses common sources for the data needed to conduct a community assessment, whether the assessment is focused or comprehensive. The accuracy, completeness, and reliability issues that must be addressed to ensure a valid assessment are discussed throughout the chapter.

■ OVERVIEW OF DATA SOURCES

There are three major sources of data for a community assessment. The first source is the data routinely collected by local, state, and federal agencies. These data are easily accessible via the web at little cost. Data collection is conducted with standardized instruments and the programs collecting these data conduct ongoing reviews examining accuracy, completeness, and reliability. Examples of routinely collected data are demographic data from the U.S. Census, vital statistics data gathered from birth and death certificates and other mandatory reporting systems, and morbidity data from national health surveys.

The second major source of data is archival materials that contain data collected for other purposes and may be useful for a community assessment. Surveys and studies conducted in the community by local or state service or governmental agencies, by educational institutions, or by nonprofit organizations may provide excellent information. Other examples of existing data are published documents; annual reports; newspapers; transcripts of programs, forums, or hearings; minutes of public meetings; and prior assessments, such as community health needs assessments conducted by nonprofit hospitals as part of mandatory reporting. As some of these data were collected for purposes other than community assessment, not all the data may be useful or complete. In addition to assessing the accuracy and reliability of the data, evaluating the credibility of the data source is important especially when retrieving data from the web. To evaluate credibility, consider applying the American Library Association's (2017) criteria for evaluating a website on authority, objectivity, accuracy, currency, and primary or secondary source. Archival data may provide information and perspectives not available elsewhere. The data have already been collected, so costs are low for the use of these data.

The third major source of data for a community assessment is original data collected specifically for the assessment. These are the data collected by windshield surveys, participant observation, key informant interviews, surveys, and/or focus groups with community residents. These data can be critical in assessing an aggregate or identifying a problem for which little or no other current, good-quality information is available. The community assessment team collects these data, so completeness, accuracy, and reliability can be reviewed and evaluated as part of the assessment process. However, because these are original data collected specifically for the community assessment, the data will be costlier and more time-consuming to obtain than data already available. Data collection must be designed, planned, and carried out, and the data must be analyzed. Time and funds must be allocated for these purposes.

■ TYPES OF DATA

One way of thinking about the data used in a community assessment is to classify the data as either numerical or nonnumerical (Patton, 2015). Both types of data have their place in a community assessment, but each type is collected and analyzed differently. In planning a community assessment, it is important to consider what will be useful comparison data as well as sources of data to ensure the assessment is balanced by considering both problems and strengths of the community.

Numerical Data

Numerical data are obtained and aggregated by enumerating cases or sampling the population according to a specific set of predetermined questions or statuses and using an instrument specifically designed to collect the data. Census data, for example, are numerical data obtained by using a standardized questionnaire as the instrument. Numerical data can be analyzed statistically and displayed graphically. The data can be used to calculate rates, ratios, and other parameters of public health importance. The community assessor can use tests to determine whether a given finding is statistically significant.

The advantages of using numerical data are that the collection, analysis, and reporting of these data are carried out according to well-established and widely understood statistical methods. The validity and reliability of the instrument used for data collection can be determined, and the process used for data collection and analysis can be replicated. If the data are part of an ongoing database, the data can be compared over time and with other state and national populations. However, when used alone, numerical data are insufficient for a comprehensive community assessment. A community is a tangible place in which real people live. Enumeration-based data alone cannot capture the values and beliefs of a community's culture or life in its neighborhoods.

Nonnumerical Data

Nonnumerical data are verbal, visual, aural, and olfactory data. These data are collected by such methods as interviewing individuals or groups of people about their knowledge, experiences, feelings, opinions, or beliefs; observing community contexts, people's behavior, or organizational processes; analyzing written documents or web/social media postings; and analyzing results of spatial mapping. Rather than using a predetermined set of questions, nonnumerical data are often collected inductively, using open-ended questions and making firsthand observations. The analysis is usually a written report detailing findings. The report may be a summary of field notes or a windshield survey; a detailed narrative description, including excerpts or case examples; or a more formal analysis of thematic content.

The advantages of using nonnumerical data are that these data provide depth and detail to the community assessment and are often the sole evidence that can be developed regarding critical parameters of the assessment. Using nonnumerical data may be the only way to adequately study the values and beliefs of the community's culture, analyze the organizational processes that determine community functioning, or describe the everyday contexts of neighborhood life.

The accuracy, completeness, and reliability of the findings, however, depend on the skill and rigor of the individuals collecting and analyzing the data. Many of the questions studied are inductively developed, so replicating the study is usually not possible. Nonnumerical data, when used alone, are just as insufficient for a comprehensive community assessment as are numerical data. Although they provide depth, detail, and unique information, nonnumerical data cannot provide the statistical "backbone" needed for a community assessment.

Comparison Data

It is worthwhile to think about the data for a community assessment specifically in terms of the comparisons that might be useful. The meaning of the assessment findings can be clarified by making appropriate comparisons. Using an epidemiological perspective, comparisons of past and present demographic data provide one set of comparisons that may be applicable to the assessment, whereas comparisons across local, state, national, or global data, as well as data including economic and social determinants of health, may provide additional meaning. In planning what data to collect, it will be helpful to decide what comparisons will be useful and collect the data accordingly.

Pertinent and Balanced Data

This chapter outlines multiple categories and sources of data for community assessments, recognizing that consulting all of them for a given assessment is neither feasible nor desirable. Community assessment does not involve collecting data without a plan; rather, it is a selective process focused on the data that are determined to be the most pertinent to the community and purpose of the assessment. Using a framework to guide the assessment will assist in determining what data will be pertinent for the assessment being planned. Assessment frameworks and models are discussed in Chapter 4.

Although the traditional purpose of assessment was to identify problems and needs, assessments are increasingly used to identify strengths and assets yielding a more balanced picture of the community and its residents (McKnight, 2010; Morgan & Ziglio, 2007). For example, the problems of a neighborhood may be only a partial reflection of the actual situation. Consulting residents and making an inventory of local associations and institutions may also reveal powerful resources for problem solving and community building (Brownson, Baker, Leet, Gillespie, & True, 2011). Collecting data about how things get done in the community, that is, the perceived trust between community members and agencies is another example (Sharpe, Greaney, Lee, & Royce, 2000). If the assessment can identify such strengths and assets, they can be considered in planning more appropriate, cost-effective interventions.

■ SOURCES OF DATA FOR A COMMUNITY ASSESSMENT

This chapter is organized around a systems framework, within an ecological perspective, to group and order the data sources discussed. Data sources for the people of the community and their physical environment are considered first, followed by data sources for health and social services, economic life, safety, transportation, government, communication, education, and recreation. The chapter concludes by considering data sources for cultural values, beliefs, and religions, as well as sources to assess community-related global health concerns because these are needed to portray the people of the community. The data sources discussed in this chapter are summarized at the end of the chapter.

Data Sources About the People of the Community

Several sources of data and information about the people of a community need to be accessed by the advanced public/community health nurse. Minimally, data should be obtained from sources about demographics, vital statistics, and health behavior.

Demographics

Knowledge of the demographic distribution and socioeconomic status of the community helps the advanced public/community health nurse identify aggregates at various levels of risk for disease and injury.

DATA FROM THE U.S. BUREAU OF THE CENSUS

The Census Bureau, a division of the U.S. Bureau of Commerce and one of 10 U.S. statistical agencies, is a critical source of information to understand the demographic characteristics of our country. The U.S. Census, which was mandated by our Constitution, has been conducted every 10 years since 1790, with the last census conducted in 2010. Between decennial censuses, numerous surveys are conducted to analyze trends. Information is provided on births, deaths, immigration, and emigration. The population is described by gender, age, education, occupation, residence, income, ethnic origin, and geographic area. Information about age, race, marital status, and household size is obtained from everyone. Detailed answers on occupation, income, and household facilities are sought from a smaller sample. All information is presented as enumerations, so that if percentages or rates are needed for an assessment, they must be calculated.

Statistical information is presented in a hierarchical geographic format. For example, population statistics are provided for the United States as a whole; by region (Northeast, Midwest, South, West), division (states within regions), state, county, and county subdivisions; cities, towns, and a geographic entity called a *census tract*. A census tract, which is intended to be a permanent statistical area that allows for continuity and demographic comparisons over time, is a small area consisting of between 1,200 and 8,000 people, with an optimum size of 4,000 people (U.S. Census Bureau, n.d.). The census also provides descriptions of metropolitan areas that consist of a large population nucleus along with adjacent counties that have grown together and show significant economic and social links. A careful review of the demographic and socioeconomic data available in the census can help to pinpoint or identify previously obscure aggregates of persons with needs differing from the mainstream community. Knowing that a community, for example, has a concentration of female heads of household, children younger than 6 years, incomes below the poverty level, or a growing elderly population assists the advanced public/community health nurse in anticipating the potential or actual problems that may be present.

It is imperative to compare community data with prior census reports to identify trends. Table 5.1 provides an example of census data compiled for Baltimore, Maryland, comparing 2000 to 2010 data. In addition, by comparing community data with neighboring communities, distinctive characteristics can be identified. Using Baltimore as an example, 55 neighborhoods within the city differ not only by demographic characteristics but also ultimately by health data (Baltimore Neighborhood Indicators Alliance, n.d.). Examining characteristics of neighborhoods within a city can be useful in identifying local health disparities. The details about use of data for community diagnoses are provided in Chapter 8.

QUALITY OF THE CENSUS DATA

The quality of the U.S. Census data is of utmost importance because census data provide the latest information about the U.S. population, but are also influential in the decisions of multiple entities, including the appointment of congressional seats as mandated in

TABLE 5.1 Case Example: Comparison of Census Data for Baltimore, Maryland

	2000 Census		2010 Census		Change
	Count	Percentage	Count	Percentage	Percentage
Total Population	651,155	100	626,664	100	−3.8
Race					
White	205,980	31.6	184,097	29.4	−10.6
Black or African American	418,950	64.3	401,204	64.0	−4.2
American Indian and Alaska Native	2,100	0.3	2,271	0.4	8.1
Asian	9,985	1.5	14,551	2.3	45.7
Native Hawaiian and other Pacific Islander	220	0.0	274	0.0	24.5
Some other race	4,365	0.7	11,312	1.8	159.2
Two or more races	9,555	1.5	12,955	2.1	35.6
Hispanic or Latino (of any race)	11,060	1.7	25,960	4.1	134.7
Total Housing Units	300,475	100	296,685	100	−1.3
Housing occupancy					
Occupied housing units	257,995	85.9	249,903	84.2	−3.1
Vacant housing units	42,480	14.1	46,782	15.8	10.1

Source: City of Baltimore, Department of Planning. (n.d.). *City of Baltimore: 2000 to 2010 decennial census comparison.* Retrieved from http://planning.baltimorecity.gov/sites/default/files/Citywide%20Demographics%202000-2010.pdf

the Constitution. The Census Bureau published updated standards of operation in 2013 with the goal of ensuring the quality, integrity, and credibility of all statistical activities (U.S. Department of Commerce Economics and Statistics Administration [USDCESA], 2013).

Despite the prescribed rigor in enumerating the total population, there are always challenges in counting vulnerable groups within the population. The homeless are one example. Although the census does include enumerations at soup kitchens, regularly scheduled mobile food vans, and targeted nonsheltered outdoor locations, a 2010 special report on the population that uses emergency and transitional shelters stressed that the data were not to be misconstrued as an enumeration of the homeless because of the difficulty in locating all homeless people (Smith, Holmberg, & Jones-Puthoff, 2012). Although the census is intended to count everyone living in the United States, undocumented populations pose another challenge especially at times when individuals may feel threatened by deportation. The terminology that is used for identification of these populations is *foreign born* in contrast to *native born* to help differentiate groups.

Shifting definitions of race and ethnicity as well as the stability of race self-identification are two other challenges affecting the validity and reliability of census data (USDCESA, 2012). With the 2000 census, respondents could identify themselves as multiple races rather than having to choose a single race. The classification is based on revised criteria from the Office of Management and Budget, which mandated that race and Hispanic origin (ethnicity) should be separate and distinct concepts and should be asked in two different questions (Office of Management and Budget, 1997). The number of individuals who reported more than one race was 9.0 million people in 2010, or 2.9% of the total population, whereas the number was 6.8 million people, or 2.4% of the population in 2000 (USDCESA, 2012). Another concern is whether self-identification of race and ethnicity changes over time. A study examining changes from 2000 to 2010 found that 9.8 million people (6.1%) self-reported a different race (Liebler, Porter, Fernandez, Noon, & Einnis, 2017).

ACCESS TO CENSUS DATA

Census data are available directly from the Census Bureau's home page, which has many access points for retrieving data. Printed reports from the decennial and economic censuses are also available in the Library of Congress, along with decennial census publications from 1790 onward.

Publications using census data are in PDF format and data tables can be retrieved using interactive data-access tools. There are additional links to websites containing census data and statistics. State Data Centers make census data even more accessible; these centers are found in every state and the District of Columbia, Puerto Rico, Guam, the U.S. Virgin Islands, and the Northern Mariana Islands. The centers are usually state or local government agencies, libraries, and academic centers. In addition to other services, many of these centers have prepared county, zip code, neighborhood, or census tract profiles to look at very specific areas.

ADDITIONAL DATA AVAILABLE THROUGH THE U.S. CENSUS BUREAU

The American Community Survey is also conducted by the U.S. Bureau of the Census on an annual basis for purposes of updating social and economic needs of a community. This survey contains information about jobs and occupations, educational attainment, veterans, whether people own or rent their home, and other topics. American Fact-Finder, which combines the Economic Census, the American Community Survey, and the decennial census, provides updated information about the United States, Puerto Rico, and the Island Areas.

Vital Statistics

Each state has mandatory reporting laws for the vital events of births, deaths, marriages, and divorces. These events must be reported by hospitals, government agencies, and other entities and legally registered with a county or city, usually a division within a local health department.

REPORTING SYSTEMS

The National Center for Health Statistics' (NCHS) national vital statistics system is a major source of the U.S. official health statistics that describe births, deaths, marriages, divorces, and fetal deaths. These data are provided through vital registration systems in 57 jurisdictions that have a contract with NCHS and are legally responsible for the registration of the vital events. The 57 jurisdictions include 50 states, five territories (Puerto Rico, U.S. Virgin Islands, Guam, American Samoa, and the Northern Mariana Islands), the District of Columbia, and New York City. In many states, vital statistics departments are part of the local and state health department (National Research Council, 2009).

Standard forms, which were revised in 2003 by NCHS, are used by states for data collection. Information obtained from the birth certificates allows the collection of significant birth data contributing to a better understanding of birth rates, fertility rates, percentage of low-birth-weight babies, and characteristics of the parents. Death certificates include demographic data and geographic information about where the deaths occurred. These data allow an increased understanding of characteristics of people dying, life expectancy, and comparisons of death statistics among countries. The cause of each death, which is listed on the registration form, provides helpful information in ascertaining both morbidity and mortality. The cause of death is coded according to the *International Classification of Diseases (ICD-10)* as endorsed and published by the World Health Organization (2016). Disease-specific mortality rates assist in identifying health problems in the population and targeting them for interventions.

Inaccuracies can occur with these data, however, and are of some concern. Underreporting of extremely low-birth-weight infants, for example, is a source of mortality inaccuracy because of the confusion as to whether it is an infant death, impacting infant mortality rates, or a fetal death (National Research Council, 2009). According the NCHS, *fetal death* refers to the spontaneous intrauterine death of a fetus at any time during pregnancy and most states report fetal deaths as death that occur at 20 weeks of gestation or more and/or 350 g birth weight.

The registration for births and deaths in the United States is very complete. There are checks built into the system. Efforts by NCHS to improve the collection of data and support states have included implementing web-based electronic birth (EBRS) and death registration systems, as well as through using the 2003 revised standard certificates in all jurisdictions. These systems, including the Electronic Verification of Vital Events (EVVE) and the State and Territorial Exchange of Vital Events (STEVE), have improved the timeliness of data collection, allowing the transfer of data among states and integrating the statistics with public health surveillance systems (National Research Council, 2009).

Although the NCHS completed state funding for development and implementation of a web-based electronic birth registration system (EBRS), similar progress has not been made with electronic death registration systems (EDRS; NCHS, 2015). This problem exists despite the fact that the NCHS began to automate the entry, classification, and retrieval of cause-of-death information reported on death certificates through the Mortality Medical Data System in 1967. The reported cause of death has always been problematic in vital statistics data as well. A study of hospitals in Missouri with high inpatient death rates found that 45.8% of death certificates indicated an underlying cause of death inconsistent with Centers for Disease Control and Prevention's (CDC) Guidelines for Death Certificate completion, an overreporting of cardiovascular disease, and an inaccurate reporting of deaths related to cancer (Lloyd et al., 2017). Hospitals in New York City have also been shown to overreport cardiovascular disease, so much so that interventions have been tried to remedy the error (Madsen et al., 2012).

One promising improvement is that the NCHS now records multiple causes of death; chronic problems are listed even if the problems did not directly cause the death. These data have been shown to provide a more complete picture than if only one underlying cause of death is listed (Fedeli et al., 2015). The Multiple Cause of Death database contains mortality and population counts for all U.S. counties and is available through the CDC's comprehensive WONDER database.

Vital statistics can be used to provide information about mortality trends over time. These data are frequently used as outcome data demonstrating the success or failure of a community intervention. For example, high death rates from cardiovascular disease may provide supporting evidence for instituting a program of cholesterol screening and nutrition education. A decrease in mortality from cardiovascular disease over the next 5 years might suggest the success of such a program. Examination of several years of data may provide information as to whether the higher local level is an isolated occurrence or a pattern over time.

Maternal and infant death rates are of particular interest to the advanced public/community health nurse because they are often preventable. The Linked Birth and Infant Death Data Set provides the opportunity to explore the relationships between infant death and risk factors present at birth. These files link information from the birth certificate to information about the death certificate for all infants who die younger than 1 year. Information, such as birth weight, prenatal care utilization, and mother's age found on the birth certificate, can be linked to information from the death certificate, including cause of death and age at death.

PUBLIC HEALTH SURVEILLANCE DATA

The CDC is a federal agency responsible for protecting the health of the nation and supporting health-promotion, prevention, and preparedness activities in the nation. One responsibility is that of public health surveillance, which is the collection, analysis, and use of data to target public health prevention efforts. The CDC and Council of State and Territorial Epidemiologists determine which conditions are nationally notifiable. The National Notifiable Diseases Surveillance System (NNDSS) is a nationwide collaboration that enables all levels of public health—local, state, territorial, federal, and international—to share notifiable disease-related health information.

Each state or territory is responsible for collecting data on infectious and noninfectious diseases specified by law and they then voluntarily report these data to the CDC. Healthcare providers, hospitals, laboratories, and others are responsible to report these conditions within their jurisdiction according to legislation, regulation, and other rules (Adams et al., 2016). The National Electronic Disease Surveillance System facilitates the acceptance of electronic data exchanges between the healthcare system to public health departments and those health departments to the CDC for the NNDSS.

A list of the nationally notifiable infectious diseases is provided in Table 5.2. Noninfectious notifiable diseases include diseases such as cancer, asbestosis, and silicosis,

TABLE 5.2 Nationally Notifiable Infectious Diseases 2017, United States

Anthrax	Diphtheria	Leptospirosis	Shigellosis
Arboviral diseases: Chikungunya virus, California serogroup viruses, Eastern equine encephalitis virus, Powassan virus, St. Louis encephalitis virus, West Nile virus, Western equine encephalitis	Ehrlichiosis and anaplasmosis: *Anaplasma phagocytophilum* infection, *Ehrlichia chaffeensis* infection, *Ehrlichia ewingii* infection, undetermined human ehrlichiosis/anaplasmosis	Listeriosis	Smallpox
		Lyme disease	Spotted fever rickettsiosis
		Malaria	Streptococcal toxic shock syndrome
		Measles	Syphilis: primary, secondary, early latent, late latent, late with clinical manifestations
		Meningococcal disease	
	Giardiasis	Mumps	
	Gonorrhea	Novel influenza A virus infections	Tetanus
Babesiosis	*Haemophilus influenzae*, invasive disease	Pertussis	Toxic shock syndrome (other than streptococcal)
Botulism: food-borne, infant, wound, other	Hansen's disease	Plague	Trichinellosis
Brucellosis	Hantavirus: non-Hantavirus pulmonary syndrome, pulmonary syndrome	Poliomyelitis, paralytic poliovirus infection, nonparalytic	Tuberculosis
Campylobacteriosis			Tularemia
Chancroid	Hemolytic uremic syndrome, postdiarrheal	Psittacosis	Typhoid fever
Chlamydia trachomatis infection	Hepatitis A: acute	Q fever: acute, chronic	Vancomycin-intermediate *Staphylococcus aureus* and vancomycin-resistant *S. aureus*
Cholera	Hepatitis B: acute, chronic, perinatal infection	Rabies: animal, human	Varicella, varicella deaths
Coccidioidomycosis	Hepatitis C: acute, chronic	Rubella	Vibriosis
Congenital syphilis	HIV infection	Rubella, congenital syndrome	Viral hemorrhagic fever: Crimean–Congo hemorrhagic fever virus, Ebola virus, Lassa virus, Lujo virus, Marburg virus
Cryptosporidiosis	Influenza-associated pediatric mortality	Salmonellosis	
Cyclosporiasis	Invasive pneumococcal disease	Severe acute respiratory syndrome–associated coronavirus	New World arenavirus: Guanarito virus, Junin virus, Machupo virus, Sabia virus
Dengue virus infections: dengue, dengue-like illness, severe dengue	Legionellosis	Shiga toxin-producing *Escherichia coli*	Yellow fever
			Zika virus disease and infection: congenital disease, noncongenital disease, congenital infection, noncongenital infection

Source: Centers for Disease Control and Prevention. (2017). *National Notifiable Diseases Surveillance System*. Retrieved from https://wwwn.cdc.gov/nndss/conditions/notifiable/2017/infectious-diseases

as well as harmful exposures such as carbon monoxide poisoning and elevated lead levels in children and adults. Based on these lists and the data received, the CDC Division of Health Informatics and Surveillance and the CDC programs prepare annual summaries of infectious and noninfectious diseases and conditions, which are published in the *Morbidity and Mortality Weekly Report (MMWR)*. In addition, data for selected nationally notifiable diseases reported by the 50 states, New York City, the District of Columbia, and the U.S. territories are collated and published weekly in the *MMWR*. Data published in *MMWR* are also accessible in various machine-readable formats, which can be found on the CDC WONDER website.

Although these reports can be useful for understanding infectious disease and trends in our country, there are obvious limitations of the data. The reporting is likely to be incomplete depending on the reporting state and the infectious disease or condition. These limitations influence how the data can be interpreted. The quality and completeness of data might depend on diagnostic facilities, public awareness, priorities of the state and local officials, or changes in methods of public health surveillance, such as new diagnostic tools or new infectious disease or condition entities.

There are several additional limitations to some data. Some diseases on the national list are not designated as reportable on the state level, so that occurrence data reported by the CDC represent totals only from reporting states and territories (Adams et al., 2016). Another factor is that the list of reportable diseases can change depending on the prevalence of the disease. Some diseases may be eliminated from the national list at the suggestion of public health officials and CDC staff because of a decline, whereas other diseases may be added with the emergence of a new disease. Therefore, the actual number of notifiable diseases does fluctuate over time and across jurisdictions. Another issue relates to a common epidemiological issue: that of defining a case. For reporting purposes, uniform criteria for nationally notifiable infectious and noninfectious conditions are provided, although there is the possibility that definitions vary among states, so they are not always counting the same thing.

The Surveillance, Epidemiology, and End Results (SEER) Program is a project of the National Cancer Institute that collects data from designated population-based cancer registries from approximately 12 regions defined within states, six metropolitan areas throughout the country, and two tribes. The goals of the program are to report cancer incidence, stage of cancer at time of diagnosis, mortality, and survival data. In addition, the program monitors trends to identify changes in forms of cancer, provide information about changes in the extent of disease at diagnosis, identify trends in therapy and patient survival, and promote studies designed to identify factors amenable to cancer interventions. The SEER website allows the practitioner to identify cancer statistics and develop customized graphs and tables. The National Program of Cancer Registries, as a part of the CDC, also provides databases that include cancer incidence and population data for 45 states and the District of Columbia, providing information about 94.5% of the U.S. population.

NATIONAL SURVEYS

In addition to data collected through reporting systems, data on morbidity can be obtained from a variety of public health surveys. These surveys use national samples or collect institutional records nationwide to provide accurate information about the incidence and trends in selected conditions and in healthcare utilization. Although local- and state-level data are not reported for all surveys, the data from all surveys can be used to identify problems that may be prevalent in the community. These and other national surveys are briefly described in Table 5.3 and in the following text.

TABLE 5.3 Sample of National Public Health Surveys

Type of Data	Agency, Database, and Description
Morbidity, health behavior	**Centers for Disease Control and Prevention** *National Health Interview Survey* The National Health Interview Survey is a cross-sectional survey that provides the main source of health information about the civilian, noninstitutionalized population (adult and children) of the United States. It neither includes patients in long-term care facilities, persons on active duty with the armed forces, persons incarcerated in the prison system, nor U.S. nationals living in foreign countries. This household interview has been conducted annually since 1957, and is used to monitor trends in illness and disability, as well as to track progress in achieving national health objectives. It consists of basic health and demographic items, and new or supplemental questions related to current health topics that are added each year. Types of data include chronic conditions, including asthma and diabetes; access to and use of healthcare services; health insurance coverage; health-related behaviors such as smoking, alcohol use, and physical activity; measures of functioning and activity limitations; and immunizations. *National Health and Nutrition Examination Survey* The National Health and Nutrition Examination Survey is a survey begun in the early 1960s and is designed to assess the health and nutritional status of adults and children in the United States. It is a major program of the National Center for Health Statistics, which is a part of the Centers for Disease Control and Prevention. It examines a nationally representative sample of about 5,000 people per year and combines interviews and physical examinations. **National Institute on Drug Abuse** *National Survey of Drug Use and Health* The National Survey on Drug Use and Health, which is sponsored by the Substance Abuse and Mental Health Services Administration (SAMHSA), an agency in the U.S. Department of Health and Human Services, is the primary source of information about the prevalence, patterns, and consequences of alcohol, tobacco, and illegal drug use and abuse and mental disorders in noninsitutionalized U.S. civilians aged 12 years and older. It is an annual nationwide survey involving interviews with approximately 70,000 randomly selected individuals.
Health behavior, national and community data	**Centers for Disease Control and Prevention** *National Immunization Surveys* Three surveys conducted by the National Center for Immunization and Respiratory Diseases of the CDC to monitor vaccination coverage among children 19 to 35 months, teens 13 to 17 years, and flu vaccinations for children aged 6 months to 17 years. *Youth Risk Behavior Surveillance System, Division of Adolescent Health, CDC* Biennially monitors priority health risk behaviors (alcohol and drug use, sexual behavior, injury, tobacco use, dietary behaviors, inadequate physical activity) of a nationally representative sample of ninth- through 12th-grade students. *Behavioral Risk Factor Surveillance System* (CDC) A health-related telephone survey that collects state data about adult U.S. residents regarding their health-related risk behaviors, chronic health conditions, and use of preventive services. Established in 1984 with 15 states, BRFSS now collects data in all 50 states as well as the District of Columbia and three U.S. territories.

(continued)

TABLE 5.3 Sample of National Public Health Surveys *(continued)*

Type of Data	Agency, Database, and Description
Morbidity, healthcare utilization	**NCHS** The National Hospital Care Survey integrates what was collected in three previous surveys: National Hospital Discharge Survey, National Hospital Ambulatory Medical Care Survey, and information about emergency department visits formerly collected through the Drug Abuse Warning Network. Focuses on 581 hospitals to examine the quality of healthcare, disparities, and trends affecting hospitals and healthcare organizations. Other NCHS surveys include the National Survey of Ambulatory Surgery; National Survey of Family Growth; National Study of Long-Term Care Providers, which includes survey data on the residential care community and adult day services sectors; and administrative data on the home health, nursing home, and hospice sectors.
Morbidity, healthcare utilization	**SAMHSA** The National Mental Health Services Survey is an annual survey of all known mental health treatment facilities in the United States, both public and private. Treatment Episode Data Set includes demographic characteristics and substance abuse problems of admissions to treatment facilities in the United States. National Survey of Substance Abuse Treatment Services provides an overview of annual census data of all substance abuse treatment facilities in the United States, both public and private.
Violence/crime	**United States Department of Justice, Bureau of Justice Statistics** *National Crime Victimization Survey* An annual household survey that provides a picture of crime incidents, victims, and trends.

BRFSS, Behavioral Risk Factor Surveillance System; CDC, Centers for Disease Control and Prevention.

ACCESS TO MORBIDITY AND MORTALITY DATA

The NCHS disseminates information and data through its home page on the web, electronic media, and major publications. The home page provides a wide range of statistical data about health status and the use of healthcare in the United States. The website provides links to CDC WONDER data-retrieval systems, as well as CDC's WISQARS™ (Web-Based Injury Statistics Query and Reporting System), an interactive, online database that provides fatal and nonfatal injury, violent death, and cost-of-injury data from a variety of trusted sources.

Major publications include *Health, United States; Health E-Stats; Data Briefs; National Health Statistics Reports; National Vital Statistics Reports; Vital and Health Statistics Series; Life Tables;* and the *Early Releases of Selected Estimates* from the National Health Interview Survey. NCHS reports are listed in the *Catalog of Publications. The Morbidity and Mortality Weekly Report* series provides provisional data based on weekly reports to the CDC by state health departments.

Although the focus thus far has been on national data, some sources of data focus on state and county data. State-level data can be obtained from the Kaiser Family Foundation, whereas County Rankings provides data about specific counties. County Rankings, a collaboration between the University of Wisconsin and the Robert Wood Johnson Foundation, provides valuable local data for communities and ranks the health of counties on the basis of 35 measures (five health outcomes and 30 health factors).

Health Behavior Data

Examination of health behaviors provides a perspective on the lifestyles of the people of a community that may be invaluable when change is desired. The National Health Interview Survey (NHIS), the National Health and Nutrition Examination Survey (NHANES), and the National Household Survey on Drug Abuse are several of the large ongoing public health surveys that provide data on health behaviors at the national level (see Table 5.3). The NHIS survey also includes items to measure progress toward achieving the objectives set in *Healthy People 2020*. *Healthy People 2020* tracks approximately 1,200 objectives organized into 42 topic areas and specifically focused leading health indicators. A midcourse review for the first half of the decade allows a glimpse of the progress made toward the achievement of *Healthy People 2020* objectives and describes progress needed in the second half of the decade.

Health behavior surveys that provide community data as well as national-level data include the Behavioral Risk Factor Surveillance System (BRFSS), Youth Risk Behavior Surveillance System (YRBSS), and National Immunization Survey. In response to the need for data on personal health behaviors on a state-specific basis, the CDC established the BRFSS in 1984. This is a telephone survey developed and conducted to monitor state-level prevalence of major health-related risk behavior, chronic health conditions, and use of preventive services among 400,000 adults each year in all 50 states, the District of Columbia, and three U.S. territories. The states collect the prevalence data to help monitor progress in achieving health objectives as well as to plan and implement programs focused on prevention and health promotion. Prevalence data can be explored by location or topic using charts, graphs, and maps.

The YRBSS consists of national, state, territorial, and tribal governments, and local school-based surveys of representative samples of ninth- through 12th- grade students. This national survey, conducted by the CDC, was originally developed in 1990 to monitor health risk behaviors among youth. The survey currently measures health risk behaviors that result in unintentional and intentional injuries; tobacco use; alcohol and other drug use; sexual behavior related to unintended pregnancy and sexually transmitted diseases, including HIV; unhealthy dietary behavior; and inadequate physical activity. It also assesses the prevalence of obesity, asthma, and other priority health topics. A probability sample of schools and students in the ninth through the 12th grades is determined, and the school-based survey is conducted biennially in these schools during the spring.

The National Immunization Survey was initiated by the CDC in 1994; it currently consists of three surveys to monitor vaccination coverage among children aged 19 to 35 months and teens aged 13 to 17 years, and flu vaccinations for children aged 6 months to 17 years. Data are gathered through telephone interviews with parents or guardians in all 50 states, the District of Columbia, and some U.S. territories. With the parents' permission, a questionnaire is also mailed to each child's vaccination provider(s) to collect specific vaccination information (e.g., number of doses, dates of administration, and other administrative data).

A challenge faced in conducting these surveys is avoiding response bias when questions relate to sensitive behaviors. For example, a primary concern regarding youths who respond to the YRBSS survey has been whether these adolescents will falsify their answers. Research indicates, however, that if students perceive the survey as important and that measures have been developed to protect their privacy allowing for anonymous participation, data can be gathered with credibility (CDC, 2013).

Physical Environment

The physical environment of a community provides information for the advanced public/community health nurse on many of the physical determinants of health from perspective of the social determinants of health. Physical determinants include the natural environment and climate, land use, housing and community design, as well as the built environment and infrastructure.

BOUNDARIES, CLIMATE, AND BUILT ENVIRONMENT

The physical features of place define the community and greatly influence the lifestyles and health of community residents.

Boundaries. Boundaries may be natural, as in rivers or shorelines; structural, as in highways or railroad tracks; or political, as in legally enacted congressional districts or city, township, county, and state lines. A current map, paper or electronic, from the community's website, planning board, or chamber of commerce will provide boundary information.

Information about the topography of the community further describes the physical environment. The local terrain may form internal boundaries or divisions influencing where people live and where industries, parks, and waste disposal areas are located. The terrain also affects how easily residents can get around within the community and may pose risks such as flooding. The U.S. Geological Survey, a division of the U.S. Department of the Interior, produces geological, topographical hydrologic, land use, and other specialized maps by county, state, and region. The topographic maps show the shape and elevation of the terrain together with natural and man-made features. Both the U.S. Geological Survey and CDC offer interactive online mapping tools that can illustrate the geographic distribution of a topic of interest such as the location of food deserts or areas at risk for flooding.

Climate. The climate and daily weather have influence on the physical comfort and safety of community residents; and data on average temperature, humidity, heat indexes, wind-chill factors, and amount and types of precipitation provide important information. By comparing past and current data about weather and terrain with housing characteristics and income levels of community residents, the advanced public/community health nurse can identify potential need for such services as heat assistance, cooling centers, or flood-relief measures. Local media and weather services are sources of information about area weather. The National Oceanic and Atmospheric Administration of the U.S. Department of Commerce offers searchable weather and climate data via the National Weather Service and National Centers for Environmental Information websites. Statistics on current and past weather, temperature range, and participation rates are available at the city, county, or state level.

Built Environment. The physical design and use of land can affect the health of the community. The built environment includes elements of physical design such as land-use patterns; presence of sidewalks and walking paths, bike lanes, road, highways, and bridges; and the types and density of buildings. The zoning or planning board of local government can provide information about current and projected land use within the community;

state land-use agencies or boards may have additional information. The U.S. Census reports data about population density for all census subdivisions within the community. Complementing these, a windshield survey will provide firsthand observations. Assessing the location and extent of business enterprises, health facilities, housing, vacant lots, waste disposal/treatment areas, recreation facilities, and other areas provides a profile of how the land in the community is currently being used.

Infrastructure is a component of the built environment and traditionally refers to the roads and highways, bridges, public utilities (e.g., water, power), and public buildings serving the community. The age, condition, and funding for building, maintaining, renovating, and replacing infrastructure are significant concerns that affect the health and welfare of the community. For example, deteriorating public housing or bridges may pose safety risks for residents. Needs related to infrastructure compete with other public services, creating political controversies around establishing and changing public policy. Firsthand observations, social media reports and field notes of public meetings and hearings, and interviews with planning agencies, legislators, and community advocates will acquaint the advanced public/community health nurse with the infrastructure issues affecting the community.

Notably, many communities and states are now focusing on the built environment and conduct a health impact assessment prior to building or implementing a new project, such as a new building complex or road. Complementary, but different from a community health assessment, a health impact assessment is a systematic process that evaluates the potential effects of a proposed policy, program, or project on the health of the community, including whether those health effects would disproportionally affect segments of the population (CDC, 2016).

HOUSING CHARACTERISTICS

An important feature of the community is its housing. By traveling through the community, the nurse becomes familiar with the housing, providing further clues to the health of the community. For example, areas with well-tended yards may suggest a commitment to the neighborhood, whereas vacant and boarded buildings suggest a lack of stability or transitioning within the community. The age of the housing stock should be considered, as housing structures built before 1978 increase the risk of exposure to lead-based paint chips, lead-impregnated plaster, or lead-contaminated dust or dirt from deterioration, renovation, or remodeling. Children and pregnant women are at great risk for higher blood-lead levels when living under these conditions (U.S. Department of Housing and Urban Development, n.d.).

The U.S. Census and the biennial American Housing Survey are valuable sources of information for describing the housing characteristics of a community with much data available down to the census track. Housing units are classified according to building size, unit size, age, and density. In addition, the advanced public/community health nurse has access to information about home values, rents, vacancies, and the number of renter or owner-occupied residences. Selected additional information that may be of interest for the assessment includes plumbing facilities, house heating fuel, source of water, and sewage disposal.

An additional source of housing information is the building department or planning board of the local municipal government. Information can be obtained on new housing development, modification of housing, housing lost through demolition, and gentrification of neighborhoods. City planning departments can provide information about population mobility. Building inspectors who inspect housing prior to occupation to identify problems and respond to complaints can be helpful in providing information about changing and problem areas within the community.

Environmental Health

The goal of assessing a community's environment is to identify hazardous agents and the possible health effects of exposures to the agents. Community members may be exposed to hazardous agents in a variety of settings, whether home, school, worksite, or surrounding community areas. Exposures can occur when the hazardous agent is transported by air, water, or soil.

AIR QUALITY

The U.S. Environmental Protection Agency (EPA) maintains the Air Quality System (AQS), an extensive source of ambient air pollution data. Daily and annual reports are available for ozone levels and other airborne pollutants that are summarized at the state, local, or monitoring-station level. In addition, AQS reports include emissions and compliance data for pollution sources within the community. The accuracy and completeness of the data may be variable because data are collected from several sources and data-collection methods may differ.

The cooperating state and local agencies involved in air quality regulation and the concerned citizen groups also can be consulted as part of air quality assessment. Each state prepares and monitors implementation plans for regulating air pollutants covered by the expanded Clean Air Act of 1970, and by the 1977 and 1990 amendments (e.g., carbon monoxide, lead, nitrogen dioxide, ozone, particulates, and sulfur dioxide).

WATER QUALITY

The EPA, in cooperation with state environmental and natural resources agencies, maintains data systems for each watershed. These data systems are accessible in many ways, including by zip code, city, metropolitan area, county, or state or by source, such as stream, river, or lake. Watershed information includes data about river corridors and wetlands restoration efforts, as well as listings of areas of concern such as Superfund pollution cleanup sites and agricultural runoff. Also included are an inventory of rivers and streams in the watershed, lists of community water sources and water discharges, descriptions of land characteristics, and a roster of the active citizen-based groups. Some data may be inaccurate, incomplete, or not useful because of the use of multiple sources of data.

The EPA's Safe Drinking Water Information System is a national inventory of public water systems and their records of compliance with federal regulations for safe drinking water. Through the EPA's Envirofacts data warehouse, the advanced public/community health nurse can locate the supplier of the community's drinking water and identify whether there have been any health-based or monitoring violations during the past 10 years. The completeness of the data, however, may vary from state to state depending on the reporting system used.

A second source of data about the community's drinking water was mandated in the Safe Drinking Water Act Amendments of 1996. Every water system must provide customers an annual report listing the sources of the drinking water it supplies, the quality of the sources, whether any contaminants have been identified, and the known health effects of such contaminants. The contaminants tracked and reported are based on the EPA's National Primary Drinking Water Regulations and include microbes such as *Giardia*, coliforms, and viruses; inorganic compounds such as fluoride, lead, and mercury; organic compounds such as fluoride and benzene; drinking water disinfection by-products; and radionuclides such as radium.

In many areas, community residents obtain their drinking water from private wells drawing on groundwater, streams, or cisterns. The extent of well-water use in a community can be obtained from U.S. Census data that report the source of water for each housing unit. Minimum EPA recommendations are that well water should be tested annually by a laboratory certified by the state or the EPA for coliform bacteria and nitrates, and more often and more extensively if other contaminants are suspected. The state or local health department or the agricultural extension can assist in identifying certified water-testing programs in local use. Testing is voluntary, so a comparison of interest would be the volume of testing reported by laboratories with the known extent of well-water use in the community.

WASTEWATER

In enumerating housing characteristics, the U.S. Census determines whether each unit is served by a public sewer or uses a private septic system. The municipal wastewater authority and local residents can supply further information about the extent of and any problems with sewage disposal. In areas with no public sewage system, being able to build often depends on an adequate percolation test showing that the lot can support a septic system. Planning boards and zoning committees are sources of information about drainage problems that may affect housing.

SOLID WASTE

Garbage disposal service is readily available from private contractors or the public authority in metropolitan and many suburban areas of the country. Systems for handling yard waste; recycling of cans, bottles, and paper; and disposal of worn-out appliances and furniture are in place in many areas of the country. In rural areas, these functions may be the responsibility of the householder, who must haul everything to the town disposal area. Information about arrangements for waste disposal in the community, including hazardous wastes, such as electronics, unused pharmaceuticals, used motor oil, paint cans, and insecticide packages, can be obtained from the town or city government offices.

Monitoring Hazardous Materials. The EPA maintains several reporting systems that track water discharge permits, hazardous waste sites, hazardous waste handling, and releases of toxic chemicals and compounds into the environment. Each of the following four systems has its own database that can be accessed through the EPA's Envirofacts data warehouse. The public law, data quality information, state reports, and query information are available for each database.

1. Established under the Clean Water Act, the National Pollutant Discharge Elimination System of the EPA regulates and monitors industrial, agricultural, and municipal wastewater treatment facilities nationwide. For regulated facilities, data on permits issued, permit limits, and monitoring data are collected through the Permit Compliance System of the EPA operating on local, state, tribal, and national levels.
2. The Superfund Program was established in 1980 to clean up hazardous waste sites, including abandoned warehouses, factories, and landfills. The EPA's

Superfund Enterprise Management Systems (SEMS) database in Envirofacts reports publicly releasable data on Superfund hazardous site assessment and cleanup; efforts are made to verify data before they are entered. However, not all Superfund-related data are publicly released, so some caution is needed when interpreting the data. Data are collected regionally across the nation and updated monthly for all sites on the National Priorities List (NPL) and for sites that have been investigated for potential Superfund NPL designation.

3. The Resource Conservation and Recovery Information System (RCRIS) database lists facilities that generate, transport, treat, store, or dispose of hazardous waste, as defined by federal law. Facilities handling hazardous waste are required to regularly report to state environmental agencies that then extract core data for inclusion in RCRIS. "Enforcement sensitive" data are not available to the public. Public access information about handler permit status, compliance records, and cleanup activities can be obtained by name, geographic location, industrial classification, or types of waste handled.

4. The Toxic Release Inventory tracks information about the release and/or management via recycling and treatment of more than 650 chemicals and compounds covered by the Emergency Planning and Community Right to Know Act. Facilities must report each toxic chemical they are manufacturing, processing, or otherwise using or emitting to the air, water, or placed in any type of land disposal. Information is available by facility, year, chemical, and method of release. Reports can be requested by state, facility, or customized query.

In addition to the databases just mentioned, the health implications of a community's exposure to chemicals and other hazardous waste can be mapped via the National Library of Medicine's ToxMap database. ToxMap uses data from 12 federal databases, including the EPA's Toxic Release Inventory, Superfund program, and the national cancer registry SEERS, and combines data with the health information provided by the Agency for Toxic Substances and Disease Registry. Data can be tracked to the level of census track.

Health and Social Services

The health and social services available in the community are of critical importance in maintaining health, controlling morbidity, and preventing death in community residents. An inventory of the available resources is a starting point for assessing these services and will provide useful baseline information. However, such an inventory should also include an evaluative component. Useful questions to consider include whether the identified services are adequate, accessible, acceptable, and affordable; whether there are redundant services; and whether services needed are not available. Useful sources of information are the chamber of commerce, telephone directory, existing community service directories maintained by the health department or voluntary agencies, annual reports, and community health needs assessment reports of any nonprofit hospitals in the community. Health administrators, local health professional organizations, and local and state health planning agencies are additional sources of information.

HEALTH SERVICES

Hospitals, clinics, group practices, and managed care organizations; home health and visiting nurse agencies; and nursing home and extended care facilities are examples of healthcare facilities and organizations that may be serving the community. For each of these, information about services and programs provided, fees required or reimbursements obtained, providers supplying the services, and the resources in terms of budget, space, and beds is useful for health planning. Statistics about who uses the services, how clients access the services, and whether clients are satisfied with the services are additional important information. Data about discontinued services, prior needs assessments, and current problems as identified by providers and clients also provide worthwhile background.

One essential area of the health services assessment is to record the emergency and disaster planning and facilities in the community. Important data to obtain include the location, quality, service record, and preparedness of the nearest trauma center, burn unit, poison control center, and professional and volunteer emergency services in the event of a disaster. Area healthcare facilities, the local Red Cross, and the fire department are sources of information.

The services and programs of the community or county health department are part of the health and social services assessment. Immunization and well-child clinics and screening for sexually transmitted diseases, HIV, tuberculosis, and lead may be among the programs available. Supporting the public safety, air and water quality, swimming sites, vector and animal control, and food establishment monitoring may be among the other services provided. Health department professionals are sources of information with additional information about programs and services available on the state level.

Several federal agencies provide information that may be useful for a community assessment. The Health Resources and Human Services Administration (HRSA) of the U.S. Public Health Service, consisting of six bureaus, monitors the supply of health professionals and publishes reports and studies of utilization, practice environments, and workforce projections. This agency publishes state profiles examining such issues as the supply of nurses and supports the training of health professionals. In addition, HRSA programs provide healthcare to vulnerable populations. For example, the Bureau of Primary Healthcare funds health centers in underserved communities and provides access to comprehensive primary and preventive care for low-income, uninsured populations, and those who face other barriers to healthcare. HRSA identifies health professional shortage areas (HPSAs) that lack access to primary care, mental health services, and/or dental care. The Centers for Medicare & Medicaid Services (CMS), which is part of the Department of Health and Human Services, administers health insurance programs through Medicaid, Medicare, and child health insurance programs that cover 100 million people. Several examples of surveys that monitor healthcare utilization from a federal perspective are listed in Table 5.3.

SOCIAL SERVICES

The inventory of social services in a community includes federal, state, and local agencies with programs in the community as well as private and volunteer organizations of all sizes. The locations of welfare, Medicaid, Medicare, and Social Security offices; the availability of counseling and support services; crisis intervention; child protective and youth services; and services for special populations, including immigrant, handicapped, disabled, and chronically mentally ill persons together provide a picture of how the community can support its more vulnerable residents. Food pantries, homeless shelters, adult day care, child day care, home day care, after-school care, mental health support groups, and Alcoholics Anonymous programs are other examples of social services that may be available.

As with the assessment of health services, data of importance include information about services and programs, fees, providers, and resources as well as about who uses the services, how clients access the services, and whether clients are satisfied with the services. Data about discontinued services, prior assessments, and current problems as identified by providers and clients also provide worthwhile background. Existing resource directories, social service professionals, volunteer organizations, churches and temples, and the phone directory are sources of information.

Economic Life

Census data are the first place to look for information about the labor force in a community. Accessed via American FactFinder, statistics are provided on the number of persons older than 16 years in the labor force, unemployed persons looking for work, and persons not in the labor force. In addition, the Census provides information about disability status, the number of persons in the labor force with children younger than 18 years and 6 years, the type of occupation, type of industry, type of work status (e.g., full time, part time), and commuting time and methods, as well as the type of health insurance coverage provided. Unemployment data are available from the Bureau of Labor Statistics (BLS) and the state Department of Employment provides information about the number of individuals receiving unemployment benefits; the chronically unemployed will not be reflected in the counts, however. Further sources of information about employment in the community include the local chamber of commerce, employers, as well as job openings on the web and in local newspapers.

PERSONAL INCOME

The U.S. Census collects data on household, family, and per capita income and further describes income by source, including self-employment (farm, nonfarm); wage and salary; interest, dividend, and rental income; Social Security; and public assistance. Data are also available about family income by family type and presence and age of children; the number of workers in the family; income by age, sex, and race/ethnicity; and poverty status by age, race/ethnicity, and sex. Other sources of income-related data include the interactive Food Environment Atlas by the U.S. Department of Agriculture, which estimates food insecurity within a community by mapping income, food access, prices, and food assistance programs.

BUSINESS AND INDUSTRY

Detailed descriptions of business patterns are collected by the U.S. Census and include the type of business or industry, the number of employees, employee wages, and presence of hazardous materials. The type of business is broken down further on the basis of the North American Industry Classification System into subtypes, for example, differentiating masonry, plastering, and tile work, as well as occupations within the business or industry. County-specific business patterns are available from American FactFinder by zip codes and the diversity and disability status of workers employed by area businesses. The agricultural extension service, chamber of commerce, planning board, and community farming and business groups are further sources of information about current and future economic development in the community.

OCCUPATIONAL HEALTH

U.S. civilian workers spend a quarter of their lifetimes and approximately half of their waking hours in work-related activities; in 2016, the BLS estimated 151 million individuals in the civilian workforce (BLS, 2017; Office of Disease Prevention and Health Promotion, 2017).

As a result of the passage of the Occupational Safety and Health Act in 1970, the worker fatality rate has fallen from 38 worker deaths per day in 1970 to 13 per day in 2015. In addition, work-related illness and injuries have decreased from 10.9 incidents per 100 workers in 1972 to 3.0 per 100 in 2015 (Occupational Safety and Health Administration [OSHA], 2017). OSHA, a division of the U.S. Department of Labor, oversees the health and safety of most private-sector workers and some public-sector workers; the Mine Safety and Health Administration oversees the health and safety of workers in the mining industry.

Health Standards and Hazards. Federal and state OSHA standards have been defined for many industries; OSHA conducts compliance inspections of private-sector employers, excluding those who are self-employed, family farms, and government facilities. Health and safety standards for specific industries can be located through OSHA's website. Data are also available on compliance inspections of specific business establishments and industry groups based on the North American Industry Classification System, the approach used across federal agencies for data collection and statistical purposes.

Workplace hazards include exposures to chemical, physical, ergonomic, biological, and psychosocial agents. Use of toxic chemicals by an employer may affect the health of the workers as well as the community residents. Workplace chemical exposure data are available on OSHA's website and are searchable by business establishment and zip code. Under the OSHA Hazard Communication standard, chemical manufacturers must supply a Safety Data Sheet summarizing health, safety, and toxicological information about the chemical in a user-friendly manner (OSHA, 2012). In assessing potential exposures of community residents to chemical agents, the Safety Data Sheets for chemicals used by area businesses can provide important information. However, as chemicals, technologies, and work processes evolve, potential risks to workers and community residents may yet to be determined.

Injury and Disease Reporting. The Department of Labor's BLS annually compiles data from private- sector employers on nonfatal workplace injuries and illnesses that resulted in days away from work. As these data are based on reports submitted to comply with OSHA's mandatory recordkeeping rule, the self-employed and government workers are not included. However, the self-employed and government workers, along with those in the private sector, are included in the BLS annual report on fatal occupational injuries (BLS, n.d.). National- and state-level data are available for both annual reports and include number and rates of cases by industry; details on the worker injured, including age, gender, and race/ethnicity; nature of the disabling condition; and source for producing the condition that involved one or more days away from work. Additional occupational morbidity and mortality data from sources, such as the National Institute of Occupational Safety and Health and the National Health Interview Survey, are available by searching CDC's WONDER database. Overall, musculoskeletal disorders, including sprains or strains from overexertion, account for the largest proportion of cases in private industry of work-related injuries. However, occupational illnesses/diseases are often underreported because of the long latency periods between exposure and disease diagnosis, as well as workers changing employers (Drudi, 2015).

Safety Services

This section includes information about locating data sources for the safety or protection services in a community.

FIRE PROTECTION

Information about the community's fire-protection services, personnel, resources, funding, response times, and service records may be obtained from the local fire department. Besides responding to fires, the department may provide educational programs for schools and the public, conduct safety checks, and provide window placards indicating the location of children's bedrooms. The leading causes of fire, the hazardous fire areas, and the availability of smoke alarms in the community are other important pieces of information for the assessment.

The National Fire Data Center of the U.S. Fire Administration, a division of the U.S. Department of Homeland Security, annually reports data from the National Fire Incident Reporting System. These data are reported by local fire departments and state fire marshals from all 50 states, District of Columbia, Native American Tribal Authorities, and Puerto Rico. The data are used to study the causes of fire-related injuries, deaths, and property loss. Data are available in a variety of formats on state profiles by year of fires, fire deaths and losses, and arson, together with nationwide comparison data.

POLICE PROTECTION

The police department, police commissioner, or sheriff's office, and the state police can provide information about police protection in the community. Baseline information includes the number of sworn officers and other employees and their training, department equipment and facilities, level of funding, and services provided. Service records are of interest, including calls received, response times, and arrests. The most common crimes and unsafe areas in the community are additional data of interest. Besides ensuring the public safety, the police may provide educational programs to schools and the public and other services, such as animal protection, which should be included in the assessment.

The Bureau of Justice Statistics publishes personnel reports that provide comparisons by state and local police departments and include ratios of types of officers and other personnel to the population served. Some personnel data are also available for tribal justice agencies. Bureau reports are available through the U.S. Department of Justice's home page on the Internet.

CRIME AND VIOLENCE

Crime and violence are clearly major areas of concern and need to be viewed as public health issues (Wen & Goodwin, 2016). The costs are great in terms of financial loss, pain and suffering, risk of death, psychological damage, and reduced quality of life. Social factors associated with violence include population turnover and community disruption often disproportionally affecting communities of color and contributing to health disparities (Wen & Goodwin, 2016).

Crime and violence data are available on local, state, and federal levels. Information provided by local agencies to their centralized state agency on a monthly or quarterly basis is available to the public upon request. In some localities, however, individuals may be asked to sign a Freedom of Information Act (FOIA) form before this information is released. The centralized state agencies publish crime statistics that may also be available on the Internet. News reporters frequently review the police blotters and publish crimes in local newspapers, thus providing an additional source of information.

The Bureau of Justice Statistics of the U.S. Department of Justice is responsible for the collection of data; the data collected are critical to policy makers at all three levels of government. The Bureau oversees two statistical programs to measure the magnitude, nature, and impact of crime in the nation. These programs are the Uniform Crime Reporting (UCR) Program of the Federal Bureau of Investigation (FBI) and the National Crime Victimization Survey.

The UCR Program collects information from local law enforcement agencies and the statistics collected include violent crime (e.g., murder and nonnegligent manslaughter, rape, robbery, aggravated assault) and property crime (e.g., burglary, larceny-theft, motor vehicle theft). Data are available at the state level and local level on the basis of population size. These data have been published since 1958 and are available in a publication, *Crime in the United States*, which is available on the home page of the FBI under UCR. The FBI, in collaboration with the Bureau of Justice Statistics, also allows users to build customized tables.

Data at the local level can be compared to the state and national crime statistics. One problem that may be encountered when comparing local and state crime statistics to those published by other states and by the UCR Program are that definitions of some crimes differ. The definition of *rape* for example has changed over time; UCR changed its definition in 2011.

The National Crime Victimization Survey gives a detailed picture of crime incidents, victims, and trends in the United States. A nationally representative sample of 90,000 households, with over 160,000 persons, is contacted and asked about the frequency, characteristics, and consequences of criminal victimization in the United States. Data are collected on nonfatal personal crimes (rape or sexual assault, robbery, aggravated and simple assault, and personal larceny) and household property crimes (burglary, motor vehicle theft, and other theft) both reported and not reported to police. Data are collected about both the victim and offender.

Transportation

Adequate transportation is vital to the growth and health of a community. Residents must be able to get to work and school, shop for the things they need, visit friends and family, and access healthcare. The U.S. Census collects data about how people get to work (e.g., car, bicycle, walking, public transportation), the travel time and distance to work, and the extent of carpooling they use. The U.S. Department of Transportation's Bureau of Transportation Statistics maintains a national transportation data archive. This archive includes data and reports on a range of topics, including information on the 30 largest transit systems in the United States; the type, time spent, and method of travel of American households; seat-belt use; motorcycle-helmet use; and driving under the influence.

PUBLIC TRANSPORTATION

If there is a local transit authority, route maps, schedules, and fares will provide information about the availability, affordability, and extent of public transportation. The transit authority can also provide information about trends in service and ridership and accommodations for disabled and handicapped riders. The telephone directory and Internet can provide information about the availability of taxicabs; shared-ride taxicab systems; and bus, rail, and airline services. Area radio and television stations may provide reports on traffic congestion as well as coverage of accidents. Finally, a windshield survey and interviews with community residents provide valuable supplements to this information.

MOTOR VEHICLE TRANSPORTATION

The Federal Bureau of Transportation Statistics and state departments of transportation maintain data about the number of licensed motorists and registered vehicles in the state. State departments of transportation may also collect other useful transportation statistics.

For example, some state departments of transportation maintain an inventory of state and interstate highways and locally owned county, town, and municipal routes; and the official websites contain information about up-to-date road conditions and road construction.

The National Highway Traffic and Safety Administration of the U.S. Department of Transportation maintains the Fatality Analysis Reporting System (FARS). This system contains data on all fatal traffic crashes within the 50 states, the District of Columbia, Puerto Rico, and tribal lands. Information about fatal crashes provided by state agencies is extracted and put in a standard format. Data on the person who died include age, gender, role in the crash, injury severity, restraint use, and blood alcohol estimates. Data on the vehicle and driver include vehicle type, initial and principal impact points, most harmful event, and driver's license status. The vehicle crash information includes location and time of the crash; whether it was a hit-and-run crash; whether a school bus, pedestrian, or bicycle was involved; and the number of vehicles and people involved. In addition, some data are available at the county level.

FARS data are available on the Internet by accessing the National Highway Traffic and Safety Administration home page. The state police, the state highway safety department, or the state department of transportation are agencies that maintain these data at the state level and are potential sources for individual communities within the state.

Politics and Government

The politics and government of a community are of interest to the advanced public/community health nurse because these are pivotal to community health and social welfare. It is through the public and behind-the-scenes processes of government that policy is created and implemented and reflects some of a community's values and priorities.

Community governance rests on federal and state laws and regulations, the charter for a community, and the ordinances enacted by the community's public governing body. Accessing these may be of importance as background for community assessment. Community, state, and congressional legislators and executive offices can be of assistance in accessing information and in obtaining and interpreting specific legislation affecting community health and social welfare.

Aside from the body of law underpinning community governance, most data sources for assessing community government and understanding community politics are particular to a specific community. Every locality has its own history and traditions, its own sets of interest groups and stakeholders, and its own patterns of interaction and participation or nonparticipation in community governance. Therefore, the best way to learn about a particular community is to study the community itself.

As a first step, obtaining or creating an organizational chart of the community's government is helpful for understanding the branches, departments, and lines of authority. Next, elected and appointed officials and their responsibilities can be identified, as well as key community leaders and their constituencies. A review of the community's annual report and other policy documents, ordinances, bylaws, and procedures will provide information about issues considered important in the community. Recent budgets, particularly the sections related to community health and social welfare, will give information about the financial condition of the community and the community's funding priorities. Studying the tax base and funding sources for local government and publicly supported health and social services may provide an understanding of what a community can and cannot do.

The advanced public/community health nurse can next study the ongoing processes of community politics and governance. The level of voter registration and participation in elections can be obtained from the local board of elections. The media are a steady source of information, including television and radio news, talk shows, cable/web broadcasts of public meetings, and local newspapers and magazines. The community and neighborhood groups may have home pages, distribute a newsletter, or issue periodic news releases. Politicians may have a website and hold news conferences, public receptions, town hall meetings, and/or fund-raising dinners.

Attending community meetings, forums, hearings, and legislative sessions will provide a wealth of detail about players, stakeholders, issues, and the dynamics of community interaction. The advanced public/community health nurse can keep field notes of these observations over time and develop an ongoing list of politically active organizations in the community. Key points in this assessment are to consider the following questions: How are decisions made in the community? Who are the key decision makers? Who are the stakeholders, and how are they aligned on current issues affecting the community? Conversely, who is left out of decision making? What processes serve to exclude and disenfranchise some groups in the community? Is there a silent, disengaged minority or majority? What are the trends in leadership and issues, and what changes are likely? And finally, how do the political processes of the community affect community health and social welfare?

Communication

Data on a community's communication systems provide information about how the community is linked to the state, nation, and world as well as to the environment and its people and systems. Awareness of the systems that can be used to communicate is essential to getting health messages to the public. Various types of communication include audio, video, print media, the telephone, social media, face-to-face communication, and the Internet.

MEDIA

Local radio and television are the primary sources of news for many community residents, whereas many others rely on or supplement these by reading newspapers. For each of these media, the philosophy, editorial and programming policies, and intended audience can be assessed. What is the size of the audience attracted? Are particular media directed toward specific political, religious, racial, or cultural groups? Does reported news include health topics or public service announcements? Some media run public opinion polls on issues of concern to the community. They may broadcast local governmental meetings and hearings, provide a forum for community members, run regular "call-in" shows, or "showcase" key events in the community such as holiday parades, sports playoffs, and graduations. All these serve to support the flow of information in the community.

TELEPHONE

Americans are increasingly connected to others through cell phone use. In fact, the Pew Research Center found that 95% of Americans own a cell phone of some type and 77% own a smartphone. Although cell phone users do not vary by demographics, smartphone users are more likely to vary on the basis of age, household income, and educational attainment. Only 42% of those aged 65 years and older own a smartphone and those with less than a high school education (52%), in contrast to high school graduates (69%) and college graduates (89%) own one. Income appears to be related to smartphone ownership; 64% of those who earn less than $30,000 per year own one in contrast to 93% of those earning at least $75,000. Rural residents are slightly less likely to own a smartphone (67%) in contrast to urban (77%) and suburban residents (79%; Pew Research Center, 2017a). These statistics are important in measuring the communication capability within a community. The U.S. Census provides data on cell phone use for those aged 18 years and older. Residents without phones may be isolated from the community or have difficulty getting help in an emergency. Use of landlines may be more frequent in areas of the country where cell towers are not yet available to support reliable cell phone service.

SOCIAL MEDIA/ FACE-TO-FACE COMMUNICATION

The use of social media has grown exponentially since 2005. In 2005, only 5% of Americans used some form of social media, but today seven of 10 Americans use one form of social media (e.g., Facebook, Twitter, Instagram, Pinterest, LinkedIn). Facebook is most popular, with young adults being the quickest adopters (88%), but growth is also noted among adults aged 65 years and older (36%; Pew Research Center, 2017b).

In addition to social media use, the advanced public/community health nurse should never underestimate the importance of face-to-face communication This includes informal networking with neighbors and congregating with people in public areas, such as parks, restaurants, and city centers, as well as formal communication that occurs at town meetings, organizations, church services, and school meetings. The advanced public/community health nurse should think about the following questions when planning communication efforts: Are these various venues for communication well attended? Which groups regularly participate and which do not?

Computers/Other Devices

Nearly nine of 10 Americans use the Internet (Pew Research Center, 2017c). According to the Pew Research Center, 80% of U.S. adults own desktop or laptop computers, and 75% of Americans have broadband Internet services in their homes (Pew Research Center, 2017a, 2017c). In addition, nearly half of Americans own tablet computers and around one in five owns an e-reader device (Pew Research Center, 2017a). Just as there are demographic differences with smartphone use, there are demographic differences in access to broadband Internet. Those less likely to have broadband service are racial minorities, rural residents, older residents, and those with lower levels of education and income (Pew Research Center, 2017c).

From a community perspective, it would be important to assess the availability of computers in homes, schools, and libraries. Local librarians and school administrators can provide information regarding the number of computers in libraries and schools. School administrators may be able to estimate the numbers of their students who have home access to computers. In addition, the U.S. Census reports access to the Internet via home or other locations. The currency of computer hardware and software and use of area networks by the local health department, libraries, school administrators, the local law enforcement agency, and other key community agencies are additional useful information.

Education

Education assists community members to become and remain societal contributors who are productive and employable, all of which supports the health and well-being of individuals, families, and the community. Being employed supports access to healthcare. Being educated influences health beliefs, healthcare utilization patterns, and the ability to understand and incorporate health teaching into personal health practices. The U.S. Census is the primary source for the data needed to characterize the educational status of the community. In the Social Characteristics sections of the Census, data are available about the years of school completed, school enrollment, and language spoken by census block or tract, community, city, and county. State- and national-level data are also available.

EDUCATIONAL RESOURCES

An inventory of public and private schools, libraries, and educational services for special groups, such as pregnant teens, developmentally disabled children and adults, and students with special needs, provides baseline information about educational resources in the community. The availability of vocational education, adult education, general equivalency diploma programs, English as a second language, and literacy programs may be important as well. The local board of education, school district, and individual school or library administrators are sources of data about the programs and resources, services, funding sources, and demographic information about students and other users of the services. School districts and individual schools may also publish home pages, newsletters, annual reports, and other information pertinent to the community assessment.

State departments of education collect information from public school districts statewide, and many publish annual or biennial report cards or other data sources providing detailed information about school performance. Much of this information is available online through home pages of state departments of education. State departments of education are also a primary source for information about college and university performance reports, state aid to education programs, programs supporting access to postsecondary education, and education for disabled and special needs populations.

On the federal level, the National Center for Education Statistics (NCES) collects and reports statistics outlining the condition and progress of education in the United States. The *Condition of Education* is a congressionally mandated report that is provided to Congress each year and available on the NCES website. Another annual report is the *Indicators of School Crime and Safety*, which covers topics such as victimization, teacher injury, bullying and cyberbullying, school conditions, fights, weapons, availability and student use of drugs and alcohol, student perceptions of personal safety at school, and criminal incidents at postsecondary institutions. NCES also collects and reports information about the academic performance of the nation's students as well as the literacy level of the adult population.

Besides the analysis of statistical data and reports, assessing the community's educational resources includes visits to the institutions of interest by the advanced public/community health nurse. Administrators, teachers, parents, and the students themselves are all sources of information, as are firsthand observations. What is the condition of the buildings and playgrounds, and what resources are available for the students? Are administrators and teachers available to parents and community residents for consultation? What is the atmosphere of hallways and classrooms? What is the level of parent participation in the parent–teacher organization, and what issues are of concern? What is the attendance at school and sporting events? Are there safety or violence problems within or around the school? Do students come to school adequately fed and clothed? What health education does the curriculum include? What school health services are offered? Is there an assigned school nurse and/or one on site? What are the primary health needs of the students enrolled? What are the absenteeism rate and the graduation rate from high school? Field notes on these and related questions provide additional useful information for community assessment.

Recreation

Understanding how community residents use their leisure time is an important aspect of community assessment. Participating in family leisure and social activities, community social and service groups, entertainment and the arts, and outdoor recreation, exercise, and sports are common kinds of leisure activities that support health and well-being, both for the people involved and for the total community. Not all groups in the community, however, may have access to these activities.

RECREATIONAL RESOURCES

An inventory of park and recreational facilities and programs, community social and service groups and sports leagues, and entertainment and art venues provide baseline information about recreational resources in a community. Community media, the park district or community recreation department, the local library, and community residents are all sources of data, as are firsthand observations. State departments of natural resources and tourism can provide additional information about recreational destinations that attract community residents.

The inventory of public facilities identifies what resources are available, locations, accessibility, affordability, and how they are being developed, maintained, and funded. Visits to the sites of interest provide the opportunity to interview staff and users and to assess the condition, upkeep, and safety of the available resources. When are these facilities open, and how do people get there? Who uses them, and who does not? What programs are offered? Are special groups provided for, such as older or disabled residents, residents with special needs, or children out of school for the summer? Is there an easily accessible community directory of social and service groups and sports leagues? How do people join and participate in such groups? Are the facilities and services affordable for all segments of the population?

There are usually many other venues for recreation in a community besides public recreational resources. These may include bowling alleys, golf courses, health clubs, movie theaters, shopping malls, galleries, sports arenas, coffeehouses, pool halls, bars, social clubs, or restaurants where residents congregate and spend time. Even crack houses and certain street corners may be recreation venues for some residents.

For home entertainment, there may be game/media rental stores, bookstores, or libraries supplying media consumers can borrow, rent, or buy. The community may support special events such as basketball playoffs, health fairs, church bazaars, ethnic festivals, parades, or holiday celebrations. These items can play a role in defining quality of life in the community. Field notes assessing these provide additional information for a community assessment.

NEIGHBORHOOD LIFE

The advanced public/community health nurse can also assess the recreational life of the community firsthand during the process of visiting neighborhoods in the community. Do residents sit on porches or stoops and chat with passersby, or are shades drawn and doors closed? Are people out and about jogging or walking their dogs, or are the streets empty? If the streets are empty, is it simply because people are away at work or school, or is it because the streets are unsafe for everyday exercise and sociability? Are there locations in rural areas where people congregate?

Culture, Values, and Beliefs

Culture influences a community's values, beliefs, and behavior. Culture is learned knowledge acquired over time that people use to generate behavior and interpret experience. A value suggests the assigned worth or importance of a given practice (Purnell, 2013). For example, when community members vote for or against a new refugee center, they may be reflecting the value their culture places on inclusiveness. Values are tied to social and religious beliefs about a variety of issues. including but not limited to economics, technology, health, religion, family, and marriage. The advanced public/community health nurse needs to gather data on the culture of a community to better understand the determinants of how they care for their children; eat; cope with stress; deal with death; respond to healthcare providers; and value the past, present, and future (Purnell, 2013).

The census report for race, ethnicity, ancestry, and language is an excellent starting point for gathering cultural data. Racial groups include "White," "Black or African American," "American Indian or Alaskan Native," "Asian," or "Native Hawaiian or Other Pacific Islander," as well as multiracial combinations. Ethnicity is reported for community members of Hispanic or Latino origin and reported by origin groups, such as Mexican, Cuban, or Puerto Rican. Ancestry is the self-identified origin, heritage, or place of birth of the person, of his or her parents, or ancestors before arriving in the United States. This entry includes single ancestry or multiple ancestries. The language spoken at home and the ability to speak English are asked of all persons ages 5 years and older.

The community library, historical society, or historical museum often provides insight into the cultural roots of a community. Usually, the materials in the collection are those provided by citizens over the years, thus giving an indication of what individuals valued and wanted preserved for future generations. It is important to understand the influence of early attitudes and values on the present.

Individuals working in and serving the community are sources of community values and beliefs. Long-established bartenders, hairdressers, restaurant owners and servers, healthcare providers, and store managers and clerks interface daily with members of the community and may offer very candid insights. Faith leaders, teachers, administrators, school board members, and local politicians can provide information about issues that the community regards as important and how community members perceive quality of life.

Global Health

In conducting an assessment, it is critical to compare data. For example, an advanced public/community health nurse compares local data to state- and national-level data to identify trends, assets, and problem areas. Thus far focus has been primarily on a domestic assessment, but there is often a need to look even broader. Some advanced public/community health nurses conduct assessments from a global perspective because their work is focused on another country. Others may be working within an organization, such as nongovernmental organizations (NGOs), or may need to focus on a target immigrant population within the United States. Several resources are useful in gathering information about a specific country other than the United States. These resources include the Central Intelligence Agency, the World Health Organization, and the World Bank. In addition, information gathered by NGOs that serves the various countries is invaluable because assessments are often performed to better understand the need for specific services or to evaluate programs to determine whether they are meeting specific needs.

■ SUMMARY

A comprehensive discussion on locating sources of data for a community assessment has been presented in this chapter. The systems framework was used to organize the chapter content, which may also be used to guide the community assessment process, as well as an ecological perspective. The local and national data sources focused on the subsystems, including the people, the physical environment, environmental health, health and social services, economic life, safety services, transportation, politics and government, communication, and education; additional data sources provided an ecological, global perspective. Data sources are summarized at the end of the chapter. Throughout the chapter, advantages and disadvantages of data sources were presented.

■ SUGGESTED CLINICAL OR PRACTICUM ACTIVITIES

1. Meet with someone in the local office that is responsible for collecting and compiling vital statistics. Discuss the issues related to collecting accurate and complete vital statistics data.
2. Review the long form of the birth certificate. What data on this form may be useful for conducting a community assessment?
3. Compile a list of the most useful sources of data for your community assessment. Meet with your preceptor or an advanced public/community health nurse who is knowledgeable about the community to review the data sources.

Summary of Community Assessment Data Sources

Community Subsystem	Data Source
Community Population	
Demographics	*U.S. Census*, Bureau of the Census, U.S. Department of Commerce
	Enumerates and conducts intercensal estimates to provide information about births, deaths, immigration, and emigration and describes the gender, age, occupation, residence, income, ethnic origin, and geographic area of the population
Vital statistics	Local and state health department data-collection programs
	National Vital Statistics System, National Center for Health Statistics (CDC)
	Collects state vital statistics and publishes data on births, deaths, fetal deaths, abortions, marriages, and divorces in the United States
	Linked Birth and Infant Death Data, National Center for Health Statistics (CDC)
	Links information from birth and death certificates for 98% of infants dying before the age of 1 year
	Multiple Cause of Death database, CDC Wonder (CDC)
	On the basis of death certificates, this database provides county-level, national, and population data by age groups, race, ethnicity, gender, state, county, underlying cause of death and multiple cause of death
	National Electronic Disease Surveillance System, Epidemiology Office (CDC)
	Collects state communicable disease records and publishes summaries of 60 notifiable conditions
	National Center for HIV/AIDS, Viral Hepatitis, STD, and TB Prevention, AtlasPlus (CDC)
	Uses HIV, viral hepatitis, STD, and TB data to create maps, charts, and detailed reports, and analyze trends and patterns
	Surveillance, Epidemiology, and End Results; National Cancer Institute
	Collects data from 11 designated population-based cancer registries throughout the nation that receive data from state cancer registries
Physical Environment	
Boundaries and terrain	Current map from community's homepage, planning board, or chamber of commerce
	Local library; state department of natural resources
	U.S. Geological Survey, U.S. Department of the Interior
	Topographic maps show terrain with natural and man-made features; state and county fact sheets report on each state's earth resources and hazards, including air and water quality and effects of global change
Climate	Local media weather service, library, chamber of commerce
	National Weather Service, National Oceanic and Atmospheric Administration, U.S. Department of Commerce
	Current weather and climate data by locality with annualized and 10-year comparisons
	National Centers for Environmental Information, National Oceanic and Atmospheric Administration, U.S. Department of Commerce
	Weather data archive, with climate summaries for every state

(continued)

Summary of Community Assessment Data Sources *(continued)*

Community Subsystem	Data Source
Physical Environment *(continued)*	
Built environment	Local zoning or planning board; state land-use agencies
	U.S. Census, Bureau of the Census, U.S. Department of Commerce
	Population density data
	Windshield survey, public meetings and hearings, interviews with planning agencies and legislators
Housing characteristics	*U.S. Census, American Housing Survey*, Bureau of the Census, U.S. Department of Commerce
	Housing characteristics data
	Windshield survey
	Local building department or planning board; interviews with local city planners, building inspectors; tax records; local registry of deeds
Environmental Health	*Envirofacts Warehouse* (EPA)
	Gateway to environmental health databases, including legislation
Air quality	*Air Quality System* (EPA)
	Airborne pollution data reported from monitoring stations and point sources; reports for major identified point sources and annual summaries by monitoring station are available
	Air Data (EPA)
	Data gateway to outdoor air quality data collected from state, local, and tribal monitoring agencies across the United States
	State air quality implementation plan; cooperating state and local agencies regulating air quality; citizens' groups
Water quality	*Healthy Watersheds Data* (EPA)
	Uses data from state environmental and natural resources agencies to inventory rivers and streams, community water sources and discharges, wetlands in each watershed
	Safe Drinking Water Information System (EPA)
	National inventory of public water systems and their compliance with federal regulations
	Local public water system annual report
	Ambient Water Quality (EPA)
	Databases on water pollution by state, including fish advisories, coastal recreational waters
	National Contaminant Occurrence (EPA)
	Database on water-contaminant incidents
	U.S. Census, Bureau of the Census, U.S. Department of Commerce
	Data on each housing unit, well-water use
	State or local health department, agricultural extension service lists of water-testing programs

(continued)

Summary of Community Assessment Data Sources *(continued)*

Community Subsystem	Data Source
Environmental Health *(continued)*	
Wastewater	*U.S. Census,* Bureau of the Census, U.S. Department of Commerce
	Data on sewer service to housing units
	Public wastewater authority
	Local planning and zoning boards
Solid waste	Private and public garbage disposal and recycling services
	Town or city government offices
Monitoring hazardous waste	*National Pollutant Discharge Elimination System* (EPA)
	Monitors industrial and municipal wastewater treatment facilities nationwide; data on permits issued and monitoring data
	Superfund Enterprise Management Systems (EPA)
	Searchable inventory of active and archived hazardous waste sites in the Superfund program; includes sites that are on, in the assessment phase, or are proposed to be on the National Priorities List
	Resource Conservation and Recovery Information System (EPA)
	Database of facilities that generate, transport, treat, store, or dispose of hazardous waste; handlers permit status, compliance record, cleanup activities by name, location, industrial classification, or chemical
	Toxic Release Inventory (EPA)
	Database of information about transfers and release of 650 chemicals covered by the Emergency Planning and Community Right to Know Act; reporting is mandatory; can be searched by facility, year, chemical, and method of release
	Integrated Risk Information System (EPA)
	Database of information related to chronic noncarcinogenic and carcinogenic effects of chemicals in the environment
	ToxMap (National Library of Medicine)
	Uses data from 12 federal databases to map chemical and other hazardous exposures in a community and combines with health information from the Agency for Toxic Substances and Disease Registry
Health and Social Services	
Service agencies and workforce	Chamber of commerce, telephone directory, community service directories, annual reports; health administrators, health professional organizations, local and state health planning agencies; Red Cross
	Health Resources and Human Services Administration, U.S. Public Health Service
	Reports and studies of utilization, practice environments, and workforce projections for health professionals; publishes state profiles of health resources

(continued)

Summary of Community Assessment Data Sources *(continued)*

Community Subsystem	Data Source
Health and Social Services *(continued)*	
Healthcare workforce, Medicare, Medicaid	*Bureau of Primary Health Care,* U.S. Public Health Service
	Reports on health professional shortage areas by state, county, or metropolitan region, with demographic and health indicator profiles of underserved populations
	Health Care Financing Administration, U.S. Department of Health and Human Services
	Current regulations and enrollments in Medicare, Medicaid, and managed care for people without health insurance by state and county
Economic Life	
Employment	*U.S. Census, American FactFinder,* Bureau of the Census, U.S. Department of Commerce
	Data on employment, unemployment, disability status, occupation, type of health insurance provided, and other characteristics of the workforce
	Bureau of Labor Statistics, state department of employment for current unemployment data
	Local job postings on Internet, newspapers, and employers
Income	*U.S. Census,* Bureau of the Census, U.S. Department of Commerce
	Data on household, family, and per capita income; income by source; family income; income by age, race, ethnicity, and gender; poverty status
	Food Environment Atlas, U.S. Department of Agriculture
	Data on food insecurity within a community, mapping income, food access, and process
Business and industry	*U.S. Census, American FactFinder,* Bureau of the Census, U.S. Department of Commerce
	Data detailing characteristics of business and industry, including type of business, number and diversity of those employed, occupations, payroll, and presence of hazardous materials
	Agricultural extension service, chamber of commerce, planning board, community farming, and business groups
Occupational health standards	*Occupational Safety and Health Administration,* U.S. Department of Labor
	OSHA health and safety standards for specific industries
	Data on inspections of specific business and industry groups and chemical exposures are also available
	Safety Data Sheets on chemicals summarize health, safety, and toxicological information
Occupational injury and disease reporting	*Illness, Injuries, and Fatalities Program,* Bureau of Labor Statistics, U.S. Department of Labor
	Data on nonfatal illnesses and injuries of private sector employees; data on fatal injuries of the self-employed and private and government workers
	State department of worker compensation

(continued)

Summary of Community Assessment Data Sources *(continued)*

Community Subsystem	Data Source
Safety Services	
Fire protection	Local fire department
	National Fire Data Center, U.S. Fire Administration, Department of Homeland Security
	Local and state fire data for state profiles and national comparisons of fire occurrences, fire deaths and losses, and arson
Police protection	Local police department, police commissioner's or sheriff's office, state police
	Bureau of Justice Statistics, U.S. Department of Justice
	Personnel reports providing comparisons by state and local police department
Crime and violence	Local and centralized state agencies, police blotters, local newspapers
	Uniform Crime Reporting Program, Bureau of Justice Statistics and Federal Bureau of Investigation, U.S. Department of Justice
	Data available on violent and property crimes at local, state, and national level based on the data from state and local law enforcement agencies
	National Crime Victimization Survey, Bureau of Justice Statistics, U.S. Department of Justice
	Annual survey of households on nonfatal and household property crimes; data include whether reported to police, characteristics of victim and offender, and victim's experience with justice system
Transportation	
Pubic and motor vehicle transportation	*U.S. Census*, Bureau of the Census, U.S. Department of Commerce
	Data about mode for transportation to work, travel time and distance, carpooling
	Bureau of Transportation Statistics, U.S. Department of Transportation
	Data on large transit systems; household travel, including type, method of travel and time spent; use of safety belts and motorcycle helmets; driving under the influence
	Fatality Analysis Reporting System, National Highway Traffic and Safety Administration, U.S. Department of Transportation
	Reports on all fatal crashes within 50 states, the District of Columbia, Puerto Rico, and tribal lands using data from state police and state departments of transportation
	Local or regional transit authority route maps and schedules; telephone directory; radio and television traffic reports; windshield survey
	State department of transportation license and vehicle registration data
Politics and Government	Community, state, and congressional legislators and executive offices for local charter and ordinances, federal and state laws and regulations
	Organizational chart of community government
	Interviews with elected and appointed officials, reviews of annual reports, policy documents, bylaws, policies and procedures, budgets
	Interviews with key community leaders, board of elections voter registration data, review of local media, field notes of political events, community meetings, and forums

(continued)

Summary of Community Assessment Data Sources *(continued)*

Community Subsystem	Data Source
Communication	Review of audio, video, and print media
	U.S. Census, Bureau of the Census, U.S. Department of Commerce
	Data on type of phone access in housing units (landline, cell) and Internet access
	Local phone, cable, and Internet providers
	Participant observation of face-to-face communication
	Interviews with local librarian and school administrators about computer access and use
	Community home page and social media presence
Education	*U.S. Census*, Bureau of the Census, U.S. Department of Commerce
	Data available on years of school completed, school enrollment, and language spoken
	Local board of education, school district offices, and school and library administrators; teachers, parents, and students
	School district newsletters, annual reports, home pages
	State department of education
	National Center for Education Statistics, U.S. Department of Education
	Database listing all public elementary and secondary schools based on surveys of state education departments; includes enrollments, graduations, school lunch program participation, student–teacher ratios, racial/ethnic composition, and other measures; also produces annual survey on *Indicators of School Crime and Safety,* with data on a variety of topics including on victimization, teacher injury, bullying, student's use of substances
Recreation	Park district or community recreation department; community audio, video, and print media; local library; community residents; firsthand observations
Culture, values, and beliefs	*U.S. Census*, Bureau of the Census, U.S. Department of Commerce
	Data on race, ethnicity, ancestry, and language
	Community historical society or historical museum
	State or local human rights commission
	Key informants working in and serving the community: long-established bartenders, hairdressers, restaurant owners and servers, healthcare providers, store clerks
	Interviews with faith leaders, teachers, administrators, school board members, local politicians, and other community leaders

CDC, Centers for Disease Control and Prevention; EPA, Environmental Proection Agency; OSHA, Occupational Safety and Health Administration; STD, sexually transmitted disease; TB, tuberculosis.

REFERENCES

Adams, D. A., Thomas, K. R., Jajosky, R., Foster, L., Sharp, P., Onweh, D. H., ... Anderson, W. J. (2016). Summary of notifiable infectious diseases and conditions–United States, 2014. *Morbidity and Mortality Weekly Report, 63*(54), 1–152. doi:http://dx.doi.org/10.15585/mmwr.mm6354a1

American Library Association. (2017). Evaluating websites. Retrieved from http://www.ala.org

Baltimore Neighborhood Indicators Alliance. (n.d.). *Baltimore neighborhood indicators.* Retrieved from http://bniajfi.org/about_bnia/

Brownson, R. C., Baker, E. A., Leet, T. L., Gillespie, K. N., & True, W. R. (2011). *Evidence-based public health* (2nd ed.). New York, NY: Oxford University Press.

Bureau of Labor Statistics. (n.d.). Injuries, illnesses, and fatalities. Retrieved from https://www.bls.gov/iif/

Bureau of Labor Statistics. (2017). *Labor force statistics from the current population survey: Employment status of the civilian noninstitutional population, 1946 to date.* Retrieved from https://www.bls.gov/cps/cpsaat01.htm

Centers for Disease Control and Prevention. (2013). Methodology of the Youth Behavior Surveillance System. *Morbidity and Mortality Weekly Report, 62*(1), 1–25.

Centers for Disease Control and Prevention. (2016). *Health impact assessment.* Retrieved from https://www.cdc.gov/healthyplaces/hia.htm

Centers for Disease Control and Prevention. (2017). *National Notifiable Diseases Surveillance System.* Retrieved from https://www.cdc.gov/nndss/conditions/notifiable/2017/infectious-diseases/

City of Baltimore, Department of Planning. (n.d.). *City of Baltimore: 2000 to 2010 decennial census comparison.* Retrieved from http://planning.baltimorecity.gov/sites/default/files/Citywide%20Demographics%202000-2010.pdf

Drudi, D. (2015, December). The quest for meaningful and accurate occupational health and safety statistics. *Monthly Labor Review.* Retrieved from https://www.bls.gov/opub/mlr/2015/article/the-quest-for-meaningful-and-accurate-occupational-health-and-safety-statistics.htm

Fedeli, U., Zoppini, G., Goldoni, C. A., Avossa, F., Mastrangelo, G., & Saugo, M. (2015). Multiple causes of death analysis of chronic diseases: the example of diabetes. *Population Health Metrics, 13*, 21. http://doi.org/10.1186/s12963-015-0056-y

Liebler, C. A., Porter, S. R., Fernandez, L. E., Noon, J. M., & Ennis, S. R. (2017). America's churning races: Race and ethnicity response changes between census 2000 and the 2010 census. *Demography, 54*, 259–284.

Lloyd, J., Jahanpour, E., Angell, B., Ward, C., Hunter, A., Baysinger, C., & Turabelidze, G. (2017). Using national inpatient death rates as a benchmark to identify hospitals with inaccurate causes of death reporting-Missouri, 2009-2012. *and Mortality Weekly Report, 66*(1), 19–22.

Madsen, A., Thihalolipavan, S., Maduro, G., Zimmerman, R., Koppaka, R., Li, W., ... Begier, E. (2012). An intervention to improve cause-of-death reporting in New York City hospitals, 2009–2010. *Preventive Chronic Disease, 9*, E157. doi:10.5888/pcd9.120071

McKnight, J. (2010). Asset mapping in community. In A. Morgan, E. Ziglio & M. Davies (Eds.), *Health assets in a global context* (pp. 59–76). New York, NY: Springer Publishing.

Morgan, A., & Ziglio, E. (2007). Revitalizing the evidence base for public health: An assets model. *Promotion & Education, 14*(Suppl. 2), S17–S22. doi:10.1177/10253823070140020701x

National Center for Health Statistics. (2015). National vital statistics improvements. Retrieved from https://www.cdc.gov/nchs/data/factsheets/factsheet_nvss_improvements.pdf

National Notifiable Diseases Surveillance System. (2017). Retrieved from https://wwwn.cdc.gov/nndss/conditions/notifiable/2017/infectious-diseases/

National Research Council (US) Committee on National Statistics. (2009). *Vital statistics: Summary of a workshop. The U.S. vital statistics system: The role of state and local health departments.* Washington, DC: National Academies Press. Retrieved from https://www.ncbi.nlm.nih.gov/books/NBK219870/

Occupational Safety and Health Administration. (2012). *Hazard communication standard: Safety data sheets* (OSHA Publication No. DSG BR-34514). Washington, DC: Author. Retrieved from https://www.osha.gov/Publications/OSHA3514.html

Occupational Safety and Health Administration. (2017). *OSHA data & statistics: Commonly used statistics.* Retrieved from https://www.osha.gov/oshstats/commonstats.html

Office of Disease Prevention and Health Promotion. (2017). *Occupational health and safety.* Retrieved from https://www.healthypeople.gov/2020/topics-objectives/topic/occupational-safety-and-health

Office of Management and Budget. (1997). Revisions to the standards for the classification of federal data on race and ethnicity. *Federal Register, 62*(210), 58782. Retrieved from https://www.gpo.gov/fdsys/pkg/FR-1997-10-30/pdf/97-28653.pdf

Patton, M. Q. (2015). *Qualitative evaluation and research methods: Integrating theory and practice* (4th ed.). Newbury Park, CA: Sage.

Pew Research Center. (2017a). Mobile fact sheet. Retrieved from http://www.pewinternet.org/fact-sheet/mobile/

Pew Research Center. (2017b). Social media fact sheet. Retrieved from http://www.pewinternet.org/fact-sheet/social-media/

Pew Research Center. (2017c). Internet fact sheet. Retrieved from http://www.pewinternet.org/fact-sheet/internet-broadband/

Purnell, L. D. (2013). Transcultural diversity and healthcare. In L. D. Purnell (Ed.), *Transcultural health care: A culturally competent approach* (pp. 3–14). Philadelphia, PA: F. A. Davis.

Sharpe, P. A., Greaney, M. L., Lee, P. R., & Royce, S. W. (2000). Assets-oriented community assessment. *Public Health Reports, 115*, 205–211.

Smith, A. S., Holmberg, C., & Jones-Puthoff, M. (2012). *The emergency and transitional shelter population: 2010* (U.S. Department of Commerce Economics and Statistical Administration No. C2010SR-02). Retrieved from https://www.census.gov/prod/cen2010/reports/c2010sr-02.pdf

U.S. Census Bureau. (n.d.). *Geographic terms and concepts-census tract.* Retrieved from https://www.census.gov/geo/reference/gtc/gtc_ct.html

U.S. Department of Commerce Economics and Statistics Administration, United States Census Bureau. (2012). *The two or more races population: 2010 census briefs.* Retrieved from https://www.census.gov/prod/cen2010/briefs/c2010br-13.pdf

U.S. Department of Commerce Economics and Statistics Administration, United States Census Bureau. (2013). *U.S census bureau statistical quality standards.* Retrieved from https://www.census.gov/content/dam/Census/about/about-the-bureau/policies_and_notices/quality/statistical-quality-standards/Quality_Standards.pdf

U.S. Department of Housing and Urban Development. (n.d.). *Healthy homes and lead hazard control.* Retrieved from https://www.hud.gov

Wen, L. S., & Goodwin, K. E. (2016). Violence is a public health issue. *Journal of Public Health Management & Practice, 22*, 503–505.

World Health Organization. (2016). *International classification of diseases (ICD-10); international statistical classification of diseases and related health problems (ICD-10;* tenth revision, 4th ed.). Geneva, Switzerland: Author. Retrieved from http://www.who.int/classifications/icd/en

CHAPTER 6

Using Methods of Data Collection

Diane B. McNaughton and Julia Muennich Cowell

◼ STUDY EXERCISES

1. What are the possible methods of data collection for community assessment in advanced public/community health nursing practice?
2. Which factors should be considered before embarking on a data-collection project?
3. Which factors determine the data-collection methods to be used?
4. What steps can be taken to ensure the quality of the data collected?
5. What are the indicators that data collection is complete?

Data collection is an integral part of every activity of public/community health nurses. The data collection procedures go beyond the assessment of individuals to the assessment of communities. There are numerous approaches to data collection for community assessment that provide elegant explanations of community health status. These approaches include participant observation, windshield/walking survey, focus groups, key informant interviews, the Delphi process, use of archival material, and use of the literature.

Data-collection activities are supported by processes that ensure *maximum* control for quality data. The preliminary process involves careful planning. Planning includes a review of the purpose for data collection. There is a wide range of purposes that can direct data collection for community assessment (McKenzie, Neiger, & Thackeray, 2016). For example, data may be needed for preintervention purposes, to develop health-risk profiles, to evaluate health-promotion needs, or for specialized studies focused on special grant opportunities. Data may also be needed to determine community leadership or community readiness for a program. In the implementation phase, data are needed to track and monitor key process and outcome variables.

By clarifying the purpose of data collection, several subsequent factors become clear, including the method, qualitative or quantitative approaches, sampling techniques, and data management and analysis procedures. The data-collection method is determined by the purpose of the assessment, the model or framework guiding the assessment, and the design of the assessment (McNaughton, Cowell, & Fogg, 2014).

Planning includes determination of the personnel necessary for data collection and the necessary training to ensure competency. In all cases, training in collection methods is essential, irrespective of whether data are collected by professional staff, paraprofessionals, or technicians.

This chapter reviews a variety of data-collection methods. The process involved with each of the data-collection methods is described in detail. The quality of a community assessment is partially determined by the validity and reliability of the data-collection process. Two examples of validity and reliability questions: Do the tools used in data collection measure what is intended? Are those measures utilized without errors?

■ PARTICIPANT OBSERVATION

Participant observation is a data-collection method to assist nurses in learning more about a community, social setting, or a group of people. Just as careful observation is an important component of assessing an individual's health status, observation is also essential in gathering information about a community.

A unique aspect of observation is that the observer purposefully sets out to understand social settings and conditions without manipulating them in any way. The intent of the observer is to gather information through the senses about events that occur naturally (Patton, 2014). Data do not have to be limited to what is observed visually. In fact, experiencing the setting using the senses of hearing, touch, smell, and taste can introduce one to a community and help one experience its life more realistically. An important aspect of observation is to learn from the surroundings and to refrain from influencing them by asking questions or probing.

Purposes of Observational Strategies

Observational strategies can be used for many purposes ranging from community assessment to formal research projects. Observation can assist nurses and others in gaining more in-depth information about a community or group of people and is particularly useful in settings the nurse is not familiar with. Observation can be used to answer questions such as: What is the character of the community? What is its economic base? What do its people do for leisure? What type of foods do people enjoy eating? Do people enjoy gathering together? Is there evidence of community pride or spirit? Do people comfortably walk the streets or do they tend to isolate themselves in their homes? What health hazards are present? Observation should be used to identify both strengths and problem areas in neighborhoods. Although discovering problems in a community can provide a course of action for the nurse, community strengths can be used to address problems.

Observation methods can complement quantitative methods. For example, a community report may indicate that there are 15 places of worship within the community's boundaries. Observation of location, size, religion/denomination, age of building, and signage can expand your understanding of the diversity of beliefs and resources within a community.

Preparation for Use of Participant Observation

Many decisions need to be made before embarking on an observational project. If a team is conducting the participant observations, team management planning must include the determination of length of time, the locations where observations will take place, and the exact focus of the observations. When several people are involved, written guidelines are established regarding what to observe (e.g., environmental conditions, interpersonal interaction). The team members should together review the results of their observations. Using a team approach can add to the validity of the findings.

Just as in research, observation should be directed by a question or theoretical framework. A research question or guiding framework specifies the focus and location of the observation. Planning includes determining whether the project will entail observational methods alone or will include other methods. Observational strategies can strengthen and enlighten the findings of other methods, such as surveys. Planning should also determine whether the aims of the project are best fulfilled by using unobtrusive or participant observational strategies.

Purposive sampling techniques are used for data collection. Purposive sampling involves careful selection of the setting or persons to be observed before data collection (Waltz, Strickland, & Lenz, 2017). For example, if an understanding is sought about nurse–client interactions in a public/community health nursing clinic, observations may be limited to nurses who have at least 1 year of experience in the department, or decisions may be made to observe interactions with special populations such as teenaged clients or clients attending a sexually transmitted infections (STIs) clinic.

After many of these decisions are made, the site or sites are selected and strategies are identified to gain entry. *Gaining entry* refers to the process of acquiring permission to observe in a setting and being accepted into the setting by those being observed. In some public settings, it is not necessary to gain permission from others to observe public activities. However, in some situations (such as schools), institutional permission is needed along with the permission of the persons being observed.

Data-Recording Techniques

An important component of observational methods is systematic recording of the data. Methods for recording data are observation checklists, field notes, a journal, and/or audio or visual recordings. The decision as to which method to use should be made after careful thought. Cost and funding constraints often limit the use of audio or visual recordings. However, such recordings can provide a permanent, objective record of the current project and can be analyzed again in the future as an existing data set. The potential influence of cameras and tape recorders on the behavior of the persons being observed should also be considered. Some people who would otherwise permit observation of themselves will refuse when a camera is involved or may alter their behavior in some way. All these issues need to be considered when deciding how data should be recorded.

An essential part of any observational data-collection activity is the recording of field notes and maintenance of an analytic journal. Field notes are used to record observations, whereas the analytic journal provides a place to write analytic thoughts (Waltz et al., 2017). Field notes should be written as soon as possible after the observation while the memory of the setting is still fresh. It should be decided beforehand what will be important to include in the field notes. Important information to include: date and time of observation, place, who was present, what activities occurred, what interactions transpired between participants, what participants said, and what the setting looked like. Observational experiences can often be interesting and exciting but may be sensory intensive and may have to be limited to only short periods (1–2 hours at a time).

Data Analysis

Data analysis begins with the first observational experience and the initial analytic thoughts of the public/community health nurse (as recorded in the field notes and journal). Handwritten field notes should be transferred to typewritten form soon after the observation. Although this is a time-consuming procedure for the observer, there are benefits to transcribing one's own field notes. Transcribing one's own notes provides an opportunity to carefully read them and become "immersed" in the data. This immersion enhances familiarity and understanding of the data. Data can be managed and analyzed using the assistance of a computer software program such as Dedoose (2015).

Issues With Participant Observation

In the participant observation method of data collection, the assessor participates in the social group being observed. In unobtrusive approaches, the researcher will primarily observe and refrain from frequent interaction with others. Data collected from participant observation are subject to bias of the participant observer; however, community members may be more trusting if the observer is a participant. Data collected from unobtrusive measures may be threatened by reactivity of community participants.

■ WINDSHIELD/WALKING SURVEY

The windshield/walking survey is a data-collection method that takes place as one drives and/or walks throughout a neighborhood (Stanhope & Lancaster, 2016). Observations are made using sight, hearing, taste, smell, and touch. The broad community overview afforded by a windshield/walking survey is a good first step in conducting a community assessment to learn about the community as a whole. If the community is large, the data may be collected over several sessions both driving and walking. If data collection for the survey is done by a team, the work can be distributed among the members, assigning them certain parts of the geographical area.

Purposes of a Windshield/Walking Survey

The basic purpose of the windshield/walking survey is to gather data and information about a community's strengths and weaknesses through use of the senses. This type of survey can also be conducted from the point of view of individuals, groups, or special populations to identify specific problems or situations. The windshield/walking survey provides a wide array of subjective data collected through personal observation of the community.

Observations may be used as indicators of the need for more data. For example, if an area of possible toxic contamination is observed, you will need to explore other sources of data to determine whether the site has already been identified and what action is being taken to eliminate the environmental hazard. Other indicators of the need for additional data include housing conditions, odors, evidence of air or water pollution, potential safety hazards, evidence of community deterioration, and inadequate community services such as grocery stores.

Preparation for Use of a Windshield/Walking Survey

Once the community being surveyed is defined geographically, the total community, such as a county or a city, may be used for the survey, or a subsection of several census tracts or a mile radius may be selected. The size of the area as well as the location (urban or rural) will dictate whether the survey is conducted by means of a drive, a walk, or a combination of the two.

In the use of any subjective data-collection method, past personal experience can bias interpretation of observations, so a planned guided tour of the identified area minimizes the threat. Survey questions are formulated to guide observations, and a data-collection strategy is identified to minimize the threat or bias and guide the assessment.

Two processes characterize a health assessment of individuals: a physical examination (PE) and a health history. The same processes are employed in community assessment, and the windshield/walking survey parallels the PE. The PE is dependent on the senses, as is the windshield/walking survey. The PE and the health history typically follow the systems of the body. The windshield/walking survey may follow the community's systems: its economy, environmental, transportation, social organizations, services, communication, recreation, and the people who are part of the community. A community assessment framework is helpful in guiding a comprehensive data-collection plan, as indicated in Table 6.1.

Data-Recording Techniques

A variety of methods are available to collect community observation data: audio recordings, photography, and field notes. Audio recording spontaneous reactions to the guided questions is one way to record reactions; field notes are another. A second rater using the same questions provides for a comparison of reactions and limits the possibility of bias in the interpretation. Careful analysis of the data is crucial and dependent on the quality of the notes or recordings.

A map of the area being surveyed is a useful tool for recording observations when driving and walking around a community. Locations of various items, such as activities, buildings, services, and potential hazards, can be recorded for future reference and to make one familiar with the total community.

Table 6.1 provides a useful template for the construction of a tool to be used for data collection. Each category may be listed on a page to provide space for detailed notes about each area of the framework.

OBSERVATIONS FROM SIGHT

Nurses observe the environment of the community by identifying the general repair of the streets and sidewalks. The condition of traffic signs and stop lights is noted. The age and quality of the housing and architecture, as well as the condition of other structures, are observed. Identification of the location of industrial sites (manufacturing or rural) warrants a safety evaluation related to emissions as well as the presence of traffic. The amount of traffic, as well as the age and condition of cars, is noted.

Social organizations and services are noted in terms of proximity to residences. The distance between services and primary sources of transportation are identified, such as public transportation or automobiles. Services of interest include governmental, healthcare, commercial, educational, and religious. The location of the services as well as visual cues, such as advertisements and accessibility, are noted. Commercial services, including grocery stores, hardware stores, and clothing and discount stores, are noted. Churches and schools as well as recreation resources are identified.

Media sources in the community include advertisements, websites, neighborhood publications, local television stations, radio, as well as broader market media like newspapers and television. Local media are valuable sources of information about cultural and civic events and can illuminate community problems, concerns, priorities, and values. In addition, research on media and violence has highlighted the importance of media influence on behavior (Huesmann, 2007). Many media sources are visible on a tour of a community, such as billboards and store signs.

The people of the community are observed to broadly determine age, gender, and racial distributions. The activities in which people are engaged as well as the location of activities

TABLE 6.1 Windshield/Walking Survey Data-Collection Plan

Sensory Domain	Economy	Environment	Transportation	Social Organizations	Services	Communication	Recreation	People
Sight								
Hearing								
Taste								
Smell								
Touch								

are noted. Clothing choices—style, quality, and condition—of adults and children suggest about their occupation and income level. General health status is implied by several characteristics of people observed in the community, such as obesity, mobility, and facial expressions. Friendliness of individuals may reflect perceived safety as well as social customs of the community.

Community members can participate in data collection through strategies such as Photovoice or "walk-alongs." Photovoice is a methodology in which community members use disposable cameras to take photographs of a specified topic in their community. Walk-alongs is another method for collecting community members' views on a specific topic. A walk-along is a strategy involving neighborhood walks and focused interviews/discussions with community members about a topic of interest. For example, a researcher in central England engaged leaders of walking groups in a project in which they were asked to discuss the environment where the walk occurred and how it affected the behaviors of the walking group (Kassavou, French, & Chamberlain, 2015). Environmental influences included safety and presence of sidewalks with signals at crosswalks. Groups that walked in parks were more likely to be social in nature and often included a stop for tea on the way home. Walks on race tracks focused more on reaching a walking goal without much group interaction. Discussion/interviews were audio recorded and transcribed for data analysis.

OBSERVATIONS FROM HEARING

Noise levels are important to community health. Stressful sources of noise may arise from transportation (automobile traffic, trains, or buses), industry, personal listening devices, and sports or entertainment venues. The U.S. Centers for Disease Control and Prevention (CDC, 2017a) and the National Institute of Occupational Safety and Health (www.cdc.gov/niosh/index.htm) provide an objective guide to evaluate the noise of a community (CDC, 2017a). Table 6.2 illustrates sources of noise that are commonly encountered as well as the decibel-level criteria for rating risk. Information about sources of noise and possible harmful effects can direct public/community health nurses and occupational health nurses in identifying community and work settings that may pose a health risk. Hearing loss and stress effects of noise are dependent on decibel levels, distance from the source, and time of exposure (CDC, 2017a).

OBSERVATIONS FROM TASTE

The sense of taste reveals not only preference related to experience and custom but also qualities of freshness. The advanced public/community health nurse conducts a visit to grocery stores as well as eating establishments. Observations would include evaluation of types of grocery stores (chain grocers or independent grocers), typical food choices, and freshness as well as food-preparation practices. One should explore the type of eating establishments as well as prices of staples such as eggs, milk, vegetables, and meats. A taste of local drinking water discloses possible additives or pollutants.

OBSERVATIONS FROM SMELL

Initial environmental assessments are often made by the sense of smell. Odors can indicate the quality of sanitation and garbage service. Although industrial plants can emit unpleasant odors, not all odors are harmful. However, the presence of noxious odors can make outdoor activity unpleasant and can contribute to the stress of community members.

TABLE 6.2 Everyday Sounds and Noises, Average Sound Level, and Typical Health Effects

Source	Decibel Level	Health Effects
Softest sound that can be heard	0	Sounds in this range do not typically have health effects
Normal breathing	10	
Soft whisper	30	
Normal conversation	60	
Washing machine, dishwasher	70	Sounds at this level may be annoying
Traffic noise (within car)	80–85	Sounds at this level may be very annoying
Gas-powered lawn mowers/leaf blowers	90	Hearing loss can occur after 2 hours
Motorcycles	95	Damage can occur after 50–60 minutes
Sporting event (such as football, hockey playoffs)	110	Possible hearing loss after 15 minutes
Electronic devices (TV, radio, personal listening device) at highest volume, loud entertainment venues (rock concert, nightclub, bars)	105–110	Hearing loss after 5 minutes of exposure
Firecrackers	140–150	Pain and ear injury

Source: Adapted from Centers for Disease Control and Prevention. (2017). *Loud noise can cause hearing loss.* Retrieved from www.cdc.gov/nceh/hearing_loss/what_noises_cause_hearing_loss.html

OBSERVATIONS FROM TOUCH

Although touch is integral to physical examination of individuals, touch in community assessment can relate to psychological feelings as well as physical feelings. For example, friendliness and a sense of safety promote a feeling of security and permeate neighborhoods. Great open spaces in rural areas can promote a sense of peacefulness or isolation. The feeling of safety can be enhanced or challenged by the presence of security devices, such as razor wire or burglar bars on residences, depending on the experience of the residents.

The sense of touch can be noted in climatic temperature. Extreme temperatures can produce sensory changes that are heightened or diminished. Extreme temperatures can also affect psychological feelings. Nurses working in dangerous urban communities often schedule home visiting at early morning during hot summer months to take advantage of cooler temperatures and when there is an increased perception of safety. In congested areas, smog and ozone problems produce physical stresses (eye irritation and respiratory problems) as well as psychological distress. Public/community health nurses are also concerned with weather conditions because extreme temperatures indicate the need for clothing alterations and heating and cooling needs.

Data Analysis

Data collection in the windshield/walking survey is systematic and sometimes iterative to address the issue of bias in data collection. Organization of windshield/walking survey data provides a controlled analysis and illuminates the need to extend data collection. Thus, the focus of data analysis after the windshield/walking survey is to determine what additional data are needed and where they may be located. Chapters 7 and 8 guide you toward these areas of community assessment.

Issues With the Windshield/Walking Survey

The data collected through this type of survey are subjective, so pieces of data should not be used as facts in a community assessment, unless confirmation is obtained. In addition, the windshield/walking survey data are used in combination with other types and sources of data to determine community diagnoses. Just as in nursing diagnoses of individuals and groups, one piece of data is inadequate to formulate conclusions.

■ FOCUS GROUPS

A focus group is a small group of people gathered to respond to a set of questions. Group participants are selected because they have certain characteristics or experiences in common. In a focus-group session, a moderator asks open-ended questions to the group, and the group members are encouraged to discuss their opinions among themselves. In fact, one of the unique qualities of focus groups is their interactive nature, designed to uncover opinions until no new opinions are uncovered (Tausch & Menold, 2016).

Purposes of Focus Groups

Focus-group methodology was developed on the assumption that people do not form opinions in isolation. Rather, the viewpoints of others influence opinions. Focus groups can capture some of the group influence on decision making and opinions, making them a unique data-collection strategy. Focus groups provide valuable information that other data-collection methods cannot fully capture because of their uniqueness and the fact that focus groups encourage respondents to provide their own answers to questions (rather than selecting from a group of multiple-choice responses). For advanced public/community health nurses, focus groups are a valuable data-collection method that can be used for community assessment. Focus groups can be conducted to provide a better understanding of the health beliefs and healthcare preferences of community members.

For example, Rose and Friedman (2017) used focus groups to identify the perceptions of sexual and gender minority (SGM) males about health services provided for them during adolescence. Researchers identified clear inclusion criteria for sampling, including identifications as SGM males, African American, aged between 18 and 21 and residing in the southeastern United States. The focus-group moderators used a discussion guide based on the theoretical underpinnings of social cognitive theory as well as constructs from communication theory. To obtain clear information about perceptions concerning health services, discussion questions were framed in three domains: current health information sources, perceptions of health information sources, and health information recommendation.

A moderator and a comoderator may lead the focus group. These persons should be experienced in conducting focus groups and guide the discussion by asking open-ended questions. Sometimes the moderator probes or encourages silent participants to share their thoughts. The comoderator can also ask questions and manage time. Time management is essential because participants are usually told that the focus group will last a specific length of time. The goal of the discussion is to hear opinions and not to reach consensus. It is expected that members will have differing viewpoints.

Preparation for Use of Focus Groups

Planning focus groups involves several steps. (For a complete discussion of planning focus groups, including budget considerations, see Morgan & Krueger, 1997.) First, the purpose of the focus group is clarified. Then, the interview questions guiding data collection, as well as the prompts to encourage responses, are outlined. The characteristics of people to be included in the group are outlined, and the location for the group is chosen. The location of the group is carefully selected to avoid inhibiting or unduly influencing the respondents; for example, avoid an organization with which you do not want to be associated, like the police department. Select a location that is comfortable, private, and convenient.

Experienced moderators are important, and the moderator should be unknown to the group. Supervisors or employers may wish to conduct a focus group to select the moderator. Having persons in authority, however, usually leads to bias because subordinates are inhibited and probably not honest in their responses. Material resources needed for the focus group are obtained such as a tape recorder, an adequate number of chairs and tables, and a comfortable environment that encourages discussion. Providing a light snack helps participants relax and demonstrates a sense of hospitality.

Focus groups usually take place in a series, that is, data from several groups (based on the same interview format) should be taken together. Each group should consist of different members. It is possible that the character of each group will differ due to the varying personalities of the participants and their eagerness to talk. A series of groups will enable the identification of common elements among groups. Usually, three or four groups are sufficient to identify common themes. Although a series of focus groups is typically planned, new groups should be conducted until the responses of the participants are anticipated or when new information ceases to come up in the group (Morgan & Krueger, 1997).

Sampling begins by determining the target population and the characteristics of the identified group. A homogeneous group is selected. The members should be roughly the same in terms of age, cultural group, gender, and socioeconomic status. Similarity in characteristics minimizes competition or dominant behavior in the group and maximizes participation. Ideally, a focus group consists of six to 10 people (Morgan & Krueger, 1997). The group should be small enough for all members to have an opportunity to share their insights and large enough to provide some diversity of opinions. It is also best to select people who do not know each other well. Individuals are more likely to express their opinions or experiences when they are with strangers.

Data-Recording Techniques

The comoderator should take notes during the focus-group session, with the moderator listing the group's ideas on newsprint so that everyone can see the major points of the contributions. These techniques also provide a way to validate what was heard.

Audiotaping can provide an accurate account of the discourse that occurs during the focus group. Tapes can be transcribed to provide a hard set of data to be reviewed easily by several persons. Permission, usually in writing, is always obtained from participants if taping (video or audio) is used.

Data Analysis

Rose and Friedman (2017) used a computer software program (QSR NVivo, 2010) to aid data analysis. Transcripts from the tape-recorded discussions were uploaded for thematic analysis using a codebook that was based on the discussion guide. To ensure trustworthiness of the analytic process, the researchers reviewed the codes and definitions separately. Differences were then resolved through discussion about the coding with subsequent revision of the codebook. Thematic analysis provides for the emersion of patterns and themes from the data.

It is important to analyze the data thematically rather than quantitatively, irrespective of whether a computer program is used. Themes discussed by the participants should be located and explored in contrast to identifying a word and counting how many times it was used in the discussion. Thematic analysis can be approached using a coding frame (Schreier, 2014). The coding frame consists of topics to be explored in the data. For example, Rose and Friedman (2017) began looking at the data to identify the current sources of health information that the participants used. They then looked for data that explained why the sources were used among the responses to questions like: "Why did you select these sources?" "How do you feel about messages concerning sexual orientation?" The responses identified a range of recommendations to guide school health services, such as marketing the availability of services and making sure that school nurses were knowledgeable about the sexual health issues of African American SGM adolescent males.

Issues With Focus Groups

Careful planning minimizes many problems that could arise with the focus-group method of data collection. The choice of an experienced moderator will minimize reactivity problems in the focus group, and careful sample selection will maximize discussion. Location and scheduling should also be considered to maximize convenience. Care must be given to assess themes embedded in the data rather than a simple counting of responses. If no new information is emerging, the focus groups can be discontinued to avoid added expense in assessment.

■ KEY INFORMANTS

Key informants are individuals who are knowledgeable about the community and willing to share information, views, and understanding of need (Fink, 2013). Key informants are often used in community assessments because they are in positions to know the community through their expertise or experience. For example, professionals in health services are aware of major health concerns and are often able to estimate the availability of services. Police officers are aware of violence and crime patterns in communities. Teachers and school administrators provide insight into child and family health conditions and necessary resources. People working in commercial establishments like restaurants, retail settings, and entertainment settings provide insight that can span an estimation of family/community wealth, health, and lifestyle habits, as well as leisure time habits.

Purposes for Use of Key Informants

The purpose of using key informants in a community assessment is to obtain information that is not available by other methods of data collection. Subjective information about community life is the major focus of interviews with key informants. Statistical and objective data available through other methods and sources should not be the focus of contacts with key informants.

Information obtained from key informants through interviews or surveys may provide information about potential areas for further exploration or confirmation of data identified through other sources. If key informants from various facets of community life are interviewed, a broad spectrum of views and opinions can be obtained.

Preparation for Use of Key Informants

Interviews with key informants are guided by structured or unstructured questions. Again, the purpose for the assessment guides the approach. For example, if key informants are interviewed to identify willingness to participate in a new intervention, the questions would be focused on perceptions of the intervention. If the key informants were to identify broad community health needs, the interview questions would be more general. The place of the interview is determined to maximize the quality of responses. The objective is to enhance the comfort and convenience of informants, so choosing a desirable location is important.

Data-Recording Techniques

As with other types of interviews, interviews of key informants may be recorded as notes or audiotaped with permission. If a structured format for questions is used, the same basic questions may be asked of each key informant and recorded in writing during the interview. If tape-recorded, the interview may be transcribed for use with in-depth analysis later. Written surveys are also used with key informants to obtain information about a specified group of questions.

Data Analysis

Responses from key informants may be analyzed with techniques similar to those used with focus groups. The use of a computer software program will provide the structure for identifying themes in the interviews. Written responses from surveys may also be analyzed using techniques described in the section on focus groups. The major objective of data analysis of key informants' interviews is to retain the individual nature of their responses so that they may be used as additional areas to explore or to validate information obtained in the community assessment.

Issues With Key Informants

Although key informants are valuable sources of information about a community, their opinions or viewpoints represent only a portion of subjective data in a community assessment. Opinions from members of the target population will broaden the assessor's understanding of community needs, resources, and priorities. Together, subjective data from key informants and community members can shed light on or improve understanding of quantitative data.

■ DELPHI TECHNIQUE

The Delphi technique is a method for obtaining a consensus opinion from a group of people. The method originated in the 1950s at the RAND Corporation in California as a way of using the opinions of experts to forecast technological developments (Dalkey & Helmer, 1962). The three basic characteristics of the Delphi method are (a) anonymity, (b) iteration with controlled feedback, and (c) statistical group response (McMillan, King, & Tully, 2016). *Anonymity* means that the identity of respondents is kept confidential and is neither linked to individual responses nor shared with other members of the group. Therefore, each group member's opinion has equal weight, and those who are well known cannot exert undue influence or control over the responses of others.

Iteration with controlled feedback means that the data-collection process takes place in rounds (usually two to four rounds). Data collected from the first round are given to each group member with her or his response and the mean response of the group. In addition, items are prioritized in accordance with the group mean (McMillan et al., 2016). The advantage of iteration is that in successive rounds the participants can change their opinions based on the responses of the group or their own reconsideration of the matter. Iterations continue until a reasonable group consensus is obtained. *Statistical group response* refers to the reporting of a group score and a ranking for each item. Data collected through a Delphi study are reported as a group response.

Purposes of the Delphi Technique

The Delphi technique can be used for multiple purposes such as development of research priorities (Lindberg et al., 2017), development of nurse-sensitive quality indicators (Chen et al., 2017), and defining workforce competencies (Weise, Fisher, & Trollor, 2016), among others. Although the Delphi method was originally designed to solicit the opinions of experts, the process has been found to work well with lay people, given that they share a common experience to form an opinion (McMillan et al., 2016; Pike et al., 2015). Therefore, it is possible to use the Delphi technique as a data-collection method in community assessment. For example, experts in the community may be asked about concerns or to confirm responses from community residents. The purpose is to form consensus on community priorities, problems, or strengths.

Preparation for Use of the Delphi Method

The Delphi method consists of a series of steps that are repeated until consensus is achieved among the respondents. Criteria for consensus are decided during the planning phase. For example, investigators may aim for a minimum of 70% group agreement. Others have reported consensus goals ranging from 51% to 80% (Chen et al., 2017; Hasson, Keeney, & McKenna, 2000). The Delphi process begins with designing the initial questionnaire. The first questionnaire usually contains a broad question or a set of questions. The questionnaire is then pilot tested, revised, and distributed. Respondents complete the questionnaire and mail it back. The researcher collects and analyzes the responses.

The sample for a Delphi study can include as few as 10 respondents or as many as several hundred (Fink, Kosecoff, Chassin, & Brook, 1984; Malcolm, Knighting, Forbat, & Kearney, 2009). The sample should represent a larger population of individuals who possess relevant information about the issue under consideration. If the population is relatively homogeneous, a smaller sample can be used. If the population is diverse, it is best to recruit a larger number of participants (Fink et al., 1984; Malcolm et al., 2009).

Data-Recording Techniques

After the first-round analysis of responses, the researcher uses the results to develop a questionnaire with the participants' answers. By the second round, the items on the questionnaire should take a fixed-response (e.g., Likert scale) format. The questionnaire is piloted again, finalized, and distributed. With the new questionnaire, each respondent will receive a report of her or his responses to the items on the previous round in addition to the group mean and variance for each item. Individuals who disagree with the group scores or wish to challenge the group response may do so. The cycle of distributing questionnaires, obtaining responses, and providing feedback is continued until the desired level of consensus is reached.

Data Analysis

Data are analyzed using measures of central tendency (mean or median, variance) and a rank ordering of items. Data can also be analyzed conceptually using qualitative techniques such as content and thematic analysis. Findings from quantitative and qualitative analyses can be compared to determine agreement between methods.

Issues With the Delphi Method

One of the advantages of the Delphi method is that experts in various geographic locations can interact with one another to form a group opinion without actually meeting each other. The iterations with group feedback serve as the interactive component of the group process. This method avoids the potential power struggles that could erupt in a face-to-face encounter. Of course, there are disadvantages to anonymity. In this method, individuals are free to take a point of view without being accountable to it because of its anonymous nature.

Several concerns must be considered when planning a Delphi study. As with other data-collection methods in community assessment, the purpose of the assessment, the target population of respondents, the financial outlay and resources, and the time frame are important considerations. It is realistic to plan for a Delphi study that requires several months for completion, particularly if questionnaires are mailed to participants. However, use of electronic or e-Delphi methods can expedite the process and make it less cumbersome than mailed questionnaires (McMillan et al., 2016). Costs include staff time to develop the questionnaires, mailing costs, and consultant services, including statistician fees. Response rates are important in the use of the Delphi technique. Participants are usually busy, so clear instructions as well as simplified questions can maximize ease of response.

■ SURVEYS

Surveys are methods of collecting information from people through either questionnaires or face-to-face interviews. For public/community health nurses, a survey can be a valuable way to collect demographic information about a community as well as the opinions, knowledge, or experiences of community members. At the outset, using and constructing surveys may seem to be a simple task; however, many issues need to be considered when planning to collect data using surveys (Fowler & Cosenza, 2009). Before discussing these issues, the purposes and benefits of surveys in public/community health nursing practice are presented.

Purposes of Surveys

There are numerous uses of surveys in advanced public/community health nursing practice. Surveys can be used to collect data for program planning, augment community assessment data, and contribute to program evaluation. Although demographic, morbidity, and mortality data are available via government and community resources, these data may be old or incomplete. Surveys can be used to update or complete the information needed to better assess the health of a community and direct program planning.

Many valid and reliable standardized surveys are in the public domain and available via the Internet without any cost. Examples are the Youth Risk Behavior Surveillance System (YRBSS) and the National Health and Nutrition Examination Survey (NHANES); an advantage of using a subscale from one of these surveys is the availability of national population based data for comparison. Additional surveys, such as the CESD or PROMIS surveys, are also free of charge.

Surveys can be constructed and tailored to meet local needs of an agency. However, constructing a survey requires several steps to ensure success. The purpose of the survey and the minimal amount of data needed should be considered. Surveys should be simple, short, and written at a low literacy level. Intrusive questions are often unnecessary and should be avoided. Double negatives should be avoided as they are often confusing to respondents (Valente, 2002). Respondents need to know the purpose of the survey, what will be done with the data, and steps to be taken to ensure confidentiality. Once the survey is complete, it needs to be reviewed for clarity and content by a colleague and a community representative.

Paper-and-pencil questionnaires are a type of survey that can be used to assess opinions of others or to measure client attributes such as beliefs or satisfaction with a service (Donsbach & Traugott, 2008). The format of the questionnaire can include open-ended questions, such as: "What are your most pressing concerns about being a resident of this community?" Fixed response items, such as true/false, multiple-choice, or Likert scale questions, can be a part of a survey. Just like face-to-face surveys, paper-and-pencil questionnaires can be useful in collecting a wide variety of information from and about members of a community. Data from the surveys may be useful in determining the problems and strengths of a community as perceived by its members.

Preparation for Use of a Survey

Planning for conducting a survey should include determining information to be obtained and resources available in terms of personnel time and money, and development or selection of an instrument. Planning should also include determination of the method for administration of the survey and training people participating in administration.

Before deciding which survey approach to use, it is best to determine the purpose of doing the survey, the target population, the type of data that would be most helpful to obtain, and the available resources. Paper-and-pencil surveys or Internet-based surveys can be low cost and easily administered. Mailed questionnaires can be more expensive and have a major disadvantage of typically low response rates. A response rate of 70% is often considered adequate to generalize a population (Smith, 2016). However, a response rate less than 70% should not be discounted. When only a portion of a sample returns a survey, an explanation for the low response rate must be sought. People who return the survey may have an unusually strong opinion and, therefore, want to make sure that their opinions are known. It is possible that they may not truly represent the opinions of the population as a whole. Subsampling of nonrespondents may provide information that would clarify a systematic bias, such as responses of a particular demographic group not being represented.

There are strategies to enhance the return rate of mailed questionnaires (Stähli & Joye, 2016). These include offering some incentive to complete the survey such as a small gift or a dollar bill in the envelope. Reminders to complete the survey may be mailed a few weeks after the surveys have been distributed. Even a postcard announcing that a survey is coming and asking people to look for it and consider completing it may help. Surveys can also be completed by telephone. Telephone surveys can take the place of a face-to-face interview. Successful telephone surveys must be short and avoid sensitive topics. Still, many people perceive telephone surveys as annoying and may decline participation.

Ideally, when collecting survey data, the advanced public/community health nurse would like to know that responses are representative of a target group or population. In rare instances, the entire population can be accessed. In most cases, however, only a small portion of the population is sampled. The goal is to obtain a sample that is representative of the total population. This is best done through random sampling. Different methods for achieving randomization are possible. A sample of the population with a high response rate is highly desirable in surveys, so purposive, randomized sampling with strategies designed to enhance the response rate is beneficial (Hampton & Vilela, 2017).

Surveys can also be used as a mechanism for designing or tailoring interventions to specific population groups. In this case, purposive sampling would be used. Purposive sampling is a procedure in which a target group is identified by its unique characteristics and only persons from the target group would be invited to participate in a survey (Waltz et al., 2017). Public/community health nurses can use surveys to determine why people do not access services available to them (such as the Women, Infants, and Children nutrition program). Surveys can include multiple-choice items along with open-ended questions where respondents can make recommendations to improve services to better meet their needs in terms of time and location that would be most acceptable to them.

Data-Recording Technique

The technique for collecting data is the survey form or instrument. In using a printed survey or a questionnaire to be read on the telephone or face to face, the data collector needs to use a survey that is appropriate. An important aspect to selecting an instrument is to consider its reliability and validity. Reliability and validity of survey instruments are basic to the quality of the data obtained. *Reliability* refers to the degree of consistency with which an instrument measures the attribute it is intended to measure. A reliable instrument will produce similar results when administered to the same sample on different occasions. *Validity* refers to the degree to which an instrument measures what it is supposed to measure (Waltz et al., 2017). It is beyond the scope of this text to discuss the complex issues of reliability and validity of survey instruments. It is important, however, to realize that these are critical issues to consider when developing or selecting a survey. Use of established survey instruments enhances the quality of surveys because problems with questions or administration may well have been addressed. Additional information about instruments is included in Chapters 17 and 18.

Data Analysis

Analysis depends on the format of the survey questionnaire. Answers to open-ended questions should be thematically analyzed, that is, the answers should be analyzed to identify common responses or themes present in the data. This can be done with the aid of a computer software program designed to analyze qualitative data (e.g., NUDIST). Several authors have described the processes involved in qualitative data analysis (Creswell & Poth, 2017; Patton, 2014).

Results of fixed-response questionnaires can be statistically analyzed for measures of central tendency (e.g., mean, standard deviation). If demographic information is obtained, this can be correlated with the results of the survey. Many computer software programs are available to analyze survey data; or it may be helpful to recruit an expert statistician.

Issues With Surveys

There are several key issues in survey data collection. These include the reliability and validity of the questions (interview, electronic, or paper and pencil) and sampling. Although careful randomization and high response rates provide for generalization to represented populations, less expensive techniques can provide useful information that becomes a composite of a whole. If questionnaires are valid and administration methods are reliable, surveys provide a relatively inexpensive data-collection method in terms of staff time and resources.

■ ARCHIVAL DATA

Archival resources provide great assessment opportunities to describe the health status of communities or populations. Vital statistics provide the most common data. There are increasing online sources from a wide variety of agencies, including governmental sources. There are many other sources, including health and illness data from community programs such as well-child clinics, senior health fair screening, or home visiting records. The concerns about using such data include confidentiality, data quality, and data access. Detailed information about data sources is given in Chapter 5.

Purposes for Use of Archival Data

In a community assessment, archival data provide a great deal of background information about a community or population. Archival data may be used to analyze changes and trends in numerous factors, such as changes in size and composition of the population and social determinants of health such as income, educational achievement, and unemployment. Mortality and morbidity data are essential to understand the disease patterns in a specific community and how these patterns compare with the state and nation.

Preparation for Use of Archival Data

The data collector should take a systematic approach to determine what type and amount of archival data are needed before collection begins because archival data are used for many purposes in community assessments. Details about planning for data collection are given in Chapter 7.

Data-Recording Techniques

Advanced public/community health nurses have a responsibility to oversee and implement accurate recording of health data. Persons responsible for entering and archiving data should be trained on procedures for data entry and assurance of confidentiality. Accurate recording of data ensures the reliability and quality of the data set. Collaboration with an information technologist is recommended to ensure that systems are in place to capture data, to allow for interface with other systems, and for meaningful retrieval of data.

Data Analysis

Archival data may also be examined by determining rates, ratios, proportions, means, and other parameters that are helpful to understand the aggregate or group as a whole. If data sets are large, subsets of the data may be used to determine trends or changes in parts of the population being studied.

Computer programs, such as SPSS and EpiInfo, are useful tools for analyzing archival data. An epidemiologist or statistician can perform more complex analyses with publicly available data sets. For example, Marshall, Cowell, Campbell, and McNaughton (2010) worked with an epidemiologist to analyze Behavioral Risk Factor Surveillance System (BRFSS) data to determine rates of cancer screening in women with diabetes. This analysis demonstrated that diabetic women were significantly less likely to receive cervical cancer screening than nondiabetic women. These data provided evidence to direct investigation into why women do not obtain screening, and ultimately provided direction to improve healthcare services.

Issues With Archival Data

Data collection from archival sources should be systematized to the simplest processes to reduce collection error. Direct access to original data can minimize error, though use of data sets that have been cleaned and verified is also useful. Missing data are difficult to explain with archival data, yet procedures can be employed to minimize issues such as sampling bias or data-entry errors.

■ LITERATURE REVIEW

A literature review as a community assessment data-collection method provides one with the opportunity to become familiar with reported problems. Literature review is integral to community assessment in several ways. The literature can introduce the primary problems in community health as well as report relationships among variables to explain community health problems. Relevant literature may be scientific publications or articles in the lay press. Literature thus becomes data for conducting a comprehensive community assessment. Literature review approaches serve different purposes.

Purposes of Literature Review

Literature reviews may be conducted for many purposes during the community assessment process. The history of a specific community may be explored through a literature review in local libraries as well as a historical society. The availability of services, facilities, activities, and other resources may be determined by reviewing literature. Literature also provides a general background about many aspects of a community assessment. For example, if local data indicate a possible problem, a literature review about the potential problem may provide information about other factors or community characteristics to examine before a conclusion can be reached.

Preparation for Use of Literature Review

After the specific purpose of the literature review is decided, the location or locations of the literature should be determined. If access to much of the literature is through a computer search, the physical location of the literature items will not be known until the specific items are identified. If the literature is of a historical nature, local libraries and historical societies need to be visited to access most of the literature. Usually, several sources are needed to obtain adequate literature on a specific topic.

Searching the Literature and Data-Recording Techniques

The usual recording techniques for literature reviews consist of taking notes from the original sources, writing annotated bibliographies, and highlighting major points in a copy of each article. A more structured approach to recording data or information from individual pieces of literature is useful when the purpose of the literature review is to identify patterns or major findings from a body of research. Types of literature reviews are narrative, scoping, integrative, systematic, and meta-analyses.

A narrative literature review is broad. Authors select material that is of interest and is specific to the question. Authors can also limit the comprehensiveness of a narrative review. Narrative reviews can be very helpful in clinical situations (Bart, Green, Johnson, & Adams, 2006). The purpose of the scoping review is to outline and analyze literature that is guided by the research question. The scoping review generally describes the current state of knowledge about the problem and can provide a base for continued work (Pham et al., 2014). Both the narrative and scoping review reports are prepared as narratives; a scoping review also includes a matrix for comparison of findings.

Integrative literature reviews are designed to present the state of the science around a particular area (Whittemore & Knafl, 2005). The purpose of the integrative review is to summarize, critique, and synthesize the studies reviewed. The search strategy is comprehensive and includes Medical Subject Headings (MeSHs) terms. The search may include studies from a range of methods, including randomized control trials, cohort studies, or qualitative studies. The inclusive years may be limited if the focus is on current information or expansive if looking broadly. The Preferred Reporting Items for Systematic Reviews and Meta-Analyses (PRISMA) flowchart illustrates all articles reviewed, rejected, and included, based on the selection criteria. Systematic reviews typically include only randomized control trials. Meta-analyses use findings from studies to create large data sets. The integrative and systematic reviews and the meta-analyses must adhere to the Cochrane Collaboration (www.cochrane.org) and PRISMA guidelines (www.prisma-statement.org). Integrative and systematic review reports are structured so that the summary, critique, and synthesis are typically displayed in tables with narrative illuminating the comparison. The meta-analyses reports include the quantitative analytics and findings.

Cooper (1989) organized an integrative literature review into five stages of primary research: (a) problem formation, (b) data collection, (c) data evaluation, (d) analysis and interpretation, and (e) public presentation. These stages assist the reviewer in conducting rigorous and comprehensive reviews that control for as many threats to validity as possible. In the problem-formation stage, variables to be reviewed are conceptually and operationally defined. Cooper (1989) suggested that the reviewer begin abstractly and then, as necessary, narrow definitions throughout the review.

The activities included in a literature review include analysis and interpretation. Literature reviews facilitate problem identification and focus questions that are useful in assessment, and provide insight into previous research or assessment. Gathering appropriate literature, as well as careful reading and reporting, is essential (Bart et al., 2006).

In some cases, a community assessment is directed by the need that is perceived. For example, the prevalence of asthma among children in low socioeconomic communities that are non-White is higher than in other communities (U.S. Department of Health and Human Services, 2007). DePriest and Butz (2017) searched the Cumulative

Index to Nursing and Allied Health Literature (CINAHL), PubMed, and PsycINFO databases to identify and critique studies examining neighborhood-level factors and asthma prevalence in urban children. More than 180 citations were screened with 26 manuscripts meeting the inclusion criteria.

Data Analysis

After completion of the literature review, the data are analyzed to develop a total view of the findings. Conclusions may be drawn by looking for commonalities among the research studies or group of articles. Quantitative methods used in meta-analyses may be used to draw conclusions, but these methods are beyond the scope of this text and are often time-consuming to employ. Instead, the advanced public/community health nurse is encouraged to work with others in a semistructured analysis of the data collected in the systematic literature review. An example of the findings from the DePriest and Butz study (2017) is described in the following text.

The analysis identified six themes within the domains of asthma prevalence: physical (outdoor air, outdoor air related to traffic, indoor air triggers, and housing) and social factors (outdoor safety, family stress). The studies were then critiqued by organizing tables for each domain with headings given in Table 6.3. The analysis illuminated the need for increased rigor in analytic methods because most studies were cross-sectional. In addition, to identify prevalence, what is being measured must be clear. The analysis showed that socioeconomic status was the factor influencing disparities, and not place. Although this finding was clear, more research is needed to support the findings (DePriest & Butz, 2017)

Issues With Literature Review

Several important issues surface when evaluating the use of literature in community assessment. Scientific journals tend to publish only statistically significant findings. Many studies demonstrate that traditionally held hypotheses are rejected, yet the preponderance of negative results are not published. Published studies also often report on segments of the population and limit the ability to generalize findings to communities at large. These limitations suggest the need to critique the literature extensively as it relates to a specific community assessment.

■ CHOOSING DATA-COLLECTION METHODS

Data collection for community assessment is carried out in a variety of ways. Key to determining the extent of data collection and the methods of data collection is the management of data to provide for comparison across sources. Continuous comparisons from various sources will provide evidence for the need to continue data collection. If there is evidence of agreement across sources, the expense of continuing to collect more data can be limited.

The content in this section was revised in collaboration with Mallory Bejster, who was a doctor of nursing practice student in advanced public health nursing at Rush University, College of Nursing, at that time.

TABLE 6.3 Organizing Headings for Critique Across Six Themes Embedded in Domains of Prevalence, Physical, and Social Factors

Author	Study	Methods	Results	Critique	Asthma	Sex, Race + Ethnicity Socioeconomic Status

Using a Variety of Data-Collection Methods

A list of community diagnoses should be generated using a variety of sources. Such a listing can be generated by identifying an assessment framework that supports the goal of data collection (see Chapter 4 for discussion of community assessment frameworks). Using an assessment framework ensures that data collection progresses in the intended direction and assists in the identification of required data sources and collection methods. For example, a windshield survey may be appropriate if trying to identify certain factors about the built environment. However, focus groups may be the most appropriate data-collection method to understand how the built environment affects community members. In some instances, key stakeholders may have already identified a priority community issue or concern. In these cases, a variety of data-collection methods can be utilized to better understand factors contributing to the previously identified community issue or concern.

The following example is a composite of multiple community assessments in a Hispanic American community focused on identifying key factors related to the high rate of childhood obesity at a local elementary school. Before starting the community assessment, community input from key partners highlighted childhood obesity as an important issue in the community to focus on in the community assessment. This example of a focused community assessment demonstrates an effort to compare data from numerous sources using a variety of data-collection methods. The PRECEDE–PROCEED model guided the data-collection plan, including identifying the data methods and sources needed for each phase (Green & Kreuter, 2005). Table 6.4 shows a sample data-collection plan for Phase 1 of the PRECEDE–PROCEED model. Data-collection methods included a windshield/walking survey, key informant interviews, literature review, statistics from databases, a teacher

TABLE 6.4 Sample Data-Collection Plan Based on Phase 1 of the PRECEDE–PROCEED Model

Framework Element	Data Needed	Methods to Obtain Data	Sources of Data	Sources for Comparison Data
Phase 1: Social assessment/ quality-of-life issues	Social assessment (a) What has the school/community already done to promote nutrition and physical activity? (b) What are priorities of this population related to nutrition and physical activity? (c) What outcomes related to childhood obesity does this school/community hope for? (d) How can nutrition and physical activity be improved within the school/ community (barriers/ facilitators)?	Key informant interviews, teacher group discussion, literature review	School administrators, school faculty and staff, community members	Literature review (analyze for similar themes, facilitators, and possible barriers)

group discussion, and paper-and-pencil teacher and parent surveys. This example used a general-to-specific approach to data collection, where more general data were collected before moving to the more focused assessment methods within the community. Data collection began with a literature review to build a foundation of knowledge regarding factors influencing higher rates of childhood obesity in Hispanic children and gathering statistics from databases such as the National Survey of Children's Health (NSCH; Data Resource Center for Child and Adolescent Health, n.d.). From there, a windshield/walking survey was completed around the school's catchment area, and key informant interviews were conducted. As the assessment process became more community focused, a teacher group discussion took place along with paper-and-pencil surveys with the school's teachers and parents.

A structured-interview guide was used in the key informant interviews in this example. Key informants included various community residents with different connections to the school community to gain different views and perspectives. A guided group discussion with teachers took place during a faculty meeting. Paper-and-pencil surveys were designed for teachers and parents using questions like those asked in other surveys, such as a teacher survey created by Perera, Frei, Frei, Wong, and Bobe (2015) for their study regarding barriers and facilitators related to nutrition education in elementary schools, and the NSCH draft questions for the parent survey (Data Resource Center for Child and Adolescent Health, n.d.). Using previously developed survey questions and instruments can strengthen the data-collection process.

Table 6.5 shows a list of common themes from data collected through various methods and sources of information. As most community issues have multiple contributing factors at various levels of the community, the problem list was organized using the ecological perspective to examine common themes at the individual, family, organizational, and community/systems levels (CDC, 2017b). An X in a Table 6.5 column indicates sources of data and information for each problem.

Analyzing Information Obtained by Various Methods

Analysis of the collected data included reviewing the findings to look for agreement among sources and the possibility of more questions arising. For example, low levels of nutrition education were identified in the literature review, in key informant interviews, and through the teacher survey. Did these data sources highlight reasons for the limited amount of nutrition education that are congruent, or is further assessment required to discover root causes of the problem? Connections among problems in the table can also be analyzed to look for common themes. The literature review noted that Hispanic communities may have fewer places for physical activity, and the windshield/walking survey and key informant interviews confirmed this issue within this community. Could the lack of green space be connected to lower levels of physical activity noted in multiple data sources? What other problems on the list could be connected to lower levels of physical activity? Understanding connections among common themes identified in the community needs assessment is a key process in analyzing the collected data.

Choosing Data-Collection Methods

When choosing data-collection methods in community assessment, valid and reliable measures should be adopted. The data collection is iterative, and the data-collection methods are expanded until there is agreement across sources. Qualitative and quantitative data provide the most elegant evidence of community health. In the previous example, the electronic databases and the parent and teacher surveys represent data collected by quantitative

TABLE 6.5 Problem Identification Related to Childhood Obesity Across Multiple Data Sources: Ecological Perspective

Problem	Source						
	Databases	Literature	Key Informant Interviews	Observations	Parent Surveys	Teacher Surveys	Teacher Group Discussion
Comparatively high prevalence of childhood obesity in Hispanic children	X	X					
Individual Level							
Low levels of physical activity	X	X	X		X	X	X
Consumption of few fruits and vegetables	X	X	X		X		
High consumption of sugar-sweetened beverages		X			X		
Electronic use/ screen time as a deterrent to exercise					X		X
Interpersonal Level							
Higher maternal educational attainment as a protective factor	X	X					
Cultural beliefs and practices around nutrition and perceptions of body image		X	X			X	X
Organizational (School) Level							
Strengthen language in school policies to "require" instead of "recommend"			X	X			
Stronger enforcement of district policies			X	X			

(continued)

TABLE 6.5 Problem Identification Related to Childhood Obesity Across Multiple Data Sources: Ecological Perspective *(continued)*

Problem	Source						
	Databases	Literature	Key Informant Interviews	Observations	Parent Surveys	Teacher Surveys	Teacher Group Discussion
Low levels of nutrition education in school		X	X			X	
Limited recess and physical activity in school		X	X			X	
Community/Systems Level							
Limited green space in the community		X	X	X			
Neighborhood safety may limit physical activity			X		X	X	X
Limited access to fruits and vegetables in the community		X	X	X	X	X	X

methods; the literature review, key informant interviews, the guided teacher discussion, and windshield survey represent qualitative data-collection approaches. Sampling issues are present, as noted in the selection of key informants. Reliability of data-collection methods is enhanced by agreement among methods, which maximizes the quality of the data.

■ SUMMARY

The descriptions of the data-collection methods in this chapter provide beginning knowledge for the advanced public/community health nurse to employ a variety of methods in conducting a community assessment. The advanced public/community health nurse needs to be able to competently use several methods detailed in this chapter, such as participant observation, windshield/walking survey, focus groups, key informants, the Delphi method, surveys, using archival data, and literature review. The purposes, preparation for using, recording techniques, data analysis, and issues with each method were discussed.

Using more than one data-collection method contributes to the validity of the conclusions drawn from data and information. Moreover, the advanced public/community health nurse needs to develop skill with several methods because not all information about a community may be found with only one data-collection method.

The data-collection methods described in this chapter are perhaps the most often used but are not the only ones available. You are encouraged to explore other data-collection methods, especially if these are more compatible with the assessment community. For example, in some communities, participant observation may not be acceptable, but audio taping by a community member in your absence would be approved by the members of a specific group.

■ SUGGESTED CLINICAL OR PRACTICUM ACTIVITIES

1. Conduct a windshield/walking survey of your assigned community. Discuss your findings with your preceptor or an advanced public/community health nurse.
2. Develop an interview schedule and conduct interviews with two key informants who reside in your assigned community.
3. Participate, if possible, in a participant observation event or a focus group.

REFERENCES

Bart, N., Green, B. N., Johnson, C. D., & Adams, A. (2006). Writing narrative literature reviews for peer-reviewed journals: Secrets of the trade. *Journal of Chiropractic Medicine, 5*(3), 101–117. doi:10.1016/S0899-3467(07)60142-6

Centers for Disease Control and Prevention. (2017a). *Loud noise can cause hearing loss.* Retrieved from https://www.cdc.gov/nceh/hearing_loss/what_noises_cause_hearing_loss.html

Centers for Disease Control and Prevention. (2017b). *Health equity toolkit.* Retrieved from https://www.cdc.gov/nccdphp/dnpao/state-local-programs/health-equity/index.html

Chen, L., Huang, L. H., Xing, M. Y., Feng, Z. X., Shao, L. W., Zhang, M. Y., & Shao, R. Y. (2017). Using the Delphi method to develop nursing-sensitive quality indicators for the NICU. *Journal of Clinical Nursing, 26,* 502–513.

Cooper, H. M. (1989). *Integrative research: A guide for literature reviews* (2nd ed.). Newbury Park, CA: Sage.

Creswell, J. W., & Poth, C. N. (2017). *Qualitative inquiry and research design: Choosing among five approaches* (4th ed.). Thousand Oaks, CA: Sage.

Dalkey, N., & Helmer, O. (1962). *An experimental application of the Delphi Method to the use of experts.* Memorandum, RM-727-/1 Abridged. Retrieved from https://www.rand.org/pubs/research_memoranda/RM727z1.html

Data Resource Center for Child and Adolescent Health. (n.d.). *National survey of children's health.* Retrieved from https://www.childhealthdata.org/

Dedoose Software. (2015). *Dedoose: Great research made easy.* Retrieved from http://dedoose.com

DePriest, K., & Butz, A. (2017). Neighborhood-level factors related to asthma in children living in urban areas: An integrative review. *Journal of School Nursing, 33,* 8–17. doi:10.1177/1059840516674054

Donsbach, W., & Traugott, M. W. (2008). Self-administered paper questionnaires. In W. Donsbach & M. W. Traugott (Eds.), *The SAGE handbook of public opinion research* (pp. 262–270). London, UK: Sage. doi:10.4135/9781848607910.n25

Fink, A. (2013). Community health and health service needs and evidence based programs. In A. Fink (Ed.), *Evidence based public health practice* (pp. 31–66). Thousand Oaks, CA: Sage. doi:http://dx.doi.org/10.4135/9781506335100

Fink, A., Kosecoff, J., Chassin, M., & Brook, R. H. (1984). Consensus methods: Characteristics and guidelines for use. *American Journal of Public Health, 74*(9), 979–983.

Fowler, F. J., & Cosenza, C. (2009). Design and evaluation of survey questions. In L. Bickman & D. J. Rog (Eds.), *The SAGE handbook of applied social research methods* (pp. 375–412). Thousand Oaks, CA: Sage. doi:10.4135/9781483348858.n1

Green, L. W., & Kreuter, M. W. (2005). A framework for planning. In L. W. Green & M. W. Kreuter (Eds.), *Health program planning: An educational and ecological approach* (pp. 1–28). Boston, MA: McGraw-Hill.

Hampton, C., & Vilela, M. (2017). Assessing community needs and resources. Section 13: Conducting surveys. In the Center for Community Health and Development at the University of Kansas (Ed.), *The community tool box* (chapter 3). Retrieved from http://ctb.ku.edu/en/table-of-contents/assessment/assessing-community-needs-and-resources/public-records-archival-data/main. doi:10.1186/s12889-015-2600-x

Hasson, F., Keeney, S., & McKenna, H. (2000). Research guidelines for the Delphi survey technique. *Journal of Advanced Nursing, 32*(4), 1008–1015.

Huesmann, L. R. (2007). The impact of electronic media violence: Scientific theory and research. *Journal of Adolescent Health. 41*, S6–S13. doi.org/10.1016/j.jadohealth.2007.09.005

Kassavou, A., French, D. P., & Chamberlain, K. (2015). How do environmental factors influence walking in groups? A walk-along study. *Journal of Health Psychology, 20*(10), 1328–1339. doi:10.1177/1359105313511839

Lindberg, D. M., Wood, J. N., Campbell, K. A., Scribano, P. V., Laskey, A., Leventhal, J. M., … Runyan, D. (2017). Research priorities for a multi-center child abuse pediatrics network–CAPNET. *Child Abuse & Neglect, 65*, 152–157.

Malcolm, C., Knighting, K., Forbat, L., & Kearney, N. (2009). Prioritisation of future research topics for children's hospice care by its key stakeholders: A Delphi study. *Palliative Medicine, 23*, 398–405.

Marshall, J. G., Cowell, J. M., Campbell, E., & McNaughton, D. B. (2010). Regional variations in cancer screening rates found in women with diabetes. *Nursing Research, 59*(1), 34–41.

McKenzie, J. F., Neiger, B. L., & Thackeray, R. (2016). *Planning, implementing & evaluating health promotion programs: A primer* (7th ed.). San Francisco, CA: Pearson.

McMillan, S. S., King, M., & Tully, M. P. (2016). How to use the nominal group and Delphi techniques. *International Journal of Clinical Pharmacology, 38*(3), 655–662.

McNaughton, D. B., Cowell, J. M., & Fogg, L. (2014) Adaptation and feasibility of a communication intervention for Mexican immigrant mothers and children in a school setting. *Journal of School Nursing, 30*(2), 103–113. doi:10.1177/1059840513487217

Morgan, D. L., & Krueger, R. A. (1997). *The focus group kit.* Thousand Oaks, CA: Sage.

Patton, M. Q. (2014). *Qualitative research and evaluation methods: Integrating theory and practice* (4th ed.). Thousand Oaks, CA: Sage.

Perera, T., Frei, S., Frei, B., Wong, S. S., & Bobe, G. (2015). Improving nutrition education in U.S. elementary schools: Challenges and opportunities. *Journal of Education and Practice, 6*(30), 41–50.

Pham, M. T., Rajić, A., Greig, J. D., Sargeant, J. M., Papadopoulos, A., & McEwen, S. A. (2014). A scoping review of scoping reviews: Advancing the approach and enhancing the consistency. *Research Synthesis Methods, 5*, 371–385. https://doi.org/10.1002/jrsm.1123

Pike, I., Piedt, S., Davison, C. M., Russell, K., Macpherson, A. K., & Pickett, W. (2015). Youth injury prevention in Canada: Use of the Delphi method to develop recommendations. *BMC Public Health, 15*, 1274.

QSR NVivo qualitative data analysis Software: QSR International Pry Ltd. Version 9, 2010. QSR International.

Rabinowitz, P. (2016). Assessing community needs and resources. Section 19: Using public records and archival data. In the Center for Community Health and Development at the University of Kansas (Ed.), *The community tool box* (chapter 3). Retrieved from http://ctb.ku.edu/en/table-of-contents/assessment/assessing-community-needs-and-resources/public-records-archival-data/main. doi:10.1186/s12889-015-2600-x

Rose, I. D., & Friedman, D. B. (2017). Schools. *Journal of School Nursing, 33*(2), 109–115. doi:10.1177/1059840516678910

Schreier, M. (2014). Qualitative content analysis. In U. Flick (Ed.), The SAGE *handbook of qualitative data analysis* (pp. 170–182). Thousand Oaks, CA: Sage.

Smith, T. W. (2016). Survey standards. In C. Wolf, D. Joye, T. W. Smith., & Y. Fu (Eds.), *SAGE handbook of survey methodology* (pp 16–26). Thousand Oaks, CA: Sage.

Stanhope, M., & Lancaster, J. (2016). *Public health nursing: Population-centered health care in the community* (9th ed.) St. Louis, MO: Elsevier.

Stähli, M. E., & Joye, D. (2016). Incentives as a possible measure to increase response rates. In C. Wolf, D. Joye, T. W. Smith., & Y. Fu (Eds.), *SAGE handbook of survey methodology* (pp. 425–440). Thousand Oaks, CA: Sage.

Tausch, A. P., & Menold, N. (2016). Methodological aspects of focus groups in health research: Results of qualitative interviews with focus group moderators. *Global Qualitative Nursing Research,* 32333393616630466. doi:10.1177/2333393616630466

U.S. Department of Health and Human Services. (2007). *The National Asthma Education and Prevention Program Expert Panel report 3 (EPR 3): Guidelines for the diagnosis and management of asthma* (NIH publication No. 70-4051). Washington, DC: Author. Retrieved from https://www.nhlbi.nih.gov/files/docs/guidelines/asthgdln.pdf

Valente, T. W. (2002). *Evaluating health promotion programs*. New York, NY: Oxford University Press.

Waltz, C. F., Strickland, O. L., & Lenz, E. R. (2017). *Measurement in nursing and health research* (5th ed.). New York, NY: Springer Publishing.

Weise, J., Fisher, K. R., & Trollor, J. (2016). Utility of a modified online Delphi method to define workforce competencies: Lessons from the intellectual disability mental health core competencies project. *Journal of Policy and Practice in Intellectual Disabilities, 13*(1), 15–22.

Whittemore, R., & Knafl, K. (2005). The integrative review: Updated methodology. *Journal of Advanced Nursing, 52*, 546–553.

CHAPTER 7

Planning and Conducting a Community Assessment

■ STUDY EXERCISES

1. Why is it important to develop a plan for conducting a community assessment?
2. In addition to the preassessment activities described in this chapter, what other activities would you want to complete before beginning an assessment?
3. How would you go about developing a team for conducting a community assessment?
4. What components should be included in a plan for conducting a community assessment? Using these components, develop a plan for conducting an assessment of a specific community.
5. How can community members be involved in conducting a community assessment? What roles can they fill?
6. How are professional team members involved in planning and conducting a community assessment?

Planning theory is based on the premise that it is better to plan than to not plan. The advantages of planning for conducting a community assessment are many. In addition to forcing the public/community health nurse to identify what will be done and when, the organization for which the community assessment is being done must commit resources if the assessment plan is formally presented and approved for funding. The commitment of resources provides support for using the results of the community assessment to plan community health improvements. As addressed in Section I of this book, requirements of the Patient Protection and Affordable Care Act (ACA, 2010) and the Public Health Accreditation Board (PHAB, 2016) have provided incentives for nonprofit hospitals and their public health partners to commit resources and to work collaboratively in identifying and addressing the health needs of their communities. These requirements provide new opportunities for advanced public/community health nurses to assume leading roles in planning and conducting local community assessments.

Notably, community assessment and planning tools have become a focus of discussion in the health-related literature. For example, Schifferdecker et al. (2016) provided an in-depth review of tools to help hospitals meet requirements for planning and implementing community health assessments and community health improvement plans. Of course, ad hoc community assessments may still be conducted but may not provide adequate depth of information for the focus required in advanced public/community health nursing practice.

Planning how and when the community assessment will be completed allows the advanced practice public/community health nurse to structure other assignments and tasks around the projected time frame for assessment activities. Adjustments may need to be made during the assessment process, but these can be made more easily with an overall plan. Another advantage of planning the community assessment is that others can better understand the process and contribute to the efforts. Individuals and groups can become involved early in the activities. The plan for conducting the community assessment should, of course, include participation of community residents as well as several categories of professionals, community leaders, business leaders, and others who are integral to community life. An assessment conducted by a team will have a broader scope than one done by only a public/community health nurse.

■ PREASSESSMENT PHASE

Before the community assessment process is begun, the preassessment phase should be dedicated to the development of a plan for conducting the assessment (Witkin & Altschuld, 1995). Such a plan will guide you and allow an ordered approach to an assessment done by a team. The preassessment phase includes decisions about the purpose of the assessment, how the community will be defined, and the framework to guide the data collection. Other preassessment decisions may be needed in a specific organization, such as to whom the report will be sent, which are discussed in later sections of this chapter.

Purpose of the Community Assessment

Determining the purpose and scope of the community assessment is one of the first decisions made in preassessment planning activities (Witkin & Altschuld, 1995). Chapter 3 discusses some purposes for conducting community assessments. In general, a community assessment is conducted to determine the health status of a community. For the advanced practice public/community health nurse, knowledge of the health status of the community is essential for competent practice in any role or position.

For the team in the community, there is usually an impetus to conduct a community assessment. In addition to the ACA and PHAB community assessment requirements, some state health departments require or support local health departments to conduct community assessments of their service areas (Centers for Disease Control and Prevention [CDC], 2015). Another reason for many organizations to undertake community assessment projects is to provide a basis for grant proposals. Often organizations that fund projects and services require that a problem, condition, or need be demonstrated in the proposal (CDC, 2015; Witkin & Altschuld, 1995). The community assessment provides not only the information about the problem or condition but also the data about the target population, risk factors, and other information that may be used as rationale for the funding request.

Framing the Assessment

The preassessment plan should include defining the community and identifying the framework or model to guide the assessment.

DEFINING THE COMMUNITY

The focus of the assessment is on a specific community; thus, a logical place to begin is by defining the community. Two aspects of this definition are desirable. The first aspect is to draw on the literature for a definition of *community*. As indicated in Chapter 3, numerous definitions of community are available and provide a rich field for the advanced practice public/community health nurse to explore. A definition provides a first step in grounding the community assessment in theoretical concepts. Of course, a community assessment could be conducted without theory, concepts, or frameworks, but it would be a different product than one expected by standards of practice for an advanced practice public/ community health nurse (American Nurses Association [ANA], 2013; Levin et al., 2008). The application of theory and concepts provides the advanced practice public/community health nurse with much more knowledge than a cookbook approach to filling in blanks on a data-collection form.

The second aspect of defining the community to be assessed is to identify the physical community, if this is appropriate. Often, a geopolitical entity, such as a county, city, township, or state, is the target of a community assessment and delineating the boundaries is an important early step in the community assessment process. An agreement on a written description of the community will facilitate the work to be done if the community does not have physical boundaries. An example of a community description is provided at the end of this chapter.

IDENTIFYING THE COMMUNITY ASSESSMENT FRAMEWORK OR MODEL

The definition of community is important as one part of identifying the framework or model to guide the community assessment. The framework guides and provides the philosophical orientation of the community assessment. This orientation captures some of the values, beliefs, and purpose of the community assessment, the community, and the assessor. Criteria for choosing a framework or model are discussed in Chapter 4.

Following the adoption of the definition of community and the community assessment framework, the preassessment phase should continue with the activities that are described next and that become part of the preassessment plan.

■ PREASSESSMENT ACTIVITIES

A number of activities should be completed before the community assessment is begun. Team building may be an early preassessment activity if team members have not worked together or would benefit from closer working relationships. In this section, other preassessment activities discussed are developing the timeline, identifying sources of data and methods of data collection, estimating time and resource needs, dividing responsibilities among team members, requesting information, and identifying key informants. As with any large project, adjustments will usually need to be made during the activities. However, with a written plan, team members have a greater chance of independently carrying out their assignments and also offering suggested changes during the course of the assessment activities.

One long-standing approach used to make the preassessment plan available for all team members is to write it on newsprint and tape the pages on a wall. Updates on the timeline or assignments may be made in different-colored markers so that all can be quickly brought up to date on the progress of the project. Another contemporary strategy is to utilize a shared computer program, such as Dropbox or Google Drive, which will allow easy access from multiple devices and real-time edits and updates by team members as the project moves forward.

Building the Team

As discussed in Chapter 1, an interdisciplinary team is a great asset for conducting a community assessment. The composition of a team used to conduct a community assessment, addressed in Chapter 3, will vary with the purpose, scope, and other aspects of the work to be completed. In practice, teams do not always know how to work well together. In addition, team members may not identify with the team enough to complete their tasks unless team building and team orientation events are conducted (West, 2012).

This section provides some practical suggestions for team-building activities that may be used before and during the community assessment process. Some of the activities may even be fun, which is one component that helps a team to work well together. Three activities described later in this chapter for team building are learning about each others' disciplines, improving listening skills, and role-playing interviews. Other activities described in Chapter 3, in other publications (Manion, Lorimer, & Leander, 1996; Mears, 1994), and on websites (e.g., vorkspace.com/blog/index.php/13-top-team-building-activities) may be used. Community members who are team members need to be included in these activities to the extent that they have the time and interest to be involved.

West (2012) proposed that effective teams should focus on their objectives, reviewing ways to achieve them by working together, a process referred to as *task reflexivity*. In addition, he noted that well-being of the team members should be promoted by reflecting on ways to support them, resolve conflicts, and understand the social and emotional climate of the team, or its "social reflexivity." The advanced practice public/community health nurse should facilitate reviews that inform the next steps related to the team's objectives and ways of working together to promote overall team effectiveness. One example of a team-assessment tool is displayed in Figure 7.1 and the score sheet is found in Figure 7.2. Clearly, the advanced practice public/community health nurse who has had experience in organizing and leading interdisciplinary teams will be at an advantage in implementing the activities to develop teamwork skills.

TEAMWORK SKILLS

Effective teamwork requires more than personality attributes; teamwork requires motivation, knowledge, and skills for working in teams (West, 2012). These skills include a set of team processes that support accurate exchange of information among members, effective flow of information to a decision maker, and accurate decision making (Brannick, Salas, & Prince, 1997). Effective teamwork in the helping professions is based on communication, collaboration, shared decision making, cooperation, consistency, conflict prevention, conflict resolution, and mutual support (Garner & Orelove, 1994; Rahn, 2016). Teamwork includes team members' preferences for working in teams; whether they have an individualist or collective approach to working with others; their basic social skills such as listening, speaking, and cooperating; and their team-working skills such as collaboration.

Although teamwork is presented as the preferred structure for approaching many complex situations, such as a community assessment, there are many barriers to forming and maintaining an effective team. Specialization in the health and social services professions has resulted in high levels of knowledge and competence in narrow fields of study. Therefore, overlapping of expertise may result, but each profession may have little knowledge of others' fields and scopes of practice. The structure of human service organizations

This assessment (Figure 7.1) was developed to help teams identify areas for improvement. Complete the assessment by rating each item according to the following legend. After completing the entire assessment, total your score, section by section, and fill in the answers on the separate score sheet (see Figure 7.2). Identify the section with the greatest opportunity for improvement. Focus on the problem areas in that section before beginning improvements in other sections.

Legend   5 = Almost always   3 = Sometimes   1 = Almost never

            4 = Frequently   2 = Occasionally   NA = Not applicable

Goals (40 possible points)

_____ 1. Our goals are in writing.

_____ 2. Our goals are clear and specific.

_____ 3. Our work assignments are in writing.

_____ 4. Our roles are clear.

_____ 5. We assign time frames for accomplishing goals.

_____ 6. Our goals support the strategic direction of the organization.

_____ 7. We follow-up to ensure that goals are accomplished.

_____ 8. We recognize our accomplishments and celebrate them.

_____ Total

Communication (50 possible points)

_____ 1. We are comfortable asking for what we want from others.

_____ 2. We are polite, courteous, and friendly to each other.

_____ 3. We communicate effectively during stressful situations.

_____ 4. We confront issues.

_____ 5. We are specific and work focused, not personal, when we express our needs.

_____ 6. We initiate communication to solve problems.

_____ 7. There is an environment of openness and trust.

_____ 8. We listen and try to understand the other person's point of view.

_____ 9. We do not engage in gossip.

_____ 10. We respect confidentiality.

_____ Total

Working together (60 possible points)

_____ 1. We value differences on the team.

_____ 2. We maintain each other's self-esteem.

_____ 3. We demonstrate sensitivity to each other's feelings, problems, and needs.

_____ 4. We use a good problem-solving method.

FIGURE 7.1   Team assessment tool.

Source: Becker-Reems, E. D. (1994). *Self-managed work teams in health care organizations*. Chicago, IL: AHA. Copyright © 1994 by American Hospital Publishing, Inc., an American Hospital Association company.

_____ 5. We use a good decision-making method.

_____ 6. We have the necessary skills to function effectively.

_____ 7. Training is readily available.

_____ 8. We evaluate our effectiveness regularly.

_____ 9. We make improvements in the way we function.

_____ 10. We welcome new employees to our team.

_____ 11. We have a good orientation process.

_____ 12. We have the information we need to be effective.

_____ Total

Leadership (60 possible points)

_____ 1. We have a clear vision of where we are going.

_____ 2. We each share the responsibilities of leadership.

_____ 3. Our leader is visible and available.

_____ 4. Coaching is effective.

_____ 5. Our leader expresses enthusiasm and commitment.

_____ 6. Our leader encourages everyone's participation.

_____ 7. Our leader invites feedback on his or her performance.

_____ 8. Our leader provides specific feedback on our work.

_____ 9. Our leader acts as a role model for the team.

_____ 10. Our leader is committed to customer satisfaction.

_____ 11. Our leader models a commitment to quality.

_____ 12. Our leader involves us with other teams when our work will affect theirs.

_____ Total

Meetings (45 possible points)

_____ 1. Our meetings start on time.

_____ 2. We have an agenda.

_____ 3. We accomplish our purpose before we adjourn.

_____ 4. We come to meetings prepared.

_____ 5. We avoid unrelated discussion.

_____ 6. Everyone participates in our meetings.

_____ 7. We document our meetings.

_____ 8. We have regular, informative meetings.

_____ 9. We end our meetings on time.

_____ Total

FIGURE 7.1 *(continued)*

Instructions: Total your score for each section on the team assessment and transfer those numbers to this score sheet. Figure the percentage for each section. Any section below 50% is in strong need of improvement. A rating of 80% or higher is very positive. (A score of 3 or less for any individual question indicates an area for improvement.)

Goals

Total: _____

Possible: __40__

Percentage: _____ (Divide total by possible; multiply by 100.)

Communication

Total: _____

Possible: __50__

Percentage: _____ (Divide total by possible; multiply by 100.)

Working together

Total: _____

Possible: __60__

Percentage: _____ (Divide total by possible; multiply by 100.)

Leadership

Total: _____

Possible: __60__

Percentage: _____ (Divide total by possible; multiply by 100.)

Meetings

Total: _____

Possible: __45__

Percentage: _____ (Divide total by possible; multiply by 100.)

Grand total (Add totals from all sections.)

Grand

Total: _____

Possible: __225__

Percentage: _____ (Divide total by possible; multiply by 100.)

FIGURE 7.2 Team assessment score sheet.

Source: Becker-Reems, E. D. (1994). *Self-managed work teams in health care organizations*. Chicago, IL: AHA. Copyright © 1994 by American Hospital Publishing, Inc., an American Hospital Association company.

may contain barriers for teamwork by continuing to be organized on hierarchical, departmental models. These types of models generally do not offer employees the opportunity to learn to function in teams. Often, teams are impeded in their functioning because of unclearly defined roles and expectations. Team decision making may be hampered by confusion or rigidity about authority and power structures within the team (Garner & Orelove, 1994; Rahn, 2016).

The development of skills for teamwork is ongoing but may be enhanced by the use of group activities and exercises before the work is begun. Starting with the agreed-upon goal to complete the community assessment provides one organizing element for the team to begin to work together.

RECRUITING AND RETAINING COMMUNITY MEMBERS

The model proposed in this chapter is for involvement of community members; it is not a community-initiated and community-led model of community assessment. Chapter 4 contains examples of community assessment frameworks that are community initiated and led. Most communities are accustomed to professionals telling them what they need, so involvement of community members requires a reorientation of both the community and professionals (Minkler, 2012). Seeking community involvement may not be the goal for every community assessment; also, it may not be the method of choice for every advanced practice public/community health nurse. This is just one of the many approaches that might be used successfully in working with communities. In addition to membership on the community assessment team, community members need to be involved in other aspects of the community assessment. These aspects are discussed and illustrated throughout the text.

OBTAINING APPROPRIATE REPRESENTATIVES

Locating appropriate persons to represent the community requires knowledge of the community and the numerous subgroups. Without this knowledge, the advanced practice public/community health nurse is left with recruiting anyone who volunteers to serve as a member of the community assessment team. One approach is to draw from the voter registration rolls and invite interested individuals to join the assessment team. Invitations may be mailed to registered voters by a random method, by selected zip codes, by geographic location, or by other method. This approach allows for a representative group but may result in underrepresentation by noncitizens and recent community emigrants. Non–English-speaking community residents may be excluded from community assessment efforts unless special efforts are made to gain their viewpoints.

Another approach is to ask community organizations to select representatives from their own memberships. One must keep in mind that volunteers may be least representative of the community-at-large (Sawyer, 1995). Whatever method is used, attempts should be made to obtain some representation from the major sectors of the community, for example, major ethnic and racial groups, religious communities, gender, and age groups.

KEEPING COMMUNITY MEMBERS INVOLVED

Keeping community members involved may be difficult, especially if the assessment activities are spaced over a long period of time. If funds are available, remuneration for travel, meals, and childcare may be provided to community volunteers. If low-income individuals are involved, a stipend may assist them to remain part of the team effort.

Giving support and specific assignments provides structure and limits to the demands made on community members. However, providing for choices in assignments may make the experience more meaningful and manageable for community members. With increasing use of communication technology, for example, mobile devices and personal computers, community members may be able to be involved more easily through a wide range of social media platforms, including Facebook, Twitter, Internet forums, blogs, networking sites, and podcasts. This expanding use of technology is one approach to building a community that has shown promise in recent decades (Gilchrist, 2009). Completion of assignments and contributions to meetings no longer needs to be face to face.

LEARNING ABOUT OTHER DISCIPLINES

One way to begin to function as a team is to get to know about each others' disciplines. An effective technique may be to have each person describe someone else's discipline, including educational preparation, licensing, major components of practice, and continuing-education requirements for continued licensing. Gaining this knowledge will require a literature review, inquiry of a licensing board, and/or an interview of someone in practice. Active acquisition of information will usually result in more interest and greater learning than if the individual tells about his or her own discipline during a team meeting.

IMPROVING LISTENING SKILLS

Exercises that foster careful listening skills are often helpful in beginning team-building attempts. One such exercise is conducted with team members grouped in trios. One member is an observer while the other two members engage in verbal communication. One member makes a statement and the other member must repeat in his or her own words what the other individual has said. The observer's job is to confirm that the second person's statement was correct. If the second person's interpretation was not correct, the statements are repeated until there is an accurate interpretation. Each person plays another role until each has had an opportunity to play all three roles. Discussion with the total team after the exercise is helpful to identify common problems and ways to improve listening skills.

Although this may seem like an easy and straightforward exercise, difficulty may be encountered because of the tendency for one to read more into a statement than the other person intended or to interpret a statement from one's own perspective. This exercise may not pose many challenges for individuals in the same discipline. However, people from different disciplines often do not use the same jargon and may encounter the need to use a common vocabulary.

ROLE-PLAYING INTERVIEWS

Another exercise for team members is to role-play a scene they identify as particularly difficult. This scene may be an interview with a group that is opposed to a specific project or an organization that rarely cooperates with others. Each person takes the role of someone in the opposition group or organization. A scenario is presented in writing for each role and the question under discussion is given to each participant in writing. After the allotted time for the role-play, a discussion of the exercise centers around how the real situation may be handled using what occurred during the role-play. Often, insights occur that will be helpful in planning strategies.

A second type of role-play is rehearsal of a specific activity that is anticipated to be difficult for one or more team members. The activity may be approaching a high-level official, asking for funding from a source that asks many pointed questions, or obtaining information from someone who is very negative about sharing public information. One team member plays the person from whom something is requested. Other team members take turns asking for the desired information, while the other team members critique each role-play scene. A combination of approaches may be tried in order to develop an optimal approach.

A modification of the role-play just mentioned is to videotape each person during his or her presentation. Review of each tape may be instructive to both the individual and the other team members. When this technique is used, it is sometimes helpful to have a consultant present to assist with suggestions for improvement.

Identifying Data Sources and Data-Collection Methods

Chapters 5 and 6 provide extensive descriptions of data sources and data-collection methods. Of the available sources and methods, the community assessment team will need to identify which are pertinent for the purpose and scope of the assessment project. Before beginning the assessment, team members may not be knowledgeable about what is available, so changes may be needed in these parts of the preassessment plan as the assessment is implemented.

In general, the data sources should be readily accessible and free or low cost for use if the budget for the assessment is limited. The use of reliable sources of data contributes to the acceptability of the final product. Data-collection methods should be matched with team skills, if possible. For example, if team members have skills in using the computer, Internet searches could be used to contribute to the data collection. Teams conducting community health assessments to meet ACA or PHAB requirements frequently benefit from the participation of skilled data analysts and technicians who work for the healthcare and/or public health system. If specific skills are needed but not possessed by any team members (e.g., interviewing key informants), training sessions may be needed before data collection begins. This type of preassessment activity could be added to the timeline.

Developing a Timeline

In developing a timeline, it is often best to work backward from the date of completion. If the completed product is needed by December 15, 1 week will be needed to edit, format, and proof the final document. All data need to be analyzed and synthesized by December 1 in order to allow enough time to write the report and meet the proofing deadline. If 4 hours per week for 12 weeks are available to obtain all the data, data collection should start on September 1. A sample timeline is displayed in Figure 7.3. It is always helpful to keep in mind the old adage: Everything takes twice as long as you think it will.

Preassessment planning	███															
Data collection			███	███	███	███	███	███	███							
Analysis									███	███						
Synthesis										███	███					
Writing report												███	███			
Typing														███	███	
Verbal reports																
Weeks	1	2	3	4	5	6	7	8	9	10	11	12	13	14	15	16

FIGURE 7.3 Sample timeline for conducting a community assessment.

A detailed schedule for specific types and methods of data acquisition should be spelled out for implementation during the 12 weeks of data collection. For example, in the first week, appointments with key informants (i.e., knowledgeable community residents) should be made because they may not have time immediately available to meet with the data collector. Any data that must be obtained by mail or with special permission should be identified early in the process so that requests can be made as soon as possible. Many states have an open information law that requires that certain types of information be made available upon request through the Freedom of Information Act (FOIA), but the process often takes several weeks. Often, requests must be written and sent to the specific office for processing. If data and information can be obtained without this time-consuming process, these alternative sources should be used. For example, there are public sources of data, such as the county health rankings (www.countyhealthrankings.org), which provide comprehensive and reliable data. This and other data sources are described in detail in Chapter 5.

ALLOCATING TIME FOR MEETINGS

The advanced practice public/community health nurse, when developing the timeline, should allow time for team meetings as well as meeting individually with team members who may have difficulty in completing assigned tasks or have questions about their specific assignments. The public/community health nurse, as the community assessment coordinator, may need to take on additional tasks if others are unable to complete theirs. These additional time demands should be accounted for in assignment allocations. Time to prepare progress reports for the organization or to meet with an administrator should be included in the timeline. It is time well spent to keep others informed and committed to continuing assistance as needed.

Any timeline may require adjustments throughout a project. In order to avoid unnecessary adjustments, adequate time needs to be allowed for specific activities in the original plan. Overly optimistic time frames can create discouragement among team members as deadlines are continuously missed, and the timeline becomes only a piece of paper. Involving team members in developing the original timeline may create not only a more realistic plan but also a commitment of team members to meet the time goals.

Community members may not be able to attend team meetings held during daytime working hours. Early morning or late afternoon meetings may be necessary to accommodate the community members' schedules. Keeping community members involved often requires a delicate balancing act between the team's needs and the volunteers' schedule flexibility. For example, individuals who do not work outside their homes may be more flexible than community members employed full time. The viewpoints of both are important, and various methods, such as use of technology, need to be explored to have the involvement of a variety of community members.

PLANNING DISSEMINATION ACTIVITIES

The timeline may also include activities to disseminate the final community assessment findings. Either written or verbal reports may be needed, depending on the purpose and scope of the assessment (Jacobs, Jones, Gabella, Spring, & Brownson, 2012). Some dissemination activities may take a great deal of time and/or be spaced over a long time period, so planning for dissemination of the assessment should be included in the timeline if the community assessment report is to be adequately disseminated.

If the assessment was conducted for a community organization, the members of the organization should be offered a verbal and a written report. For the local health department, a

---

BOX 7.1   OUTLINE FOR ORAL PRESENTATION OF A COMMUNITY ASSESSMENT

I. Description and history of the community
II. Framework or model used to guide the assessment
III. How the assessment was conducted
    A. Methods of data collection and sources of data
    B. Team members
IV. Results of data analysis and synthesis
    A. Major findings about the community by framework category
    B. Community diagnoses
V. Conclusions
VI. Summary

---

written report that is also available as an e-document may suffice because the state health department will expect that the findings will be used throughout the following years for project proposals, planning efforts, and collaborative work with community groups.

Community assessments are important pieces of information for employees in many agencies. If a verbal report is given and videotaped, the videotape could be used in new employee orientation. The written report could also be made available to all employees, such as public health nurses and home health aides, who will need the information to more effectively conduct their jobs.

One example of a unique approach to dissemination was to invite community members and professionals to a town hall forum after the project was completed. An advanced practice public/community health nurse, who was the director of community outreach at a community hospital, coordinated the assessment. Another approach was to present the findings to various community groups at their monthly or special meetings. This is a good approach for the advanced practice public/community health nurse who works in a community nursing center (CNC) or a federally qualified health center (FQHC) that has a goal of involving the community in projects to improve the health of the total community. An oral presentation could include points such as those outlined in Box 7.1. These examples of dissemination activities require long lead times for planning and implementation and, thus, need to be thought through carefully and added to the timeline for the community assessment.

Estimating Time and Resources

Another aspect of preassessment activities is to estimate time and resources needed to conduct the assessment. The timeline will provide some guidance for the time requirements. In addition, time estimates need to include who on the assessment team has time and skills to do which tasks. For example, staff public/community health nurses are often very skilled at interviewing key informants and could be assigned to these contacts as time permits.

The questions and format for key informant interviews need to be determined before interviews begin. This activity should be included in the preassessment planning and before data collection is begun. Questions, such as those in Box 7.2, are generic but could be tailored for a specific community assessment. For example, when using the epidemiologic triangle as the community assessment framework, you could organize specific questions

---

BOX 7.2   SAMPLE QUESTIONS FOR KEY INFORMANTS

1. What are the biggest changes you have seen in the county (or community) in the past 5 years?
2. What are the biggest decisions facing the county for the next 5 years?
3. If you could make changes in the services available to the county residents, what changes would you make?
4. What are the greatest strengths of this county?
5. What do you think most needs to be changed in this county?
6. How well do you think people work together to make this county a better place for everyone?
7. How do you think people could work better together?
8. What are the major health problems in the community?
9. What is being done to address these problems?
10. Who would you say knows a lot about what goes on around the county?

---

around the three components of the framework: host, agent, and environment. Examples of questions about the environment are as follows:

- What are positive aspects of the community physical environment?
- What aspects of the physical environment need to be addressed?
- What plans does the community have for improving the quality of the water and air?

Resources needed for the assessment include, in addition to personnel time, access to telephones, libraries, information in the agency and community, the Internet, a copy machine, and a computer. Some expendable supplies will be needed, but will usually be ordinary office supplies, such as paper, pens, notebooks, and computer supplies.

To estimate supplies needed, use a rough rule of thumb for every team member at the customary usage rate. For example, if the agency has a history of using one pen per worker per week, use this kind of information to calculate the supplies needed. More paper and copying time will be needed when the report is duplicated for distribution to community groups, team members, agency administrators, and others. Some groups have been able to obtain external funding for printing the community assessment document. If the document is to be widely distributed, a professional quality product is especially desirable. Such a professional quality document can also be widely disseminated electronically as a portable document format (PDF) file.

Although a community assessment process consultant may not be available in the agency, one may be helpful when contacted by telephone or computer. Such consultants may be found in the state health department, a nearby university school of nursing or school of public health, or a consulting firm. Usually, assistance from public agencies can be obtained without payment. Extensive consultation, such as having someone to conduct and/or write most of the report, will require payment for the consultant's time and often other items. A private consulting firm almost always charges for services but will usually provide a written prospectus of the proposed work and fees upon request.

If funding is being sought to conduct the assessment, the information about resources needs to be detailed in order for a budget to be prepared. Chapter 13 contains information about developing budgets for program plans. The approaches are also applicable for developing a budget for conducting a community assessment.

Dividing Work Among Team Members

Organizing the division of work by aspects of the conceptual framework will provide guidance to focus and narrow the assessment. All possible information cannot be obtained, so the community assessment plan should provide the parameters of the assessment in terms of volume of data and information to be collected. Often, during the analysis phase of the assessment, gaps and inconsistencies in data and information appear that require further work (Anderson & McFarlane, 2015). This approach may slow the analysis and synthesis phases of the community assessment, but time for additional data collection should be allocated in the plan timeline.

Dividing the work among team members should be done in a systematic manner in order to ensure that all aspects of the work are assigned and individuals complete their assignments. A division of work that allows individuals to volunteer for specific assignments is preferred to the coordinator's assigning work without obtaining individuals' preferences. Assignment of data collection categories to individuals or small groups of individuals by areas of expertise makes sense if the work is to be completed quickly. For example, a data category on environment could be assigned to someone in environmental health. This individual will usually have readily available data about the quality of air and water, or know where to quickly find such information. During the planning phase, team members should be encouraged to provide information about available data and how to obtain them.

If at all possible, the team should regularly meet face to face to discuss assignments. At times, individuals may volunteer for jobs they do not have skills to complete, for example, a community member who has not done literature searches. It may be best to ask two people to work together in these instances. With this approach, the unskilled person can learn new skills and the other person will have the satisfaction of helping someone to become a better worker. Providing opportunities for development of skills in teamwork is a great benefit of working together.

The work division is best communicated by putting everything in writing and distributing it after the organizing meeting. This written summary should contain names of individuals for each task, a target deadline, and a brief description of the task. The advanced practice public/community health nurse who is leading the community assessment effort should be available to assist each team member as the work proceeds and call the team together for periodic updates and adjustments in the schedule or for other needed changes.

Requesting Information From Government Sources

Individuals who are responsible for requesting data and information from government sources may need to be directed to these sources and given information on how to contact them. Although much information is available in libraries and on the Internet, some data and information may be considered sensitive and require a written request to obtain. These requests should be made only when there is no other alternative because the time required to obtain the information is usually long.

Often team members know individuals in government offices who can be helpful in obtaining data in a timely manner. These contacts should be used in the place of written requests whenever possible. If data can be obtained in no other way, written requests should be made as soon as possible in the community assessment process. Most telephone directories and websites contain the titles, addresses, and telephone numbers of government offices. Usually, a letter written to the head of the department or office that compiles the data will be adequate, but a phone call to obtain the exact name and title of the correct individual is well worth the time and effort. If a specific protocol must be followed to obtain information, the protocol should be obtained. A request via an email message will be possible for many government offices.

Identifying Key Informants

The team will be very helpful in compiling names and telephone numbers of key informants. Five to 10 key informants will be adequate as an initial database for the community assessment, if the community is not too large. Other key informants may be added if need is discovered later in the process. The obvious key informants are community leaders, for example, elected officials, school district officials, clergy, law enforcement officials, and prominent citizens. However, lay leaders should not be overlooked, especially within minority groups who make up the community. Lay leaders may include church deacons, officers in community and school organizations, activists, elder residents, and informal group leaders.

One technique for identifying key informants involves asking several people who they see as community leaders. If someone's name is mentioned two or three times, that individual should be considered as a key informant. The people who are interviewed could also be asked who they see as community leaders. If it is not possible to conduct face-to-face or telephonic interviews with all key informants, they could be sent short, written interview forms to complete and return. This technique may not get a 100% return, but the information will be useful in obtaining a broader view of the community and issues.

Often programs are planned to relieve a problem in a minority community, but members of the community have never been included in identifying and/or verifying the problem. The involvement of several community residents may be accomplished by the use of group sessions. Focus groups, the Delphi process, and the nominal group process are approaches that have been used successfully to obtain a great deal of information from groups of individuals (Grove, Burns, & Gray, 2013; Krueger, 1988). Planning these events requires time and expertise. The local university may be a resource for training on how to implement such group approaches to data collection.

Writing the Preassessment Plan

The preassessment plan can be written as a draft document while the activities described earlier are being carried out and decisions made. A plan that contains the final decisions and agreements among team members provides guidance for everyone and may make implementation easier. Box 7.3 contains the outline for components to be included in the preassessment plan.

BOX 7.3   OUTLINE FOR A COMMUNITY ASSESSMENT PREASSESSMENT PLAN

   I. Purpose and scope of the community assessment
  II. Framework for the community assessment
     A. Definition of community
     B. Community assessment framework
 III. Sources of data
 IV. Methods of data collection
  V. Timeline for completing the assessment
 VI. Resources needed to complete assessment
VII. Work assignments

■ USING A FRAMEWORK OR MODEL TO GUIDE THE COMMUNITY ASSESSMENT PROCESS

A framework or model, such as described in Chapter 4, provides a guide for organizing the data collection for the community assessment. Using a specific framework, the advanced practice public/community health nurse can determine the categories of data needed and, to some extent, how and where to obtain the data. It may be helpful to develop a data-collection matrix during preassessment planning. An example of the format for a data-collection matrix is given in Table 7.1.

Adding details to the matrix, such as the specific type of demographic data to collect and who is responsible for collecting the data, will make it more useful for the team. The matrix could also be used as part of the monitoring tools to track progress on data collection. Such a matrix could be constructed using a computer program for a spreadsheet so that updating the matrix is an easy task.

Allocating Time

An allotment of time for each data-collection section will provide information to calculate the amount of money needed for personnel to complete this phase of the community assessment. For example, 8 hours may be needed to gather all the information about the host (people) for the epidemiologic framework, but the timeline will allow only 6 hours. Planning for how the task can be completed in 6 hours will require some thought and ideas from other team members. Adjustments may also be made after data collection has started. Often, the first assessment takes longer; and a new assessor takes longer to complete each task.

Organizing by Model Components

Arranging the data-collection tasks by components of the community assessment framework or model will provide an early structure for organizing the tasks to be completed. Often, the written description of the framework delineates what data are to be included in each category; for example, the core of the community assessment wheel represents the community residents (Anderson & McFarlane, 2015). If this kind of detail is lacking in the

TABLE 7.1 Data-Collection Matrix Using an Epidemiologic Framework

Framework Element	Data	Source	Method
Host (people)	Demographics	Census	Internet or CD-ROM search
Agent	Morbidity data	Reports	Internet search or health department
Environment	Toxic waste sites	Website	Record search

Note: Additional columns may be added to indicate the team member assigned to collect the specific data and the date for completion.

literature (see Chapter 4 for examples), the preassessment phase will allow the assessor time to decide what data elements fit into each framework category.

Lack of organization creates chaos as soon as a large volume of data begins to accumulate. Although in the long run, examining relationships among the various components of the framework or model will facilitate putting the data together, the assessor must make some sense of the volumes of data for each component individually. This step will be facilitated by the organization of data by category.

Irrespective of whether a manual or computerized system for data organization is used, the key to successful organization is to use the system consistently and make it available for all team members to use. Training in use of a computer software program may be necessary if team members are not familiar with the program chosen for data organization.

■ CONDUCTING THE DATA-COLLECTION PHASE OF THE COMMUNITY ASSESSMENT

The data-collection phase of the community assessment is the one that usually takes the longest amount of time to complete. In addition, most nurses feel comfortable collecting data because this is similar to the first step of the nursing process. One word of caution at this stage of work is to avoid the pitfall of data overload. This situation comes about when the nurse (or other team member) believes that an assessment is not complete until every possible piece of data is collected, catalogued, and safely set aside for the analysis. The next sections address organizing data and acquiring adequate data.

Getting Started

A thorough community assessment should begin with an overview of the community. If it is a geopolitical community, a windshield or walking survey is a good place to begin. Chapter 6 provides a data-collection framework for a windshield survey. The guide in Box 7.4 is a suggested template that is an elaboration of the windshield survey framework used to assist you in identifying the specific items for data collection. This template could be put into a document for the computer and used on a laptop, notebook, or smartphone in the car.

A map of the community may be used to provide direction for the windshield survey and to allow you to note the locations of various items of interest during the drive-around or walk-around part of the survey. Notes should also be made about areas that require additional exploration, such as ordinances about illegal dumping, locations of abandoned automobiles, and possible toxic dump sites. The notes taken during the windshield survey will provide some direction for other parts of the assessment.

A second activity in starting a community assessment should be a stop at the local library if the community has one. The librarian can direct you to books and materials about the community's history, the people, resources, housing, clubs, organizations, and other potential sources of information. Some materials may also be located online.

If the community does not have a public library, you may locate some material in a county municipal library, a community college library, a university library, a chamber of commerce, the public high school library, or the state capital. Local churches or clubs may also be repositories for historical materials. The history and current general status of a community will help you to see the community as a whole.

With the ACA requirement for nonprofit hospitals to conduct a community health needs assessment every 3 years, these assessments are readily available to the public on hospitals' websites. These community assessments can be useful as sources of information, as well as a means of verifying information and data trends.

BOX 7.4 GUIDE FOR WINDSHIELD/WALKING SURVEY

A windshield or walking survey is a method of collecting data about a community by driving and/or walking. The observations allow the nurse to collect subjective data about the sights, sounds, tastes, and smells of the community while driving slowly and walking through selected areas. A map should be used to indicate locations of important items and areas that need further exploration. It is best to conduct a survey in pairs or small groups. The following outline may be followed to provide organization to the data-collection activity.

Observations:

I. Sight
   A. What is the gender and racial distribution of people in the community?
   B. Where do you see people?
   C. What do you see people doing?
   D. How are people dressed?
   E. What types of housing units are located in the community?
   F. What kinds of schools do you see?
   G. What types of churches or religious organizations do you see?
   H. What are the local industries and businesses?
   I. What health services are seen?
   J. What other organizations are visible?
   K. What protective services are seen?
   L. Where are parks, play lots, and gardens located?
   M. Are there vacant lots and fields?
   N. Where are laundries, dry cleaners, and drugstores located?
   O. What kinds of transportation do people use?
II. Sound
   A. What do you hear in the community?
   B. Do you hear children playing, loud music, airplanes, heavy machinery in use, noisy automobiles?
   C. Can you hear sounds of birds or other animals?
III. Taste
   A. Where do people shop for food?
   B. What are the prices of one quart of milk, a dozen eggs, and a loaf of bread?
   C. Do the produce and meat appear fresh?
   D. What type of drinking and eating establishments do you see?
   E. How does the water taste?
IV. Smell
   A. How does the area smell?
   B. Are there any industrial emissions?
   C. Are garbage cans visible?
   D. Is debris present?
V. Touch
   A. Are fences used to delineate boundaries? What natural boundaries define each area?
   B. What is the atmosphere in local shops?
   C. How do you feel walking on the streets?
   D. Do residents say anything to you?

Organizing Data by Framework or Model

A filing system or a mechanism to physically sort data into categories is useful from the beginning of the project. A notebook with dividers or computer files or folders separated by category and subcategories of the community assessment framework will provide adequate organization in the early phases of data collection. Within the notebook or electronic file (e-file) folder, each team member should include notes on sources and methods of data collection, dates, and amount of time used. This detailed record will assist the coordinator as well as other team members who may need to substitute a team member during the data-collection activities. If needed, a hanging-file system or boxes can supply space for organizing larger items such as reports, books, and pamphlets.

Team members may photocopy or scan pages of a report, book, or other document and insert the pages into the appropriate place in the notebook or e-file folders. Such parts of documents must include the author, date, source document title, publication location, and publisher (American Psychological Association [APA], 2010). Lots of information and data are available on the Internet, so documents may be printed from a computer and placed in the notebook or downloaded and saved as PDF files. It is also necessary to have the sources of Internet information properly documented for inclusion in the final report.

A computer spreadsheet may be useful for organizing the data and information. A summary of each data item could be entered into the spreadsheet after it is read and abstracted at the end of each data-collection day. This approach could ease the work of writing the final report. One team member may be assigned this task if all team members are not familiar with the use of spreadsheets or other software programs chosen for use in the community assessment process.

Organizing the Community Assessment Report

A final report of the community assessment may be organized around the framework used. Box 7.5 contains a suggested outline for a community assessment paper or report. The categories of the framework are used to organize the outcomes of the data analysis. Although some results of data synthesis may be presented within the categories of the framework, most of the results of the synthesis will be expressed as the community diagnoses.

Acquiring Adequate Data

In conducting the data-collection phase of a community assessment, the dilemma is more often how to limit the volume of data rather than acquiring adequate data. However, community assessments serve various purposes, and data to fit some purposes are more difficult to acquire than others. For example, data about health behaviors are usually not available for small localities. Through studies of randomly collected samples, state health departments often conduct statewide surveys of health behaviors, for example, exercise, smoking, diet, physical examination frequency, and preventive dental care. The CDC also conducts a monthly telephone survey of a sample of adults, the Behavioral Risk Factor Surveillance System, which is done in every state (CDC, 2014). These data may or may not reflect the health behaviors of a specific community.

Original data collection from a total community or population is very expensive and time-consuming. Furthermore, questionnaires will usually need to be developed and tested, or located from other studies if the results are to be useful. Several questions put together by a team will usually not yield the desired results of reliable data.

**BOX 7.5   OUTLINE FOR ORGANIZING FINAL COMMUNITY
ASSESSMENT REPORT**

  I. Definition and description of the community
     A. Definition of *community*
        1. Formal definition
        2. Informal ways of defining *community*
     B. Description of community
        1. Physical or other boundaries
        2. Historical description of the community
     C. Description of larger community in which study community is located (e.g., county,
        state)
 II. Framework or model used to guide the community assessment
     A. Description of framework or model
     B. Rationale for use of the framework
     C. Relationship of community definition and framework
III. Methods of data collection
 IV. Sources of data
  V. Analysis of data
     A. Results of analysis by category of community assessment framework
     B. Comparison of community with larger community (e.g., state, country)
 VI. Synthesis of data
     A. Results of synthesis of data: community diagnoses
     B. Summary and conclusions

LOCATING ALTERNATIVE DATA SOURCES

Without good baseline data, the real need for a program or project cannot always be adequately documented and justified. This situation leaves the advanced practice public/community health nurse with an inadequate planning base and, thus, uncertainty about what to do next. Although the lack of data for a specific community or population cannot be totally offset, some alternative data sources may be useful for data needs.

Publications. Publications, such as *Healthy People 2020* (Office of Disease Prevention and Health Promotion, 2014), contain baseline data for the U.S. population as a whole; some baseline data are also provided for special population groups. These baseline markers are useful if no other data can be located. The caveat that data about the specific community are not available should be added to statements in which national data are used.

Surveys. In addition to statewide surveys, several large surveys are conducted on a national level by federal agencies, such as mentioned earlier and in Chapter 5. Although not specific to the local level, these surveys may be useful as a source for baseline data in writing objectives.

National surveys also provide the advanced practice public/community health nurse with cues about what to explore on the local level in terms of potential problems, trends, and other indicators of health status of the community. A review of one of the comprehensive data sources may serve as a beginning list of data categories to include in the data-collection plan. Chapter 5 has extensive references for comprehensive data sources, such as the Behavioral Risk Factor Surveillance System and surveys conducted by the National Center for Health Statistics. These types of sources are available on the Internet.

Other Community Assessments. A helpful document to review is a community or needs assessment compiled by the local health department, a local planning council, or a local hospital. Such documents may not be complete but provide a valuable beginning database. In addition, they may be useful in verifying subjective data and confirming data trends. If data are already available in a tabulated form, the team need not feel compelled to collect the same data from the original sources unless data accuracy is questioned.

Team Members' Ideas. Another resource for a beginning list of data sources is the team. Each team member is probably aware of some data sources and should be encouraged to contribute this information during early team meetings. A comprehensive list of data sources will take some time to develop and may require more than one team meeting for completion.

Organizing Data Collection

Once the pre-assessment plan is completed, the data collection may begin. Specific time allotted for data collection may be used more productively if telephone calls are made to be certain that documents are available. The data collector may need to make an appointment with a reference librarian in order to have some uninterrupted time to obtain information about the location of specific data. If data are being collected from public agencies, appointments with the appropriate persons will save valuable time and probably decrease frustration.

CONTACTING INDIVIDUALS

At times, individuals at public institutions do not promptly return telephone calls or the game of telephone tag goes on for days. This is especially frustrating when there is a short time period to complete a community assessment. Some alternative approaches to this dilemma may be helpful. Ask a secretary or receptionist if there is anyone else who may be able to help with the request. Often, there are others who know about or can locate data. Attempt to locate the data in written form whenever possible. A report, a news-paper article, a state document, or minutes of a meeting may contain the needed information. If the data are extremely important to the study, ask for assistance from someone in the individual's office or a colleague of the individual. In this day of many alternative modes of communication, some individuals are better able to respond to email requests, a list of questions sent and returned by fax, or a mailed survey with a postage-paid envelope enclosed.

At times, all attempts to obtain local information fail. If this situation results in less than an optimal report, a summary of the attempts to obtain information and data may be included in the community assessment report. State or national data may then be used to the extent possible.

Keep in mind that information or data obtained from an individual should be data or information that cannot be obtained elsewhere. Avoid the error of making an appointment to ask questions such as "what is the population of the county?" or "how many new cases of AIDS were reported last year?" Basic data about the population, morbidity, mortality, and environmental factors should be available in documents or on the Internet. Information to be obtained from individuals includes items such as what changes in services or the health status of the community are anticipated, what trends are being observed, what services need to be funded, and pending decisions that have not been documented. Although opinions are also part of a community assessment, you will want more than opinions about a topic in order to document a problem or a trend.

ONGOING DATA COLLECTION

A key aspect to remember when conducting a community assessment is that an assessment is a picture of a community at only one point in time. Just as people constantly change, communities are always changing. Ideally, a community assessment is a continuous process that is updated every week or month, if not every day. This is not practical, so the assessor should continue to collect data after the formal assessment is completed. With a file of current data, an updated assessment may be completed in less time than needed for the original one.

■ TRANSITION CITY: A COMMUNITY ASSESSMENT

The following community assessment is an example of the final product of the community assessment process, which uses the earlier outline for the report (Box 7.5). This is the type of report that may be included in a grant proposal as an appendix or provided to an interested group that does not desire or need the detail obtained to develop the community diagnoses. Data may be appended to the report for specific groups.

Data are fictitious but represent the type of situation that may be found in real communities. Chapter 8 provides information and examples of how to analyze and synthesize data in order to formulate community diagnoses.

Definition and Description of Transition City

A community is a group of people who develop relationships as they use institutions and agencies in a physical environment (Moe, 1977). Although community may imply that people have something in common, often there are numerous communities within one municipality. Transition City is one such community that contains subcommunities within the geographic boundaries.

Located on the western edge of the state along interstate route 60, Transition City is bounded on the north by the Northern Atlantic railroad, on the east by the interstate, on the west by the state border, and on the south by the Ohio River. The physical terrain is flat with the river providing the only variety in the topography.

In the mid-1800s, Transition City was settled by merchants from the eastern United States looking for trade routes to the west. After several decades of lackluster growth, the city became a major location for the manufacture of small appliances and components for automobiles.

Transition City has seen days of boom with a population of 82,525 in 2000, and days of gloomy economic state with the population dropping to 75,805 by 2005. Currently, Transition City is recovering from an adverse economic period that has lasted for 10 years. New businesses are moving into the area, and current businesses have seen an increase in profits in the past 2 years. A total recovery seems possible.

The people of Transition City are of primarily Anglo-Saxon extraction, with the newest residents being Hispanic and African American. The changes in the population mix have come about primarily as the economy has started to recover and more jobs, especially minimum wage jobs, have become available.

Transition City is the county seat for Pleasant County, which has a population of 300,100, and four other population centers. Pleasant County has also experienced a downturn in the economic state since the early 2000s and is also making an economic comeback.

Framework Used to Guide the Community Assessment

The epidemiologic triangle was used to guide the community assessment of Transition City. Specifically, the epidemiologic triangle indicates that the host, agent, and environment interact to result in disease or injury. This model is helpful for assessing the community of Transition City for several reasons. The many changes that the city is undergoing require a model that is dynamic and allows for the rapid examination of factors. Change creates stress, which may be examined by use of the epidemiologic triangle. The compatibility of the community definition given earlier and the epidemiologic triangle is another reason for using the model.

Methods of Data Collection

Both quantitative and qualitative methods of data collection were used. A windshield survey provided visual information about the city and its environs. The Internet, literature, and archival information were searched to begin the data collection. Interviews of five key informants were conducted in various community organizations. A face-to-face survey was also administered in three public locations to 50 people during the data collection period. A group interview was conducted in one elementary school and during one PTA meeting at the same school.

Sources of Data

A major source of data was literature. Census reports; history of the city; morbidity and mortality reports; reports of injuries, crimes, and arrests, especially for driving while intoxicated; and studies completed by other organizations (e.g., the Cancer Society, the United Fund) were included in the literature.

Key informants and city residents provided qualitative data of their perceptions of city life. Newspapers, local television and radio stations, and local publications provided depth to the data about community life.

Analysis of Data

The following brief summary of each category of the epidemiologic triangle provides the highlights of the data analysis.

HOST

The population of Transition City in 2000 was 52% females with a median age of 33.1 years. The population age composition at that time was as follows: 7% younger than 5 years; 47% between 20 and 64 years; and 11% 65 years and older. Sixty percent of the Transition City population has completed at least 12 years of school, which is higher than the county level of 55%.

The people of Transition City reflect the disease profile of the county and state with heart disease, cancer, and unintentional injuries as the three leading causes of death for adults. An examination of health behaviors shows that 24% of the population report smoking, 21% report exercising regularly, and 30% report diets composed of 30% fat or less. An unknown amount of alcohol and drug use is present in the adult and adolescent groups. An estimated 41% of the adult population is overweight.

AGENT

An agent is a factor essential for a disease to occur (Gordis, 2014). In Transition City, exposure of residents to a number of agents has resulted in diseases and injuries. The leading reportable diseases are gonorrhea, chlamydia, salmonella, and strep throat infection. The number of reported cases of tuberculosis has increased 2% per year in the past 4 years. Unintentional injuries and deaths from automobile crashes have also increased in the past 5 years. Automobile crashes are now the third leading cause of death in children aged 12 to 18 years.

ENVIRONMENT

An examination of the physical environment of Transition City reveals a clean appearance with little litter and trash. Some uncollected garbage was observed in the northeast section of the city. The river has a brown color, with an occasional fish seen breaking the water surface. A cleanup campaign over the past 5 years has improved the quality of the river water and increased the fish population.

Transition City is known for its strong support for families and schools. The social environment provides health and social services, as well as clubs, organizations, support groups for people with chronic conditions, and mental health services. The increase in non–English-speaking families has created a need for more translators in all city service agencies. In the past 5 years, the proportion of children in poverty has increased by 8% compared with a 5% increase for the county and 2% for the state.

The examination of the biological environment shows that 75% of children younger than 2 years are adequately immunized compared with 90% for the county. The number of people infected with HIV has increased from 0.2% in 2005 to 2%, though the county has the lowest infection rate of the state. In the past 2 years, infestations of rats have been found in two areas of the city.

Community Diagnoses

1. Risk of outbreaks of communicable diseases among children in Transition City related to a low immunization level (75% adequately immunized) in children younger than 2 years and the closing of a clinic for low-income families in the southeast section of the city, as demonstrated in five cases of measles reported in 2015, and 10 cases of pertussis diagnosed in the first 6 months of 2016.
2. Risk of HIV infection among sexually active people in Transition City related to unprotected sex and lack of knowledge about how HIV is transmitted, as demonstrated in an increasing level of HIV infection in the city population, 10% increase in sexually transmitted diseases in the past year, and a stable level of pregnancies among adolescents.
3. Risk of community stress among the residents and agencies of Transition City related to an increase in the diversity of the population, as demonstrated in a 50% increase in the Hispanic population and a 35% increase in the African American population in the past 5 years.
4. Support for families among residents of Transition City related to values and beliefs that place a priority on family life, as demonstrated in a 20% increase in donations to community organizations past year, funding for family services, an abundance of activities for families, and city ordinances that support family life.

Summary and Conclusions

An assessment of the community of Transition City was guided by the epidemiologic triangle. Methods of data collection included a windshield survey, literature searches, interviews of key informants, a survey of residents, interviews of children and parents, and Internet searches. Sources of data were literature, reports, media, archival information, and residents of Transition City.

From the analysis and synthesis of the data and information obtained, the areas that should be addressed are the low immunization rate among children aged 2 years and younger; the risk of transmission of HIV among sexually active members of the community; and the risk of stress on the community related to an increasingly diverse population. Dealing with the adverse situations described earlier will be easier because of the community strength of support for families.

■ SUMMARY

Planning and conducting a community assessment are important functions of the advanced practice public/community health nurse. This chapter presented information for using a framework or model to guide the community assessment process as well as a discussion of developing the pre-assessment plan.

Pre-assessment activities include developing the timeline for completing the assessment, estimating time and resources needed for the assessment, dividing the work among team members, requesting information, and identifying key informants. After completion of the pre-assessment activities, the data collection phase of the community assessment may begin. Organizing data collection by the framework or model provides a format for all team members to follow.

A brief community assessment was presented as an example of assembling the summary of data and information at the end of the data collection, data analysis, and data synthesis phases of the community assessment process. A community assessment report may be more elaborated than the example presented. Data analysis and synthesis are addressed in detail in Chapter 8 to demonstrate how community diagnoses are derived.

■ SUGGESTED CLINICAL OR PRACTICUM ACTIVITIES

1. Go online to locate a recent community assessment that was conducted by a local health department or nonprofit hospital in your region. Interview at least one healthcare professional responsible for conducting the assessment about the pre-assessment planning procedures.
2. Given the information gleaned in the preceding activity, ask about the roles of nurses and advanced public/community health nurses in particular in planning for the community assessment.
3. What community members or key stakeholders were engaged in the pre-assessment planning process? What was the rationale for selecting these individuals? How would an advanced public/community health nurses engage these community members in the process?

REFERENCES

American Nurses Association. (2013). *Public health nursing: Scope and standards of practice* (2nd ed.). Silver Spring, MD: Author.

American Psychological Association. (2010). *Publication manual of the American Psychological Association* (6th ed.). Washington, DC: Author.

Anderson, E. T., & McFarlane, J. (2015). *Community as partner: Theory and practice in nursing* (7th ed.). Philadelphia, PA: Wolters Kluwer Health.

Becker-Reems, E. D. (1994). *Self-managed work teams in health care organizations.* Chicago, IL: American Hospital Publishing.

Brannick, M. T., Salas, E., & Prince, C. (Eds.). (1997). *Team performance assessment and measurement: Theory, methods, and applications.* Mahwah, NJ: Lawrence Erlbaum Associates.

Centers for Disease Control and Prevention. (2014). Behavioral risk factor surveillance system. Retrieved from https://www.cdc.gov/brfss/

Centers for Disease Control and Prevention. (2015). Drivers of health assessment & improvement planning. Retrieved from https://www.cdc.gov/stltpublichealth/cha/drivers.html

Garner, H. G., & Orelove, F. P. (Eds.). (1994). *Teamwork in human services: Models and applications across the life span.* Newton, MA: Butterworth-Heinemann.

Gilchrist, A. (2009). *The well-connected community: A networking approach to community development* (2nd ed.). Bristol, UK: The Policy Press.

Gordis, L. (2014). *Epidemiology* (5th ed.). Baltimore, MD: Elsevier Saunders.

Grove, S. K., Burns, N., & Gray, J. R. (2013). *The practice of nursing research: Appraisal, synthesis and generation of evidence* (7th ed.). Philadelphia, PA: Saunders.

Jacobs, J. A., Jones, E., Gabella, B. A., Spring, B., & Brownson, R. C. (2012). Tools for implementing an evidence-based approach in public health practice. *Preventing Chronic Disease, 9,* 110324. doi:http://dx.doi.org/10.5888/pcd9.110324. Retrieved from https://www.cdc.gov/pcd/issues/2012/11_0324.htm

Krueger, R. A. (1988). *Focus groups: A practical guide for applied research.* Newbury Park, CA: Sage.

Levin, P. F., Cary, A. H., Kulbok, P., Leffers, J., Molle, M., & Polivka, B. J. (2008). Graduate education for advanced practice public health nursing: At the crossroads. *Public Health Nursing, 25*(2), 176–193.

Manion, J., Lorimer, W., & Leander, W. J. (1996). *Team-based health care organizations: Blueprint for success.* Gaithersburg, MD: Aspen.

Mears, P. (1994). *Healthcare teams: Building continuous quality improvement.* Delray Beach, FL: St. Lucie Press.

Minkler, M. (Ed.). (2012). *Community organizing and community building for health and welfare* (3rd ed.). New Brunswick, NJ: Rutgers University Press.

Moe, E. O. (1977). Nature of today's community. In A. M. Reinhardt & M. L. Quinn (Eds.), *Current practice in family-centered community nursing* (Vol. 1, pp. 117–137). St. Louis, MO: Mosby.

Office of Disease Prevention and Health Promotion. (2014). *Healthy people 2020* [Internet]. Washington, DC. Retrieved from https://www.healthypeople.gov

Patient Protection and Affordable Care Act, Public Law 111-148. (2010). *111th United States Congress.* Washington, DC: United States Government Printing Office. Retrieved from http://www.gpo.gov/fdsys/pkg/PLAW-111publ148/pdf/PLAW-111publ148.pdf

Public Health Accreditation Board. (2016). *Accredited health departments.* Retrieved from http://www.phaboard.org/news-room/accredited-health-departments

Rahn, D. J. (2016). Transformational teamwork: Exploring the impact of nursing teamwork on nurse-sensitive quality indicators. *Journal of Nursing Care Quality, 31*(3), 262–268.

Sawyer, L. M. (1995). Community participation: Lip service? *Nursing Outlook, 43,* 17–22.

Schifferdecker, K. E., Bazos, D. A., Sutherland, K. A., Ayers LaFave, L. R., Ruggles, L., Fedrizzi, R., & Hoebeke, J. (2016). A review of tools to assist hospitals in meeting community health assessment and implementation strategy requirements. *Journal of Healthcare Management, 61*(1), 44–56.

West, M. A. (2012). *Effective teamwork: Practical lessons from organizational research.* London, UK: Wiley-Blackwell.

Witkin, B. R., & Altschuld, J. W. (1995). *Planning and conducting needs assessments.* Thousand Oaks, CA: Sage.

CHAPTER 8

Community Diagnosis: Analysis and Synthesis of Data and Information

■ **STUDY EXERCISES**

> 1. What is a community diagnosis?
> 2. Why is it important to develop community diagnoses?
> 3. Compare and contrast community diagnoses, community needs, and community problems.
> 4. How are community diagnoses developed?
> 5. State one community diagnosis for the community you are assessing.

Effective community health programs almost always begin with community diagnoses that use data to accurately identify a community's health status and strengths. As early as 1970, Freeman asserted that community diagnosis was "the keystone of community health practice" (p. 252). A community diagnosis was more than mortality rates and the distribution of illness and disability in a community. Community diagnoses comprised broad community health goals, including quality of health, prevention and treatment, and the influence of ecological and psychological factors on health and healthcare (Freeman, 1970).

This chapter provides guidance for using the data and information acquired during the data-collection phase of the community assessment process. However, the steps to developing community diagnoses remain somewhat ambiguous. Also, there are no taxonomies or comprehensive lists of community diagnoses, as with nursing diagnoses (Herdman & Kamitsuru, 2014; Martin, 2005). However, diagnoses that address a total community have been added to the North American Nursing Diagnosis Association (NANDA) list (Herdman & Kamitsuru, 2014) and the Omaha System (Martin, 2005). Community diagnoses will continue to be added as nurses work to meet the process required for testing diagnoses.

The guidance provided in this chapter will help you to establish a systematic approach to data analysis and synthesis—both complex processes. With practice, you will be able to state community diagnoses that accurately reflect data collected from a variety of sources and by various methods.

■ DEFINITION OF COMMUNITY DIAGNOSIS

To diagnose is to critically analyze the nature of something and to reach a conclusion by such an analysis. Thus, a *community diagnosis* is a hypothesis or statement of the outcome of the analysis and synthesis of the data and information acquired during data collection about a community. Community diagnoses were described in nursing as statements of risks to the population, conditions, trends, potential problems, strengths, or latent situations (Watson, 1984). Community diagnoses provide comprehensive snapshots of the condition of the community in a coherent way (Higgs & Gustafson, 1985). These snapshots are taken at one point in time, so community diagnoses require periodic updating.

Community diagnoses are stated so as to recognize that health and illness are multivariate phenomena, so solutions require that the various aspects of the diagnosis be identified before action can be taken. Risk factors, related characteristics of the environment, and other variables are bundled into the diagnostic statements so that a comprehensive picture of a situation is apparent. Causes need not be included in community diagnoses because causes are not always known or discovered during the community assessment. However, after you have completed the community assessment and are ready to plan the program, the first step will be to examine the causes or possible causes of a given diagnosis.

The following community diagnosis is an example of a risk to the population:

> Risk of contracting tuberculosis among residents of Blake County is related to (a) immigrants and refugees residing in the county not screened for tuberculosis; (b) incomplete treatment of individuals diagnosed with tuberculosis; and (c) 15% of known TB cases being HIV coinfected last year, as demonstrated in (a) a rate of tuberculosis of 13.7 per 100,000 compared with a rate of 8.2 for the Midwest region; (b) an increase of 20% in cases of tuberculosis in people ages 25 to 29 years in 2013; and (c) three new tuberculosis cases reported in children ages 5 years and younger during the first 6 months of 2015.

In addition to developing statements of adverse situations, the advanced practice public/community health nurse needs to generate diagnoses that show the assets or strengths of a community. The community uses these assets to solve problems, prevent problems, and develop solutions to fit the situation. An example of a community diagnosis that demonstrates an asset is as follows:

> Community cohesion among residents of Blake County related to (1) history of racial harmony and (2) use of mechanisms for peaceful resolution of conflicts, as demonstrated in (a) a reduction in the last 6 months by 20% in the incidence of physical fighting among adolescents aged 14 to 17 years; (b) a 10% decrease in the number of assaults in the past year; and (c) two new coalitions formed to deal with drug use in the community.

Distinguishing Between Community Diagnoses and Nursing Diagnoses

The concept of nursing diagnosis was first applied to nursing practice in care of an individual in 1950 (Miller & Keane, 1983). Nowadays, the use of nursing diagnoses is standard practice in most areas of nursing. Physicians originated the idea of community diagnosis in the 1950s (McGavran, 1956). In 1970, Freeman proposed that "The basis of community health action must be an accurate assessment of the state of health of the community as a whole" (p. 252). Freeman's ideas from 1970 are still relevant for nursing practice; however, community diagnoses did not have widespread use in public/community health nursing until the late 1980s (e.g., Anderson & McFarlane, 1988).

Nurses who use community diagnoses and nursing diagnoses follow a similar pattern of steps to arrive at conclusions, that is, collect data, analyze the data, and state the conclusion as a diagnosis (Herdman & Kamitsuru, 2014; Muecke, 1984). However, the two statements differ in several ways. Community diagnoses address a community, population, or aggregate, whereas nursing diagnoses generally deal with individuals or families who live within a community.

Community diagnoses differ from nursing diagnoses in other ways. Work with a community is often more effective with an interdisciplinary team, so community diagnoses are more general than nursing diagnoses. Many conditions and situations are included in community diagnoses that may require more than nursing interventions to solve. For example, the presence of paint containing lead is important to be explored when assessing a community, but the advanced practice public/community health nurse may not be the person to complete all the activities necessary to resolve the situation. Inspection of living quarters and initiation of plans for abatement of the sources of lead in the house may be more appropriately performed by environmental health or housing personnel. The role of public/community health nursing in the prevention and resolution of lead poisoning is primarily in activities of case finding, screening, teaching, and referral. Thus, the team members working together are important for protecting the health of a community.

Another difference between nursing diagnoses and community diagnoses is the way in which they are stated. Several approaches to stating community diagnoses are provided in the literature (Anderson & McFarlane, 2015; Helvie, 1998; Martin, 2005; Muecke, 1984). Some authors have provided examples that use a format like that of NANDA (Higgs & Gustafson, 1985). Although there is not one accepted format for stating community diagnoses, some approaches are more comprehensive than others. Later in this chapter, a suggested format and wording are presented that follow the examples provided earlier (Muecke, 1984). Two additional formats (Anderson & McFarlane, 2015; Helvie, 1998) are discussed.

A summary of the comparisons between nursing diagnoses and community diagnoses is presented in Table 8.1. One major difference is the interdisciplinary practice nature of community diagnoses as compared with a focus on nursing practice of nursing diagnoses. A second major difference is the focus of the content. Community diagnoses deal with

TABLE 8.1 Comparison of Community Diagnosis and Nursing Diagnosis

Characteristic	Community Diagnosis	Nursing Diagnosis
Definition	Statements of risk, condition, trend, potential problem, strength, or latent situation about a community or population (Watson, 1984)	"A clinical judgment about individual, family, or community responses to actual or potential health problems/life process" (NANDA, 1999, p. 651)
Client focus	Aggregate, community, population	Usually individual, group, family; may be community
Process followed	Analyze data, synthesize data, state conclusion with supporting data	Analyze data; identify health problems, risks, and strengths; and formulate diagnostic statements (Kozier, Erb, Berman, & Burke, 2000)
Nature of content	Health status of community/ population related to multiple determinants; usually interdisciplinary	Usually conditions about health or illness of individual addressed by nursing interventions
Format	Anderson and McFarlane (2015), Helvie (1998), Muecke (1984)	NANDA nursing diagnoses (1999), Omaha System (Martin, 2005)

communities, populations, or aggregates, whereas nursing diagnoses deal primarily with individuals or families.

■ IMPORTANCE OF FORMULATING COMMUNITY DIAGNOSES

In addition to the importance of community diagnoses as the basis for professional practice, formulating community diagnoses is important for several reasons. Community diagnoses help you to focus efforts for the improvement of a community's health, establish boundaries around a problem or situation, define a problem or situation using data, and provide a common understanding of the problem or situation so that team members and others can work more efficiently toward a common goal.

Focusing Efforts

After formulating community diagnoses, the advanced practice public/community health nurse is more likely to focus efforts on defined circumstances instead of vague adverse community situations (Watson, 1984). A well-formulated community diagnosis provides an initial direction for the exploration of causes of an adverse situation, trend, or strength.

Establishing Boundaries

It is often difficult to avoid addressing all the identified adverse situations during program planning and other activities based on community assessments. A community diagnosis assists the advanced practice public/community health nurse to be clear about the boundaries being addressed in a particular diagnosis. Indeed, if the community diagnosis is not written clearly, the nurse will discover that more work needs to be done before program planning can begin. One example of a boundary is the age group being addressed in the diagnosis. Other examples of boundaries are geographic, cultural, conditions such as unemployment, and situations such as community conflict.

Defining the Situation

A community diagnosis provides a beginning level of organized information about a situation that is usually not available elsewhere. Often, health workers begin to solve a problem or address a situation without an adequate statement of the problem or situation. Thus, programs planned for inadequately identified adverse situations often fail to resolve the concern. In addition, programs that do not include features to address the characteristics of the community often fail to reach the desired objectives. For example, a health-promotion program designed to reach adults who work during the day will unlikely be successful without evening and weekend hours or components offered at worksites.

Providing a Common Understanding

Another reason to formulate community diagnoses is that they allow for a common understanding of a situation before program planning tasks are begun. In interdisciplinary teamwork, a common understanding is especially important. Health team members have varied educational preparation, so terms and words do not always have the same meaning to everyone. Use of a common language for community diagnoses will facilitate communication and effective team functioning. At the very least, a written community diagnosis allows all team members equal access to the same information.

■ DIFFERENTIATING AMONG COMMUNITY DIAGNOSES, COMMUNITY NEEDS, AND COMMUNITY PROBLEMS

In the literature on community diagnoses, terms are used interchangeably for the same concept, for example, *community need* and *community problem*. This section provides an overview of the differences among community diagnoses, community needs, and community problems.

Community Needs

Much of the literature on community assessment addresses needs and/or discusses needs assessment. A *need* is defined as a gap or a discrepancy between the current state of a community or group and "what should be," that is, a desired state (Witkin & Altschuld, 1995). A needs assessment is structured to determine what the gaps are, to examine their nature and causes, and to set priorities (Witkin & Altschuld, 1995).

Another definition of need is what is required to close the gap between what the situation is now and the desired state (Witkin & Altschuld, 1995). For example, if the percentage of women who begin prenatal care in the first trimester is less than the objective for the year 2020 (Office of Disease Prevention and Health Promotion, 2014), the need is the action or activity required to increase the level of early prenatal care.

DETERMINING THE DESIRED STATE AND CLOSING THE GAP

After the gap is determined, the assessor still does not know what will close the gap. In order to determine what will close the gap, questions must be posed and answered, such as: Why are women not starting prenatal care in the first trimester? The answers to this question are probably multiple, for example, lack of access, not enough services, or no need seen for prenatal care.

Determining what is the desired state requires additional decision making. For example, if a gap exists between the current infant mortality rate of a county and the state, is the infant mortality rate of the state the "desired state"? We have health objectives for the United States, so should the desired state be the *Healthy People 2020* objective (Office of Disease Prevention and Health Promotion, 2014)? Although the national objective may be desirable, communities may need to move in increments from their current levels to that of the national goals. For example, the infant mortality target for 2020 is 4.5 deaths per 1,000 live births. A community that has an infant mortality rate of 9 will not be able to decrease the rate by 50% in a short time period. The desired state may be a rate of 6 in 5 years and then the objective of 4.5 in the next 5 years.

On the basis of what you determine is the desired state, you must next ask what program, intervention, or other activity will close the gap between the county and state infant mortality rates. These questions must be answered through the use of additional steps of the planning process, which is discussed in Section III of this book.

PURPOSES FOR CONDUCTING NEEDS ASSESSMENTS

Needs assessments are often conducted for very specific and targeted purposes, for example, as a prerequisite for receiving funding for a targeted problem. Usually, a problem or situation is already identified that requires an assessment to confirm certain hypotheses or directions for a program. The steps used to design a needs assessment include identifying stakeholders, listing expectations, identifying the importance of the findings, and designing the study (Soriano, 2013). The advanced practice public/community health nurse may be called upon to conduct a needs assessment. It is important to keep in mind that a needs assessment and community assessment use different processes and have different outcomes.

DIFFERENTIATING BETWEEN NEEDS AND COMMUNITY ASSESSMENTS

In comparison with a needs assessment, a community assessment is conducted to determine the health status of a community. The causes of the adverse situations identified in the community diagnoses are explored after the community assessment is completed and as a separate step in advanced practice. The gap may become apparent during the analysis and synthesis processes of the community assessment, but what will close the gap will not be apparent until you gain input from the community and the literature. Also, the authors take the position that the professional does not have all the answers of "what should be." The community has an important stake in determining the desired results. The community needs to be involved in setting priorities for future action.

Community diagnoses also describe assets or strengths, so no action may be required after the diagnosis is stated. Community diagnoses as summary statements about a community provide information required to understand and work with a community on its priorities.

Community Problems

In contrast to a need, a problem is a specific current situation or condition, such as a high death rate due to automobile crashes or new cases of tuberculosis, that people feel should no longer be tolerated or need no longer exist (Blum, 1981). Early descriptions of nursing assessment of community health frequently referred to community problems, problem analysis, and problem prioritization (Goeppinger, 1984). We often think of problems when writing community diagnoses because problems need to be solved, a process much practiced by nurses.

DIFFERENTIATING BETWEEN COMMUNITY DIAGNOSES AND PROBLEMS

A community diagnosis does not always present a problem or imply a solution. The description of the health status of a community gives the advanced practice public/community health nurse an idea of the current state of affairs but does not give answers to what should be done, if anything, to change the current state of affairs.

The community-diagnosis approach requires that the nurse change orientation from trying to provide immediate solutions to gaining an in-depth understanding of the community. The advanced practice public/community health nurse is unable to provide the leadership required to plan with a community to address the conditions or situations that the community wants to address without a depth of understanding. The application of the community assessment process, as presented in Section II of this book, provides you with much of the in-depth knowledge to function competently in working with communities.

The solution-minded approach often results in the wrong solution or one that is not adequate to resolve the situation or prevent the situation from getting worse. For example, the conclusion that a lack of services is the reason for a low immunization rate among preschool children may result in more services being offered without an increase in immunization rates. Often, the lack of immunizations among children is a combination of factors such as parents' perceptions that immunizations are not needed until children go to school, inconvenient service hours, and inadequate income of parents. More than one approach or intervention may be needed to address the situation of inadequate immunization levels in preschool children.

We may often think of needs and problems as negative statements about communities. Diagnoses also usually carry negative connotations, for example, cancer and hypertension. However, the term *diagnosis* is widely used in several professions as summary statements about a person's or community's situation. In addition, community diagnoses are not always negative, as has been mentioned earlier.

COMMUNITY DIAGNOSES AS HYPOTHESES

Community diagnoses are also hypotheses. Hypotheses are formal statements about the expected relationships between two or more factors in a given population (Grove, Burns, & Gray, 2013). Hypotheses are premises about a situation, not proven conclusions. However, hypotheses require data to support the stated premises. For example, nurses often identify a lack of knowledge about some self-care topic in individuals or families as a nursing diagnosis. If this diagnosis, lack of knowledge, were to be stated as a community diagnosis, the nurse would need to have a basis to posit such a conclusion. If a survey of a community, population, or aggregate had demonstrated lack of knowledge, then such a diagnosis could be justified. Often, though, the conclusion of lack of knowledge is reached without any data and based only on the assessor's assumption.

Moreover, from research into human behavior, we know that human behavior is very complex and not just the result of knowledge of a topic (Dignan & Carr, 1992; Glanz, Rimer, & Viswanath, 2015). Community diagnoses need to reflect this complexity of our current state of knowledge about human behavior as well as the community as a whole.

Furthermore, a hypothesis is never really proved or disproved, but a research study can provide support for a specific conclusion (Grove et al., 2013). A community diagnosis may be considered in a similar way. If a program developed to address a specific community diagnosis is successful in solving or improving the condition, the nurse has some proof that the hypothetical situation described in the community diagnosis was valid.

Although community diagnoses may be worded as potential disease states (e.g., risk of contracting tuberculosis), the primary goals of advanced public/community health nursing practice are the prevention of disease and injury and the promotion of health. A focus on the relationship of multiple factors and determinants of health is necessary to carry out activities to reach the practice goals. In the case of risk of contracting tuberculosis, the nurse would concentrate on identifying the causative factors for the spread of tuberculosis among the community and the characteristics of those who are at risk of contracting tuberculosis.

The advanced practice public/community health nurse is obligated to develop a balanced view of all aspects of a community to avoid branding communities as needy and problem-ridden, especially low-income communities (McKnight & Kretzmann, 2012). Knowledge of talents, strengths, skills, and abilities of community residents and the community is a necessity for the nurse who is committed to assisting a community to reach and maintain a healthy state.

■ ANALYZING AND SYNTHESIZING DATA FROM MULTIPLE SOURCES

Processes of both analysis and synthesis are needed to formulate community diagnoses. Analysis is the intellectual separation of some concept or item into parts for study. Synthesis is the combination of separate elements or parts into a coherent whole (Bloom, 1956).

Although the two processes, analysis and synthesis, are not two entirely separate mental operations, they will be treated separately to give a clearer explanation of each.

The ability to conduct analysis and synthesis at a comprehensive level requires more knowledge than can be provided in one textbook. This discussion is a beginning point so that application can be made in the clinical setting and in classroom exercises. Moreover, public/community health nursing is in its adolescence in terms of how to formulate community diagnoses. Although some scholars have been working to include community diagnoses in the taxonomy of nursing diagnoses since the 1990s (e.g., Neufeld & Harrison, 1990), this work is still in the beginning stages. Most community nursing diagnoses have not been tested for reliability and validity, nor have they been used extensively for community interventions (Helvie, 1998). However, with the implementation of the Patient Protection and Affordable Care Act (ACA, 2010) and the focus on community health assessment and population health, the Centers for Disease Control and Prevention (CDC, 2013) has reported on advances in metrics for population health outcomes, and risk and protective factors, over the past three decades. These metrics are useful to advanced practice public/community health nurses and their community partners when describing the health of a community and driving community health improvements. See Table 8.2 for recommended community health metrics.

■ ANALYZING DATA FROM MULTIPLE SOURCES

A sense of being overwhelmed is a common feeling after the data-collection step of the community assessment process is completed. An approach to deal with the volume of data is needed. One such approach is described here.

SEQUENTIAL APPROACH TO DATA ANALYSIS

The suggested approach to data analysis is to read through each category of data from the community assessment notebook or electronic filing system suggested in Chapter 7. From this examination, you are attempting to glean the most important points of a data set. The highlights of each category may be outlined on paper or in e-files as the analysis continues. Some examples from categories of data follow.

Demographic and Social Data. Almost all community assessment frameworks or models contain a category about the characteristics of the people who make up a community. Demographic and social characteristics include age, gender, race, education, income and poverty level of a defined population (see Table 8.2 for additional characteristics). These characteristics have standard definitions, so they may be compared reliably across various geopolitical entities (e.g., cities, counties, and states).

The advanced practice public/community health nurse will determine the characteristics of the population as a whole, for example, the age structure, percentage of each gender, and change in the racial composition when examining the demographic and social data of a community. Examples of questions used to address demographic data are given in Box 8.1.

A second step of this examination is to compare statistics for at least two points in time, for example, the last two decennial censuses. Comparison at two points in time allows for examination of trends, changes, and potential areas for continued close monitoring. Sample questions to be answered for this comparison are displayed in Box 8.2.

Comparing the community demographics with the next larger governmental entity, for example, county or state, is another step to be completed in the data analysis. The

TABLE 8.2 Community Health Assessment for Population Health Improvement: Most Frequently Recommended Health Metrics

Heath Outcome Metrics		Health Determinant and Correlate Metrics			
Mortality	**Morbidity**	**Healthcare (Access and Quality)**	**Health Behaviors**	**Demographics and Social Environment**	**Physical Environment**
Leading causes of death	Obesity	Health insurance coverage	Tobacco use/smoking	Age	Air quality
Infant mortality	Low birth weight	Provider rates	Physical activity	Gender	Water quality
Injury-related mortality	Hospital utilization	Asthma-related hospitalization	Nutrition	Race/ethnicity	Housing
Motor vehicle mortality	Cancer rates		Unsafe sex	Income	
Suicide, homicide	Motor vehicle injury		Alcohol use	Poverty level	
	Overall health status		Seatbelt use	Educational attainment	
	STDs		Immunizations and screenings	Employment status	
	AIDS			Foreign born	
	Tuberculosis			Homelessness	
				Language spoken at home	
				Marital status	
				Domestic violence and child abuse	
				Violence and crime	
				Social capital/ social support	

STDs, sexually transmitted diseases.
Source: Centers for Disease Control and Prevention. (2013). *Community health assessment for population health improvement: Resource of most frequently recommended health outcomes and determinants.* Atlanta, GA: Office of Surveillance, Epidemiology, and Laboratory Services.

comparison is important to provide the nurse with points of reference about how different from or similar a community is to the larger community of which it is a part. In addition, the comparison with the larger entity provides some perspective about the magnitude of changes. One example of this is the change in the number of elderly in the population. Using U.S. Census data, the Rural Health Information Hub (2018) reported that in general, rural-dwelling populations are older than populations residing in other parts of

---

BOX 8.1 SAMPLE QUESTIONS ABOUT THE DEMOGRAPHIC COMPOSITION OF A COMMUNITY

1. What is the total population?
2. What is the age structure of the community; that is, how many people and what percentage of the population are in each age group?
3. What is the gender structure of the community; that is, how many males and females are there in the total population, how many males and females are there in each age group, and what percentage is each of these numbers?
4. What is the racial composition of the community (number and percentage in each category)?

BOX 8.2 SAMPLE QUESTIONS ABOUT THE COMPARISON OF CENSUS DATA FROM TWO TIME PERIODS

1. What is the pattern of population change over the 10-year period (or other time period)? Has the population increased? If so, how much (number and percentage)? Has the population decreased? If so, how much (number and percentage)? Has the population stayed the same?
2. How has the age structure changed over the 10-year period?
3. How has the gender structure changed?
4. What changes have occurred in the racial and ethnic compositions of the community over the two periods?

---

the country. Moreover, populations of older adults increase by the degree of rurality. An example of a comparison of a county and state demographic profile for two census points is given in Table 8.3.

Another approach to use in analyzing demographic data is to construct a population pyramid (Anderson & McFarlane, 2015). A population pyramid is a bar graph that displays the age and gender composition of a population (Figure 8.1). If pyramids are constructed for two periods in time and/or for the county and state, visual changes in the population structure are readily apparent in the differences in the sizes of the bars for each age and gender group.

Vital Statistics. Another area of data that is part of most community assessment frameworks is vital statistics, which provide data about births, deaths, marriages, and divorces. As pointed out in epidemiology, raw data are more useful when converted into rates that provide a standardized way of comparing one population with another. An example of comparison of vital statistics for Blake County and New York State is given in Table 8.4. To gain a view of trends, data from several time points are needed.

Examples of questions to address in analyzing vital statistics are provided in Box 8.3. Answers to such questions assist you to focus your examination of a large amount of data. Foundational knowledge in demographics, epidemiology, biostatistics, and other sciences

TABLE 8.3 Demographic Characteristics of Blake County and New York State for 2010 and 2015

	Blake County[a]		New York State	
	2010	2015	2010	2015 *(Estimated)*
	Number/Percentage		Number/Percentage	
Total Age	59,075/100	60,517/100	19,378,102/100	19,673,174/100
Younger than 5	3,467/5.9	3,813/6.3	1,155,822/6.0	1,176,432/6.0
5–14	7,988/13.5	7,956/13.1	2,375,411/12.3	2,329,969/11.8
15–19	7,144/12.1	5,899/9.7	1,410,935/7.1	1,293,794/6.6
20–34	14,936/25.3	14,157/23.4	4,070,272/21.0	4,240,796/21.6
35–54	11,152/18.9	14,317/23.7	5,488,708/28.3	5,347,972/27.2
55–64	5,901/10	5,250/8.7	2,303,668/11.9	2,463,776/12.5
65+	8,487/14.4	9,107/15	2,617,943/13.5	2,820,435/14.3
Gender				
Female	31,006/52.5	31,653/52.3	10,000,955/51.6	10,131,373/51.5
Male	28,069/47.5	28,864/47.7	9,377,147/48.4	9,541,801/48.5
Race				
White	58,283/98.7	59,111/97.7	13,155,274/67.9	13,131,658/66.7
Black	355/0.6	810/1.3	3,334,550/17.2	3,344,602/17.0
Asian	207/0.4	316/0.5	1,579,494/8.2	1,733,149/8.8
American Indian	70/0.1	116/0.2	221,058/1.1	193,357/1.0
Other	160/0.3	164/0.3	1,720,811/8.9	1,880,258/9.5

[a]Not an actual county. Figures are adapted from a county in New York State.
Source: U.S. Census Bureau, American Factfinder. (n.d.). *Community facts*. Retrieved from https://factfinder.census.gov/faces/nav/jsf/pages/community_facts.xhtml

will provide you with more direction for formulating questions for your particular study community.

Other Framework Categories of Data. As the analysis continues through each category of the assessment framework, the nurse will notice areas that are very different from previous years' statistics and the state or national statistics. For example, the county crime rate may be decreasing faster than the state rate, or the county unemployment rate may be low compared with the state rate. These are areas for inclusion in potential community diagnoses. A list of the most outstanding differences or changes should be compiled for later use in synthesizing data.

The analysis may be concluded when the major findings are summarized by category of the assessment framework. The summary should be done in a narrative format as well as with table, graphs, figures, and other visual summaries as desired. There are no rules about when completion of the analysis is achieved, but comparison of one's findings with other assessments may be helpful in the beginning stages of learning to conduct an assessment.

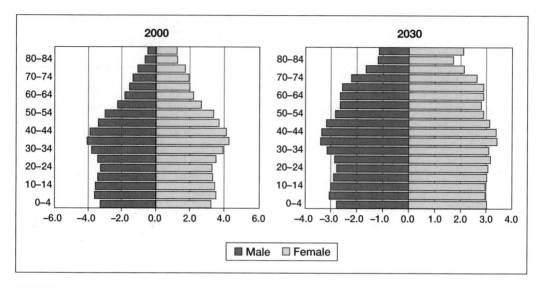

FIGURE 8.1   Population pyramids of New York State.

Source: Scardamalia, R. (2008). *New York State demographic trends.* New York State Office for the Aging, Department of State. Retrieved from https://aging.ny.gov/livableny/Documents/NewYorkStateDemographicTrends.pdf

Synthesizing Data From Multiple Sources

Analysis of all data need not be completed before synthesis is begun. Often, you will use an iterative process, going back and forth between the processes, as more questions arise. The data are collected in separate categories of the framework or model, so the tendency is to look at isolated bits of data. However, as in formulating nursing diagnoses, individual pieces of data must be put together in order to see a larger picture (Muecke, 1984). For example, if a patient complained of a distended abdomen to one nurse, no bowel movement for 2 days to the nurse's aide, and loss of appetite to a family member, but no one person knew all the symptoms, the nursing diagnosis of

TABLE 8.4 Vital Statistics for Blake County and New York State for 2014

Event	County	Rate	State	Rate
Live births	662	10.8[a]	238,000	12.1[a]
Deaths	568	9.2[a]	147,482	7.5[a]
Infant deaths	3	4.5[b]	1,068	4.5[b]
Marriages	432	7.0[a]	139,687	7.1[a]
Divorces	196	3.2[a]	57,245	2.9[a]

[a]Rate per 1,000 population.
[b]Rate per 1,000 live births.
Source: New York State Department of Health. (2016). Annual report of vital statistics of New York State 2014. Retrieved from https://www.health.ny.gov/statistics/vital_statistics/docs/vital_statistics_annual_report_2014.pdf

---

BOX 8.3   SAMPLE QUESTIONS FOR ANALYZING VITAL STATISTICS

1. What are the trends in live births for the county and the state (e.g., increasing, decreasing, or remaining stable)? If there are changes, what are the magnitudes of the changes?
2. What changes have occurred in infant death rates since the early 2000s?
3. How do the infant death rates differ for the county, the state, and the nation?
4. What patterns of change are seen in deaths at the county, state, and national levels?
5. How many marriages and divorces are there each year? What is the rate for each?

---

constipation may not be readily reached. A similar situation exists with a community diagnosis.

CONSTANT COMPARISON APPROACH TO DATA SYNTHESIS

One approach to data synthesis, constant comparison, may be useful. Using this approach, the nurse begins with a complete reading of all material collected for the assessment. Next, the nurse examines the data in each assessment framework category for data that fit with data from another category. For example, the educational level of the population is related to several health status measures such as trimester for starting prenatal care, smoking level, and obesity (Catholic Health Association of the United States, 2013; Glanz et al., 2015).

Related pieces of information must be located and pulled together in order to form community diagnoses. The fact that the infant mortality is 14 deaths per 1,000 live births does not constitute a community diagnosis of "a high infant mortality rate." Data about the areas of the community that are related to infant mortality (e.g., low birth weight, low income, inadequate prenatal care, smoking in pregnant women) need to be put together, or synthesized, to view the situation more completely. In addition, a diagnosis of risk of death among infants in Blake County is a preferred wording because interventions will be directed at the infants who are alive and those not yet born.

Once the area of a tentative community diagnosis is identified, such as risk of death among infants, related factors are identified for the specific community. Without previous knowledge of risk factors, the nurse will need to rely on literature to become familiar with some areas. For some diseases and injuries, such as leukemia, the risk factors or related factors are not known.

For some diseases, all causes are not known, for example, breast cancer. What this means, of course, is that we cannot prevent them. In these instances, the nurse is interested in the risk factors and health behaviors of the target population in order to focus programs for screening and early detection or secondary prevention (Leavell & Clarke, 1965). Factors related to increasing screening and early detection of breast cancer are found in the various categories of data. Within the demographic data, the number of women at risk by age may be found as well as the change in numbers over time. Dietary habits of the population, rates of obesity, alcohol intake, and other factors or characteristics related to breast cancer may be found in other categories of the community assessment framework.

After identifying the factors related to the risk, trend, situation, or condition, data that support the hypothesis are identified. In the example of breast cancer, the number of deaths from breast cancer is one piece of supportive data. Another is the number of women receiving a mammogram. This piece of data is pertinent because women who have not been screened are at risk for not having a cancer detected and treated early. A community diagnosis is a statement that brings together the related factors and the supportive data. This approach is explained and demonstrated in the following section.

Writing a Community Diagnosis

The format for stating community diagnoses is adapted from the work of Muecke (1984). Using this approach, a community diagnosis has four elements:

1. The conclusion of data analysis and synthesis stated as a hypothesis about an adverse situation or status, strength, trend, weakness, potential problem, or risk
2. Description of the population, community, aggregate, or group to which the conclusion applies; connected to the statement of the hypothesis with the word *among*
3. Social, environmental, cultural, economic, and other associated characteristics of the community or aggregate related to the conclusion; linked to the community description by the phrase *related to*
4. Indicators that the adverse situation or status, strength, trend, weakness, risk, or potential problem exist; linked to the associated characteristics by the phrase *as demonstrated in*

An example of a community diagnosis follows:

Risk of death *among* infants born in the Smithville community *related to* (a) 12% of infants had low birth weight (less than 2,500 g) in 2015; (b) 24% of births in 2015 were to females aged 18 years and younger; (c) 46% of the female population had incomes below the poverty level in 2015; and (d) 20% of women in 2015 had inadequate prenatal care (started after the first trimester or had an inadequate number of visits) as *demonstrated in* (a) an infant mortality rate of 12 deaths per 1,000 live births in 2015; (b) infant mortality rate of 7 for the White population and 16 for the African American population in 2015; and (c) neonatal infant mortality rate of 14 and postneonatal rate of 5 in 2015, which have increased by 10% over the past 10 years.

Using the format adapted from Muecke (1984), the first part of the diagnosis, "risk of death," is the potential adverse situation. The second part of the diagnosis (i.e., among) describes the aggregate of who is at risk. This could be specified more narrowly, such as in a more specific location of Smithville or for only postneonatal infants. If a different aggregate is used, data related to the specific aggregate should be used rather than data for the total community. The third element of the community diagnosis provides the characteristics of the community or population "related to" the risk or trend. In the last element of the diagnosis, the indicators that the situation exists are listed (i.e., as demonstrated in). All four elements together form the community diagnosis.

VARIATIONS ON WORDING AND FORMAT

The format previously suggested is appropriate for most community assessment frameworks and models. However, some modifications in wording will be needed to accommodate the conceptual and theoretical approaches of some frameworks.

Community-as-Partner Format. Anderson and McFarlane (2015) used the phrase *related to* for linking the etiological statement to the descriptive statement (i.e., a potential or actual community health problem or concern). They use *as manifested by* to indicate signs and symptoms of a diagnosis and to indicate the duration and magnitude of the problem. This phrase is similar to *as demonstrated in* as used in the suggested community diagnosis format to indicate that the adverse situation exists. An example of a community diagnosis stated in the community-as-partner framework is as follows.

High prevalence of dental caries among youngsters at Temple Elementary School in Rosemont, is *related to* the following:
- Lack of dental assessment and treatment at the Third Street Clinic
- Lack of fluoride in Rosemont's drinking water
- Low median household income and associated limited economic resources for purchasing dental care
- No dental hygiene education offered at Temple Elementary

As manifested by the following:
- No dental program at the Third Street Clinic
- City of Hampton does not have naturally occurring fluoride in the water and does not add fluoride to the water supply
- Median income is $28,247
- No health education programs are offered at Temple Elementary (Anderson & McFarlane, 2015, p. 230)

Helvie's Energy Theory. Helvie's (1998) approach to stating community diagnoses requires the use of the phrase *community energy deficit* or *community energy balance*. These phrases are reflective of his energy theory used as a framework for community assessment. Helvie used the phrase *due to*, which is similar to *related to*, and *resulting in* is similar to *as demonstrated in*. An example of a community diagnosis stated in Helvie's energy theory is as follows:

There is a community energy balance related to the employment of the adult population, due to the community's ability to provide adequate employment resulting in (a) a high percentage of the population working; (b) a low percentage of poor families; (c) a low percentage of the population below poverty level; (d) a high median income; (e) a high percentage of more affluent families; and (f) low unemployment. (Helvie, 1998, p. 227)

These examples are not meant to imply that all community assessment frameworks are the same, but only to provide a guide for drawing some parallels for using various theoretical foundations in advanced practice. Box 8.4 contains a summary of the comparisons among the three approaches to stating community diagnoses.

Diagnoses Related to Disease

The delineation of the four parts of the community diagnosis previously listed (Muecke, 1984) is applicable for other diagnoses. For the breast cancer example stated earlier, a community diagnosis is as follows.

Risk of death from breast cancer among women aged 50 years and older in Blake County *related to* (a) 42% of women are obese; (b) 10% of women have a family history of breast cancer; and (c) 15% of women aged 50 years and older were screened for

BOX 8.4   COMPARISON OF COMMUNITY DIAGNOSIS APPROACHES

Approach	Conclusion (e.g., Potential or Current Problem, Strength, Trend)	Description of Population or Aggregate	Characteristics of Population or Community	Indicators of Conclusion
Muecke (1984)	Risk of or presence of	Among	Related to	As demonstrated in
Anderson and McFarlane (2015)	Potential or actual health problem or concern	Among	Related to	As manifested by
Helvie (1998)	Community energy deficit or community energy balance	Not always stated explicitly	Due to	Resulting in

breast cancer in 2015, as *demonstrated in* a cancer death rate of 22.7 per 100,000 in Blake County, which is 10% above the national baseline for 2010.

When using any format for stating community diagnoses, explicit data should be provided as often as possible, as shown earlier. Other formats state the author's conclusions about the data (e.g., high rate of obesity), but data provide objective measures to the community diagnosis. In addition, these data make it possible for the community to decide whether the rates are too high, too low, or just right. We, as professionals, have standards and criteria to follow, but community members use their own standards and values to make decisions about what concerns are important.

Diagnoses Related to Community Strengths

Risk of contracting a disease is one area for the development of community diagnoses; several other areas should be explored. As mentioned earlier, community assets and strengths should also be identified. These may be stated as accomplishments, positive movement toward resolution of problems, and other hypotheses about beliefs, values, and cohesion. Data may be examined in relation to improving crime indicators, rehabilitation of housing, expanding employment opportunities, community organizations, and health campaigns. An example of a diagnosis of one community strength, that is, community cohesion, was stated earlier in this chapter.

Diagnoses Related to Community Improvements

Indicators of improvements in health status of the community may be found by examining mortality and morbidity data over longer periods of time. For example, changes in infant mortality rates are observed more accurately over 3-year periods rather than year to year, especially if the population base is small as in rural areas and sparsely inhabited counties. Using small populations for rate calculations makes rates unstable, and large changes may be seen in rates from year to year (Valanis, 1999).

Another area to examine for improvements is the environment (Leffers, Smith, Huffing, McDermott-Levy, & Sattler, 2016). Reports located to demonstrate improvements in air and water quality over the years should be part of the community assessment. Attempts to eliminate hazardous waste sites and improve the handling of solid wastes are other areas to explore. Improvements in the environment may also be seen in cleanup campaigns, removal of abandoned automobiles, control of rats, and regular inspections of food service establishments.

Other Areas for Diagnoses

Other areas to explore for community diagnoses are listed in Box 8.5. Each potential diagnosis must be tailored to the specific community using data from the community and must reflect the cultural values, beliefs, and practices of that community.

Other Issues for Formulating Community Diagnoses

Although you can develop community diagnoses for just about any area of a community's health status, some topics provide less precision than others for program planning. One such area is a diagnosis of a lack of services. Another issue for formulating community diagnoses is using conflicting data. These two issues, lack of services and conflicting data, are discussed in the following text.

LACK OF SERVICES

What may appear as a lack of services at first blush may in truth be some other factor, such as lack of transportation to existing service sites, acceptability of existing services, lack of providers, lack of insurance coverage, inability to pay for services, or other nuances in the service system.

Exploring whether there is a lack of services may require use of surveys, focus groups, or other data-collection methods plus examination of data from service agencies. Data about the service system capacity may be available from a local planning agency or from the state health department. If there are mandated planning agencies in your state, these data will be more readily available.

The lack of services may be a justifiable diagnosis in some instances, but the advanced practice nurse is interested in describing the health status of the community through the assessment. Identification of a lack of services points to a solution (e.g., more health services), which creates circular thinking (Kiritz, 1980). Identifying the health status indicator or trend provides more direction for action to be taken after the community assessment is completed. For example, if high rates of death due to specific diseases point to a lack of health services, other factors almost always contribute. The mere presence of health services will not ensure that people seek care for symptoms or preventive services, so a community diagnosis about lack of health services is incomplete. The lack of health services is more often appropriately listed as one of the "related to" factors in the community diagnosis.

USING CONFLICTING DATA

Another issue in developing community diagnoses is dealing with conflicting data. As discussed earlier, not all data are accurate. However, you must have some trust in data sources in order to even perform a community assessment.

The assessor facing the reality of conflicting data has several choices. One choice is to not use any of the conflicting data. Another approach is to seek an expert's opinion about the accuracy of the data. The expert opinion may be used in place of a definitive answer.

BOX 8.5 AREAS TO EXPLORE FOR COMMUNITY DIAGNOSES

Trends

Structure of demographics

Changes in values and beliefs

Educational and employment patterns of residents

Condition of housing and homelessness

Pollutants and related diseases

Esthetics of neighborhoods and community activities

Patterns of health benefits with employment

Patterns of residents receiving entitlement funds

Changing patterns of poverty

Strengths

Community cohesion

Safety of residents, crime, and public safety (e.g., community policing, traffic lights, crossing guards)

Access to government by residents

Media available in various languages

Locations and types of recreation facilities

Major areas of employment

Involvement of businesses in community life (e.g., support for working families)

Adverse Situations

Intergenerational conflict

Increasing rates of specific diseases

Lack of support for families and individuals

Increasing poverty, especially among women and children

Potential Adverse Situations

Relationship of changing disease rates to economic and social factors

Changes in healthcare providers and facilities

Patterns of health-related behaviors (e.g., smoking, exercise, diet)

Stress-management techniques used by community (e.g., drinking alcohol, risk-taking behaviors)

Changes in indicators of mental health status of community members

Community reactions to stressors (e.g., gang activity, drug sales and use, crime, increasing numbers of elderly in the community)

At times, it may be appropriate to include the conflicting data in a diagnosis or footnote to highlight the need for better data.

Probably, the most common approach used to deal with conflicting data is to consult a third, fourth, or even fifth source. The assessor may then use the data from two or more sources that agree. This approach only works, of course, when there is more than one source of the same data. Often, this is not the case. In instances of conflicting data, the assessor is often faced with making decisions without adequate time or resources to investigate all data sources. One's best judgment is called for in such situations.

■ SUMMARY

A community diagnosis is a hypothesis about the status of a community. Community diagnoses provide a broad view of a community's health status, which is needed for a comprehensive approach to work with a community as an advanced practice public/community health nurse. How community diagnoses differ from nursing diagnoses, community problems, and community needs was discussed.

Data collected from multiple sources for a community assessment require both analysis and synthesis in order to formulate community diagnoses. *Analysis* is the intellectual separation of some concept into parts, whereas *synthesis* is the combination of separate parts into a coherent whole (Bloom, 1956). An approach to each process was summarized and illustrated in this chapter. A modification of the format developed by Muecke (1984) was introduced as one format for stating community diagnoses.

The next section of the book addresses program planning, which uses community diagnoses as the basis for developing programs and services to address community situations.

■ SUGGESTED CLINICAL OR PRACTICUM ACTIVITIES

1. Locate a community assessment that was completed by a local health department or nonprofit hospital and made available to the public. Analyze the findings of the community assessment with respect to community diagnoses, community needs, and/or community problems.
2. Using your analysis from question #1, reframe two or three major findings of the community assessment as formal community diagnoses.

REFERENCES

Anderson, E. T., & McFarlane, J. (1988). *Community as client: Application of the nursing process.* Philadelphia, PA: J. B. Lippincott.

Anderson, E. T., & McFarlane, J. (2015). *Community as partner: Theory and practice in nursing* (7th ed.). Philadelphia, PA: Lippincott Williams & Wilkins.

Bloom, B. S. (Ed.). (1956). *Taxonomy of educational objectives. Handbook 1. Cognitive domain.* New York, NY: David McKay.

Blum, H. L. (1981). *Planning for health: Generics for the eighties.* New York, NY: Human Sciences Press.

Catholic Health Association of the United States. (2013). Assessing and addressing community health heeds. Discussion draft: Revised June 2013. Retrieved from https://www.chausa.org/docs/default-source/general-files/cb_assessingaddressing-pdf.pdf?sfvrsn=4

Centers for Disease Control and Prevention. (2013). *Community health assessment for population health improvement: Resource of most frequently recommended health outcomes and determinants.* Atlanta, GA: Office of Surveillance, Epidemiology, and Laboratory Services.

Dignan, M. B., & Carr, P. A. (1992). *Program planning for health education and promotion* (2nd ed.). Philadelphia, PA: Lea & Febiger.

Freeman, R. B. (1970). *Community health nursing practice*. Philadelphia, PA: Saunders.

Glanz, K., Rimer, B. K., & Viswanath, K. (Eds.). (2015). *Health behavior and health education: Theory, research, and practice* (5th ed.). San Francisco, CA: Jossey-Bass.

Goeppinger, J. (1984). Community as client: Using the nursing process to promote health. In M. Stanhope & J. Lancaster (Eds.), *Community health nursing: Process and practice for promoting health* (pp. 379–404). St. Louis, MO: C.V. Mosby.

Grove, S. K., Burns, N., & Gray, J. (2013). *The practice of nursing research: Appraisal, synthesis and generation of evidence* (7th ed.). Philadelphia, PA: Saunders.

Helvie, C. O. (1998). *Advanced practice nursing in the community*. Thousand Oaks, CA: Sage.

Herdman, T. H., & Kamitsuru, S. (Eds.). (2014). *Nursing diagnoses 2015–17: Definitions and classification* (10th ed.). West Sussex, UK: Wiley-Blackwell.

Higgs, Z. R., & Gustafson, D. D. (1985). *Community as a client: Assessment and diagnosis*. Philadelphia, PA: F. A. Davis.

Kiritz, N. J. (1980). *Program planning and proposal writing*. Los Angeles, CA: The Grantsmanship Center.

Kozier, B., Erb, G., Berman, A. J., & Burke, K. (2000). *Fundamentals of nursing: Concepts, process, and practice* (6th ed.). Upper Saddle River, NJ: Prentice Hall Health.

Leavell, H., & Clarke, E. (1965). *Preventive medicine for the doctor in the community* (3rd ed.). New York, NY: McGraw-Hill.

Leffers, J., Smith, C. M., Huffing, K., McDermott-Levy, R. & Sattler, B. (Eds.). (2016). *Environmental health in nursing*. Mount Rainier, MD: Alliance of Nurses for Healthy Environments. Retrieved from https://envirn.org/e-textbook

Martin, K. S. (2005). *The Omaha System: A key to practice, documentation, and information management* (2nd ed.). Omaha, NE: Health Connections Press.

McGavran, E. G. (1956). Scientific diagnosis and treatment of the community as a patient. *Journal of the American Medical Association, 162*(8), 723–727.

McKnight, J. L., & Kretzmann, J. P. (2012). Mapping community capacity. In M. Minkler (Ed.), *Community organizing and community building for health* (3rd ed., pp. 171–186). New Brunswick, NJ: Rutgers University Press.

Miller, B. F., & Keane, C. B. (1983). *Encyclopedia and dictionary of medicine, nursing and allied health* (3rd ed.). Philadelphia, PA: Saunders.

Muecke, M. A. (1984). Community health diagnosis in nursing. *Public Health Nursing, 1*(1), 23–35.

Neufeld, A., & Harrison, M. J. (1990). The development of nursing diagnoses for aggregates and groups. *Public Health Nursing, 7*(4), 251–255.

New York State Department of Health. (2016). Annual report of vital statistics of New York State 2014. Retrieved from https://www.health.ny.gov/statistics/vital_statistics/docs/vital_statistics_annual_report_2014.pdf

North American Nursing Diagnosis Association. (1999). *Nursing diagnosis: Definitions & classification 1999–2000*. Philadelphia, PA: Author.

Office of Disease Prevention and Health Promotion. (2014). *Healthy people 2020* . Washington, DC: Author. Retrieved from https://www.healthypeople.gov

Patient Protection and Affordable Care Act, Public Law 111–148. (2010). *111th United States Congress*. Washington, DC: United States Government Printing Office. Retrieved from http://www.gpo.gov/fdsys/pkg/PLAW-111publ148/pdf/PLAW-111publ148.pdf

Rural Health Information Hub. (2018). *Demographic changes and aging population*. Retrieved from https://www.ruralhealthinfo.org/community-health/aging/1/demographics

Scardamalia, R. (2008). *New York State demographic trends*. New York State Office for the Aging, Department of State. Retrieved from https://aging.ny.gov/livableny/Documents/NewYorkStateDemographicTrends.pdf

Soriano, F. I. (2013). *Conducting needs assessments: A multidisciplinary approach* (2nd ed.). Thousand Oaks, CA: Sage.

U.S. Census Bureau, American Factfinder. (n.d.). *Community facts*. Retrieved from https://factfinder.census.gov/faces/nav/jsf/pages/community_facts.xhtml

Valanis, B. (1999). *Epidemiology in health care* (3rd ed.). Stamford, CT: Appleton & Lange.

Watson, N. M. (1984). Community as client. In J. A. Sullivan (Ed.), *Directions in community health nursing* (pp. 69–90). Boston, MA: Blackwell.

Witkin, B. R., & Altschuld, J. W. (1995). *Planning and conducting needs assessments*. Thousand Oaks, CA: Sage.

SECTION III

Program Planning

CHAPTER 9

Overview of Program Planning

Paul L. Kuehnert

■ STUDY EXERCISES

1. Define the planning process and its four stages. How have you used this process in other aspects of your life, such as in school or in your family?
2. Identify two or three key skills that advanced practice public/community health nurses need to have to perform well when leading community-wide planning efforts around health issues. How have you seen nurses or others in community health settings demonstrate these skills?
3. Discuss the ways in which population-focused planning activities are multidisciplinary. In what ways are nurses well prepared and/or ill prepared to provide leadership in multidisciplinary activities?
4. Discuss the concept of scale in relation to planning. What are the implications of scale for involving others, from other disciplines and/or community members, in planning efforts?
5. Discuss the ethical implications of community-wide planning for scarce health-related resources. What ethical principles could be applied?

In the nearly three decades since the Institute of Medicine's landmark report *The Future of Public Health* (Institute of Medicine, 1988), public/community health nursing has moved to position its practice in the new population-focused paradigm with the core public health functions of assessment, policy development, and assurance (American Nurses Association, 2013; Bekemeier, Walker Linderman, Kneipp, & Zahner, 2015). Leaders from the public health disciplines have refined and explicated the public health core functions model to include a widely endorsed public health vision and mission statement that enumerates the 10 essential public health services listed in Box 9.1 (Centers for Disease Control and Prevention, 2014; Public Health Functions Steering Committee, American Public Health Association, 1995). The core functions model is the basis for national accreditation standards for public health agencies (Public Health Accreditation Board, 2011).

Educators from public/community health nursing (Maurer & Smith, 2013; Stanhope & Lancaster, 2016) and other public health disciplines (Gebbie & Turnock, 2006; Tilson & Gebbie, 2004) have subsequently identified a variety of practice-related skills and competencies in key areas. These include analysis, communication, policy development, program planning, and public health sciences. Skills in all these areas are needed by the multidisciplinary public health workforce to deliver the 10 essential public health services. Planning

---

BOX 9.1 ESSENTIAL PUBLIC HEALTH FUNCTIONS

- Monitor health status to identify community health problems
- Diagnose and investigate health problems and health hazards in the community
- Inform, educate, and empower people about health issues
- Mobilize community partnerships to identify and solve health problems
- Develop policies and plans that support individual and community health efforts
- Enforce laws and regulations that protect health and ensure safety
- Link people to needed personal health services and assure the provision of healthcare when otherwise unavailable
- Ensure a competent public health and personal healthcare worker
- Evaluate effectiveness, accessibility, and quality of personal and population-based health services
- Research for new insights and innovative solutions to health problems

Source: Centers for Disease Control and Prevention. (2014). The public health system and the 10 essential public health services. Retrieved from https://www.cdc.gov/nphpsp/essentialservices.html

---

and planning-related skills and competencies are prominently featured in these documents because planning is key to and links activities across the core functions.

Nurses comprise the largest discipline within the public health workforce and have a long tradition of population-focused practice (Bekemeier et al., 2015; Bigbee & Issel, 2012). As a result, nursing has unique opportunities to contribute to the successful implementation of the new public health paradigm. These opportunities flow from two factors: (a) community-as-client, one of public/community health nursing's conceptual frameworks, and (b) public/community health nursing's ability to use the community assessment process as a method to guide practice. A brief examination of these unique contributions to population-focused practice in public health provides a necessary background for this chapter's overview of planning.

■ PUBLIC/COMMUNITY HEALTH NURSING'S UNIQUE FRAMEWORK

Public/community health nursing's 100-plus-year tradition has provided the basis for the development and articulation of its unique conceptual framework of community-as-client (American Nurses Association, 2013; Bigbee & Issel, 2012; Hanchett, 1988; Higgs & Gustafson, 1985; Rodgers, 1984; Smith & Bazini-Barakat, 2003; Storfjell & Cruise, 1984; Walgren, 1984; Watson, 1984; White, 1982). This framework focuses on practice as the improvement of the health of the community-as-a-whole. The identification of community-as-client implies qualities of person and interaction for the community-as-a-whole (Schultz, 1987), so this framework provides vitality otherwise lacking to the notion of population-focused practice. Community-as-client necessitates approaching community multidimensionally as setting, unit, and target of practice (Sills & Goeppinger, 1985). Community-as-client also implies that the "'whole' of a community . . . might be different from and greater than the sum of all its parts, an entity capable of decision making and action" (Hamilton, 1983, p. 27).

The entire practice of a public/community health nursing agency, when based on the framework of community-as-client, is directed toward the community-as-a-whole. The community is not simply a passive setting in which the agency acts upon residents.

Community is a living, breathing entity that has unique social and economic features; its own history and political structure; and a set of traditions, beliefs, and mores that actively shape community members' lives. In turn, the community is redefined by the actions and interactions of its members. Like other community institutions, the public/community health nursing agency and staff are a part of the community, and the agency's purpose is shaped and reshaped by ongoing interaction with the community (Kuehnert, 1995).

■ RELATIONSHIP OF COMMUNITY ASSESSMENT TO PROGRAM PLANNING

Although the community-as-client framework provides a needed set of conceptual references that bring life to the notion of population-focused practice, the application of the community assessment process sets in motion a highly interactive, ongoing dynamic to that practice. As illustrated in Figure 9.1, three distinct community units are targeted by the public/community health nursing agency, resulting in separate but interactive foci of practice for both staff and the agency.

The community-wide focus of practice applies the community assessment practice to the community-as-a-whole, resulting in programs directed to other units of the community,

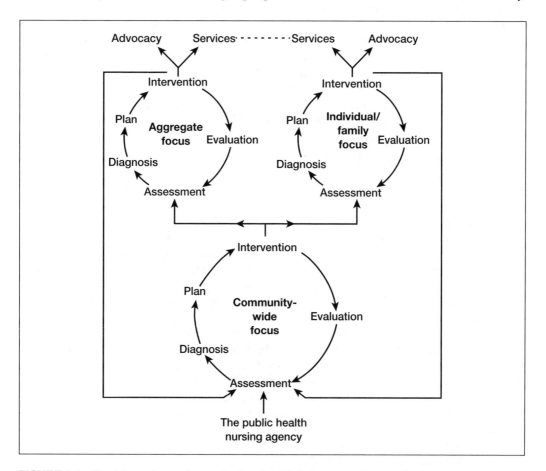

FIGURE 9.1   The interactive and organizational model of community-as-client.

Source: Adapted from Kuehnert, P. L. (1991). Community health nursing and the AIDS pandemic: Case report of one community's response. *Journal of Community Health Nursing, 8*(3), 138. Copyright © 1991, Lawrence Erlbaum Associates. Used with permission.

but with the overall target for health improvement or preservation being the community-as-a-whole. Certain high-risk subgroups or aggregates of the community and organizations, such as schools and workplaces, are targets of the aggregate or group focus of public/community health nursing practice. Individuals and their families are the third unit and target of public/community health nursing practice, particularly those at risk for poor health outcomes. The community assessment process leads to interventions that include both direct services and advocacy within each focus of practice. This process is the dynamic force that moves public/community health nursing practice forward, both within and between practice foci, leading to ongoing change in the overall direction of improved health for the community-as-a-whole (Kuehnert, 1995).

Planning is a key component of advanced public/community health nursing practice, providing a vital link between assessment and diagnosis, on the one hand, and intervention and evaluation on the other. Planning encompasses a set of skills and competencies that are vital to the successful implementation of population-focused public health practice. Although the planning process may essentially be the same whether applied to individuals, families, groups, or community-as-a-whole, the specifics vary widely depending on the focus of practice.

As in other aspects of nursing practice, ethical considerations must be fully explored when population-focused planning activities are undertaken. Conflicts between community members' perceptions of individual rights and the common good (Bellah, Madsen, Sullivan, Swidler, & Tipton, 1985, 1991), as well as differences in their perceptions of community and experiences of social justice (Beauchamp, 1985; Moccia, 1988), are often brought out and expressed forcefully during planning activities. Nurses and other leaders must be able to identify these conflicts as expressive of ethical dilemmas and work with the community members to name and seek to resolve them.

■ CONCEPTUAL FRAMEWORKS AND MODELS TO GUIDE PROGRAM PLANNING

No matter what the level or type of planning effort, the use of conceptual frameworks and models facilitates effective planning. Their use provides an overarching system of organization and a unifying approach to the various steps of the planning process. Moreover, most opportunities, problems, or needs being addressed through a planning process are multifaceted, requiring the planner to have the knowledge and ability to integrate and synthesize large volumes of data. The use of conceptual frameworks provides the means to examine several alternatives and to test various approaches without the expense of operationalizing each one (Nutt, 1984).

Neither public health in general nor public/community health nursing specifically provides a single conceptual framework or model that can be used across planning efforts. The application of nursing theories developed with individual clients in mind is inadequate (Chalmers & Kristajanson, 1989; Hamilton & Bush, 1988) and artificial when applied to community-focused planning. Public/community health nursing's community-as-client model has not yet been totally developed as a framework that can guide practice. Likewise, the use of a biomedical theory, such as epidemiology, as the sole framework for community-focused planning reduces the key underlying concept of community to a unidimensional entity (Hanchett, 1990).

The advanced practice nurse is faced with the challenge of identifying relevant conceptual frameworks to guide practice and may have difficulty finding one framework that can provide adequate guidance to planning on all scales. However, one conceptual framework may provide the basis for the nurse's community-focused practice, including planning activities, and can be cobbled together with additional models of limited scope and used to guide specific efforts or planning on various scales. This approach can be successful as long as the models are compatible and internally consistent.

The remainder of this chapter describes four separate, but related, conceptual frameworks for planning and illustrates their use in a case study. First, the Community Organization Model (Ross, 1967; Rothman & Tropman, 1987) is explained as the over-arching conceptual framework for community-focused work and planning on the community or population level. Next, Piercy's Creating Method (Piercy, 1996) approach for planning on the agency level is explained, followed by a description of the McLaughlin Model of Health Planning (McLaughlin, 1982) for the program-planning level. The Four-Step Planning Process, a comprehensive planning model based on these conceptual frameworks and the author's own practice, is defined and explained.

Community Organization Model

The Community Organization Model has been described as a set of principles that guide purposive community change (Rothman & Tropman, 1987; Weil, 2004). It arose from macro-practice of social work, dealing with "human service activity that . . . focus(es) on broader social approaches to human betterment, emphasizing such things as developing enlightened social policy, organizing the effective delivery of services, strengthening community life and preventing social ills" (Rothman & Tropman, 1987, p. 3). Although lacking fully articulated assumptions and propositions, the Community Organization Model provides a grounded approach to the community as unit and target of practice. The implicit assumptions of the model include the following:

- A community is a geopolitical entity in which people reside; combine in families, social networks, and other groups and organizations; and interact in ways to enhance the common good.
- Community well-being, or the common good, results from purposive actions by community actors.
- Community well-being is a determinant of individual well-being, and is a determinant of the well-being of other community components.
- Community well-being is affected by, and affects, its unique national and regional circumstances and its historical circumstances.
- Community organizing increases the agility of a community to solve its problems and improves community well-being (Minkler, 1990; Rothman & Tropman, 1987).

The Community Organization Model provides a framework for approaching change at the community level. The need for change is usually determined by community actors who have perceived a present or potential threat to community well-being. The Community Organization Model is inductively based and its boundaries are very wide, embracing all of community life. This model asserts that intentional problem solving, labeled *community organization*, is a special community process undertaken by community actors to solve a present or potential problem and results in enhanced community well-being.

The Community Organization Model provides three different approaches to change. These approaches (labeled Models A, B, and C by Rothman & Tropman, 1987) are differentiated according to 11 practice variables. This typology is not seen as mutually exclusive by community organization theorists (Minkler, 1990; Rothman & Tropman, 1987), and a blending of approaches is expected.

Model A, or locality development, is a process-oriented approach to problem solving that presumes that a broad cross-section of community components can and should be involved in any solutions. This model seeks to enhance the capacity of the community by emphasizing communication skills and consensus building in an interactional, democratic process.

Model B, or social planning, presumes that solutions to community problems are beyond the reach of "ordinary" members of the community and, to be solved, need the input, at least, of experts. The emphasis is on the task or the problem to be solved and finding the right solution as opposed to the process of problem solving itself, as in Model A. Community members are encouraged to participate by some social planning approaches, but more in the role of consumers or clients as opposed to active partners.

The third approach, Model C, is known as the social action approach. Social action presumes that the community is always in a state of unequal relations among members (i.e., there are "haves" and "have-nots"). Model C seeks to shift the power relations in a community to solve problems and improve well-being. It can be focused on both process and outcome, sometimes one more than the other. Community members are believed to be in conflict with each other, and participation in community organization activities by those who are oppressed by the power structure of the community is seen as vital to change.

These models of community organization, taken separately or blended, can be used by planners as a framework with which to guide and organize the planning process. Specific planning activities undertaken at different stages of the planning process should be consistent with the model of community action practice. For example, the planner's role in a locality development approach is that of an enabler-catalyst, a coordinator and teacher, whereas in the social action approach, the planner role is that of an activist or advocate. Overall guidance is provided to the planning process by incorporation of key concepts common to all organization approaches, such as empowerment, community competence, and participation (Minkler, 1990).

The Creating Strategic Planning Method

Day Piercy's Creating Strategic Planning Method (1996) is rooted in a process-oriented, developmental approach to organizational growth and change. The method focuses on the possibilities and opportunities present during organizational transitions. By focusing on what organizations want to create, it "provides a structure and process to:

- Create a vision and priorities
- Build on organizations' strengths rather than concentrating on weaknesses
- Define how to maximize opportunities rather than avert threats
- Apply entrepreneurial energy and leadership to address challenges
- Decide what you need to do to attain your goals
- Create plans that reflect community and constituent needs, the external environment and internal organizational development priorities
- Build consensus and buy-in" (Piercy, 1996, p. 7)

This method of strategic planning is rooted in the notion of creating a philosophical approach that emphasizes working with, rather than reacting to, the transitional forces affecting an organization. Creating is conceptualized as a spiraling process with four phases: creative energy, confusion, clarity, and creative action (Figure 9.2). Creative energy is the phase in which options emerge, enthusiasm and possibilities abound, and a wide variety of ideas are generated. As the complexities of the situation facing the organization emerge, along with the various possible responses and their related consequences, the confusion phase begins. If the organization allows the confusion and conflicts to be

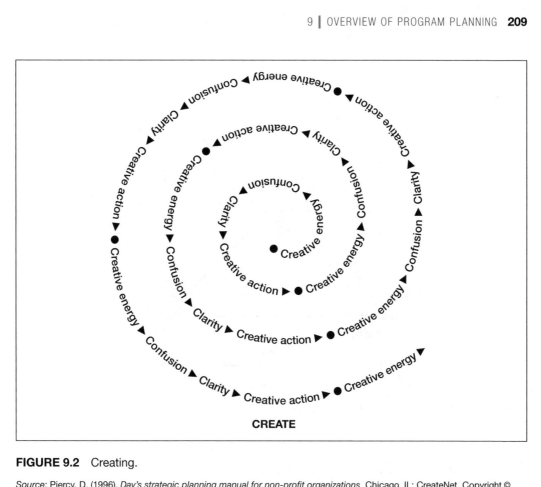

CREATE

FIGURE 9.2 Creating.

Source: Piercy, D. (1996). *Day's strategic planning manual for non-profit organizations.* Chicago, IL: CreateNet. Copyright © 1996 by Day Piercy. Used by permission.

fully expressed, a breakthrough will occur. The breakthrough heralds the clarity phase, when the organization reaches decisions about the "what" and "how to" of its next actions. As the organization enters the creative-action phase, by adopting a strategic plan component or otherwise acting on a strategic issue with which it has been wrestling, a new creative spiral is initiated even as the previous one is completed and implementation begins (Piercy, 1996).

The creating method is contrasted with reacting, when an organization's energy is mired in a focus on the organization's problems and limitations. Reacting is a negative organizational state driven by fear and in which actions are limited to blaming, idolizing, "shoulding," and assuming, as illustrated in Figure 9.3.

To end the cycle of reacting, organizations must acknowledge what is happening and detach from it. Accepting the confusion and labeling it as a necessary phase, not a state of being, allows the creative energy that has been frozen by reacting to be freed (Piercy, 1996).

The creating method of strategic planning focuses on organizational process. This type of planning results in the development of a document that articulates a vision of where the organization wants to go and what it wants to be, as well as measurable goals and objectives to attain the vision. The creating method of planning supports the viewpoint that strategic planning is an ongoing process and, the planning document provides a framework for discussions and decisions to be made during plan implementation.

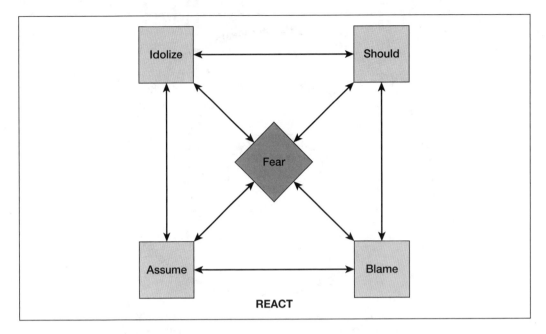

FIGURE 9.3 Reacting.

Source: Piercy, D. (1996). *Day's strategic planning manual for non-profit organizations*. Chicago, IL: CreateNet. Copyright © 1996 by Day Piercy. Used with permission.

The McLaughlin Model of Health Planning

A broad, process-oriented focus is appropriate to high-level planning scaled to an agency. A much tighter, outcome-oriented framework is needed to guide program planning. One such model was developed by McLaughlin (1982).

This community health-oriented model conceptualizes populations as clustered into groups according to where individuals would fall into one of four quadrants formed by the intersection of two axes. One, the horizontal axis, is the continuum of perceived wellness, ranging from a perception of illness to one of high-level wellness. The other, the vertical axis, is the continuum of perceived psychological readiness to act on health benefits, ranging from little to high intention to act. The intersection of the two axes form quadrants that can be used to define community health program interventions that seek to influence the corresponding population's health in a positive direction.

McLaughlin (1982) asserted that these community health programs act as cues to the population. Hence, the general cues provided by health-promotion programs may foster a response from a population with a perception of high-level wellness and a high psychological readiness to act. In contrast, another group with a self-perceived high level of wellness but with less readiness to act may be more likely to respond to cues that alter perceptions and attitudes, such as those found in early-detection and health-supervision services. Disease control and monitoring services may provide appropriate cues to limit behaviors in conflict with health for a population with self-perceived illness and with little readiness to act on health beliefs. Those with a readiness to act and a self-perception of illness or being less than well respond to cues specific to correction of health threats that are found in disease-avoidance and health-protection services (McLaughlin, 1982).

The Four-Step Planning Process

In the Four-Step Planning Process, *planning* is defined as an organized response to opportunities, challenges, or needs facing an individual, organization, or community. In the case of advanced public/community health nursing practice, *planning* is further defined as a response to the process of community assessment and diagnosis (Finnegan & Ervin, 1989), which lays the foundation for public health interventions and evaluation.

Typically, advanced practice public/community health nurses are involved in planning on at least three levels or scales: (a) for and with agencies for which they work, by developing strategic plans for the entire agency or for components of the agency; (b) for and with the community or communities in which they practice, by developing comprehensive plans around particular community health issues; and (c) for and with the agencies for which they work, by developing specific public health advocacy or service interventions, usually targeting specific subpopulations within the community.

Depending on the nurse's role in the community and the agency, the nurse may take on one or more of the following: provide central leadership to a planning effort, often with an emphasis on facilitating intra- or interagency communication and collaboration; staff an effort directly or manage staff or consultants who are providing staff-support functions to the planning effort; or be an active participant in planning-related meetings and other related activities. Planning requires an organized process of a series of intentional, time-related actions taken by a group or an individual. These actions are designed to move an idea from vision into reality. The core of the planning process itself is generic and consists of the four interdependent steps of defining, analyzing, choosing, and mapping, as illustrated in Figure 9.4. The steps are defined in the following sections.

DEFINING

During the defining stage, the planner gathers and organizes information from a variety of sources that will provide an all-sided view of the opportunity, challenge, or need to be addressed and possible responses to it. The defining stage may be simplified if the comprehensive data have already been gathered and organized, for example, when an in-depth community assessment has already been completed. The planner then focuses on gathering information about possible programmatic or policy responses. Much more comprehensive data must be gathered that describe the need, as well as information about possible policy or programmatic responses to it when, for example, only one data source may be pointing to a community need.

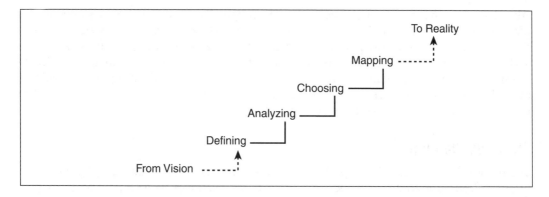

FIGURE 9.4 The Four-Step Planning Process.

In all cases, the planner also gathers information about past responses to the same or similar needs. Preliminary outcome-related goals should be identified on the basis of the results that are desired by the agency, community, or program participants.

ANALYZING

The planner enters the analyzing stage after clearly defining the dimensions of the challenge, problem, or need. During this stage, the planner critically evaluates what the various data sources reveal about the challenge or problem. In addition, the planner analyzes the information about the possible programmatic or policy responses that might be made, and the barriers to and resources available for each alternative response. The alternatives are evaluated for their consistency with an agency's mission or legislative mandate. The alternatives deemed appropriate to the agency are further analyzed in terms of their ethical, political, and economic costs and benefits. Finally, alternative responses are evaluated for their effectiveness in producing the desired outcomes.

CHOOSING

As a result of analyzing, the planner most often faces choosing from among several alternative approaches to the need, challenge, or opportunity that is to be addressed. Choosing may be relatively simple, for example, if the agency or community must choose the least costly alternative. On the other hand, choosing may be extremely difficult if two or more similar attractive alternatives are being considered, or if the choices reflect significant differences in approach and each has strong advocates. In most cases, it is helpful to have an agreed-upon set of criteria or process for choosing between alternatives before the planning process begins. After choosing an approach, the outcome-related goals should be reviewed and finalized, laying the groundwork for the final step in the planning process.

MAPPING

After a choice has been made regarding the approach to be taken and outcome-related goals have been finalized, the planner maps the final time-linked action steps to be taken before implementation begins. Steps that must be mapped include establishing necessary policy or procedural frameworks, obtaining human and material resources, and setting evaluation criteria.

USING THE FOUR-STEP PLANNING PROCESS

Although defining, analyzing, choosing, and mapping are the four broad stages in the planning process, the specific planning activities undertaken during each stage will vary according to the scale of the planning effort. Table 9.1 gives examples of these activities and how they may vary according to whether planning is being done for an agency, a community, or a specific program. Advanced practice nurses with planning responsibilities may play different roles in specific planning activities, depending on both the scale of the planning effort and their own level of skill and experience.

Strategic Planning

The highest level of planning typically undertaken by agencies is strategic planning. The organization, through the strategic-planning process, examines its own past performance, assesses internal and external opportunities and threats, envisions its future, and identifies its strategic priorities. The strategic plan, usually framed in a 3- or 5-year time period,

TABLE 9.1 Sample Planning Activities Compared by Scale

	Agency	Community	Program
Steps in Planning Process	**Strategic Planning**	**Service System Planning**	**Service Delivery Planning**
Defining . . . gather and organize data that fully describe the problem . . .	• Gather information regarding agency's history, funding, community needs and trends, ideas about future directions. • Conduct key informant interviews or focus groups.	• Obtain and organize community assessment data from a variety of sources. • Conduct consumer surveys, focus groups, and/or key informant interviews.	• Identify information regarding target service population—currently available resources, preferences, and perceived barriers. • Conduct literature review to identify possible intervention strategies.
Analyzing . . . evaluate alternative responses based on desired outcomes . . .	• Conduct planning retreat to brainstorm organizational strengths, opportunities, challenges, vision for the future, and priorities. • Draft and refine summary document(s) regarding vision, priorities, and goals.	• Facilitate meeting with community stakeholders to present summary data and tentative advocacy- or service-related action steps. • Draft and refine summary documents describing the challenge or opportunity and proposed policies or action steps to be taken by community stakeholders.	• Draft tentative program goals and objectives. • Assess cost–benefit of alternative intervention strategies.
Choosing . . . select a course of action . . .	• Circulate draft plan to board, committees, and staff for feedback. • Review feedback and prepare final draft plan	• Circulate draft to key stakeholders and decision makers. • Review feedback and prepare final draft plan, including policies and action steps.	• Circulate draft program plan among appropriate management and staff. • Review feedback and draft final program plan, including measurable goals and objectives.
Mapping . . . develop time-linked, specific markers to guide implementation and evaluation . . .	• Strategic plan by board is adopted. • Staff and committees prepare annual work plans, including the agency budget, to implement strategic plan.	• Plan and relevant policies and/or action steps adopted by community stakeholders. • Annual work plans are prepared for implementation by staff and interagency committees.	• Obtain needed human and material resources for implementation. • Prepare program work plan for program implementation, including evaluation plan.

allows the agency to position itself in the larger community of which it is a part. The plan provides a clear, self-determined, future-oriented focus to guide agency practice. Such plans are necessarily fairly broad and general in scope, and the planning process itself is often as important to the agency as the resulting document.

The advanced practice nurse's role in strategic planning depends on her or his role in the agency that is undertaking the planning effort. If she or he is a board member or a member of the management or leadership team, the nurse is likely to be an active participant in every aspect of the process. If the nurse is skilled in group facilitation and consensus building and has a leadership position in the agency, she or he may play more of a direct leadership role in the planning process. The nurse may direct the plan's overall progress, or supervise the work of an outside consultant who has been retained to facilitate the strategic plan. In either case, the nurse needs to have great familiarity with the agency, its niche, its stakeholders, its internal strengths and weaknesses, its external political and economic environment, and the community the agency serves.

COMMUNITY-WIDE PLANNING

An agency's strategic plan may identify priorities that could lead to initiation of or participation in interagency or community-wide planning efforts addressing a specific problem the community faces. Such efforts seek to identify policy changes and/or system-level service planning that will address the problem in ways that transcend single agencies. Critical to the success of such efforts is the active involvement by a diverse array of individuals and agencies to ensure accurate assessment of need and buy-in from these same key stakeholders in the planned solution(s). Often, such efforts establish ongoing means by which implementation can be monitored, and problems that arise during implementation can be addressed.

Depending on the nurse's role both in the community and in the specific community agency, as well as the nurse's personal skills and leadership abilities, the advanced practice nurse's role in these efforts may vary widely. If, for example, the nurse is in a leadership position in the community's health department and the community is seeking to address a health-related problem, the nurse is likely to play a key role. The nurse may also provide staff support to such an effort or may supervise staff or a consultant staffing the planning effort.

The nurse can be key to the success of a collaborative planning venture by modeling full, active participation in the planning effort, regardless of the specific role. Vitally important to such collaborative efforts are excellent communications skills, the ability to draw out and articulate a vision of the common interests of the collaborators, and skillful application of negotiating techniques. Also, key to successful collaborations is the consistent involvement of each participant and the assurance that consistency will continue into any ongoing efforts during implementation.

PROGRAM PLANNING

Program planning may flow from either an agency's strategic plan or from community-wide planning efforts that have identified specific service gaps. Although strategic and community-wide planning are both highly process oriented, program planning is much more specific and detail oriented. Key to successful program planning is extensive knowledge of the program's potential client or customer population, the program's perceived needs and available resources, and barriers to actively engaging them in the program. In addition, program planning requires knowledge of the broader community's resources, experience of serving the target population, and experience at the national and regional levels using the specific or similar interventions. Program planning is usually closely related to, and often shaped by internal agency processes to obtain resources for implementation. It may also be tied to obtaining external funding, such as grants awarded by public or private sources.

The advanced practice public/community health nurse's role in program planning will depend on her or his role in the agency. The nurse may be responsible for managing the entire process from beginning to end, followed by managing implementation and ongoing evaluation of the program. Successful program planning depends on the nurse's ability to integrate knowledge of the intervention and the client population, along with careful attention to details.

■ CASE STUDY: THE AIDS FOUNDATION OF CHICAGO

In late 1985, the AIDS Foundation of Chicago (AFC) was established to coordinate local response to the AIDS crisis. At the time, there were only a few hundred confirmed cases of AIDS in Chicago, virtually no private or government funds earmarked for prevention or care, and only a handful of social services and health agencies willing to provide care for those infected. Some 12,000 cases of AIDS were reported in the Chicago area over the ensuing 9 years, and the fund-raising, advocacy, and service coordination efforts of the AFC, although not keeping pace with the overwhelming array of needs, ensured that a growing set of resources were made available to people with AIDS.

Plans, Policy, and Service Initiatives

By 1994, the AFC had grown to be the largest AIDS organization in the Midwest, with an annual budget of more than $6 million and a staff of 20. It pursued its mission of providing leadership in marshaling public and private resources to care for people living with HIV/AIDS and to prevent the further spread of the epidemic through advocacy, fund-raising, grant making, and service coordination/coalition building (AFC, 1995). Programmatically, this translated into key initiatives. For example, in 1994, AFC administered more than $3 million in federal CARE (Caregiver Advise, Record, Enable) Act funds for case management, transportation, housing, emergency assistance, primary care, mental healthcare, child care, and nutrition services. AFC coordinated a metropolitan area-wide HIV/AIDS case management system for more than 4,000 unduplicated clients through nearly 50 local agencies. AFC's staff provided ongoing leadership and support to a wide variety of collaborative service planning and coordination initiatives conceived and implemented by its 120-member Service Providers Council (SPC). AFC initiated statewide advocacy efforts for sound AIDS-related public policies and increased public support for AIDS-related programs and services at all levels of government. AFC raised and distributed more than $1 million in grants through an aggressive fund-raising program aimed at increasing private sector support for AIDS programs and services among individuals and institutions.

In 1994, an advanced practice public/community health nurse joined the staff of AFC as its associate director. As an advanced practice nurse in a multidisciplinary, private, nonprofit agency, he was part of the senior management team of the AFC. The nurse participated in all aspects and provided leadership to some aspects of a number of planning initiatives that AFC undertook during an 18-month period. These planning initiatives included an AFC 3-year strategic plan, a Metro Chicago 5-year HIV/AIDS housing plan, and a Metro Chicago rent subsidy program plan for low-income persons with HIV/AIDS.

This case study describes these initiatives and the role that the advanced practice public/community health nurse played in each as an illustration of the planning models, methods, approaches, and role of the advanced practice nurse as discussed in this chapter. Key comparisons among the three planning efforts are summarized in Table 9.2.

TABLE 9.2 AIDS Foundation of Chicago (AFC) Planning Activities Compared by Scale

Key Comparisons	Agency	Community	Program
	3-Year Strategic Plan	Metro Chicago Comprehensive AIDS Housing Plan	Metro Chicago Rent-Subsidy Program for Low-Income Persons With HIV
Problem	Routine organizational growth and development	Growing demand for housing with minimal, short-term growth in AIDS funding	Uneven distribution of rent-subsidy funding to eligible persons with HIV in the nine-county region
Planning unit	AFC strategic planning committee and the board of directors	Ad hoc committee of consumers and service providers	AFC program department
Process	Consultant-facilitated board retreats and committee meetings	• Consultant-facilitated public meetings • Consumer survey • Consumer focus groups • Service provider interviews and site visits • Need/resource analysis	• Consumer focus groups • Meetings with rent subsidy service providers • Meetings with Department of Health staff • Written proposal for funding
Advanced practice nurse role	• Participant • Staffing working subcommittees	• Coordination of entire project • Oversight of consultants	• Leadership/management of entire effort • Grant writer
Outcome	Written plan with mission/vision statement, 3-year priorities, and related goals and objectives in eight areas of the organization's life	Written plan with consumer survey findings, need/resource analysis, and four recommendations for implementation over 5 years	• Creation of centrally coordinated rent-subsidy program for low-income individuals disabled with HIV • $1.4 million funding secured for the initial 1-year period
Sample goal statement	"Work to ensure the further development of a comprehensive, integrated system of HIV/AIDS services (by) support(ing) the continued development of a comprehensive continuum of housing services"	"Increase the supply of independent housing units"	"Provide 100 ongoing rent subsidies to eligible clients residing in DuPage County, West Suburban Cook County, and designated community areas on the west side of Chicago"

Strategic Planning

The AFC's board of directors decided to undertake its first long-range planning process as the organization approached its 10th anniversary. The decision came after a 3-year period during which the foundation experienced exponential growth in programs, staff, and budget. An 18-member strategic planning committee was convened that included present and past members of the board of directors, AFC management staff, and members of the foundation's SPC executive committee. The strategic planning committee met with a

consultant/facilitator a total of eight times during the 10-month planning period and provided overall direction to the process. On the basis of Piercy's Creating Method (1996), the
process deliberately sought extensive input from the foundation's diverse constituencies.
To gather data about perceptions of the foundation, the consultant and staff from AFC conducted a series of interviews with local and national funding sources, representatives from
other advocacy organizations, local and state government officials, foundation donors,
and members of the SPC.

Two half-day retreat sessions followed the data-gathering process and involved members of the board of directors, the SPC's executive committee, and the staff. During these
sessions, participants reviewed the AFC's history and accomplishments, processed
the data gathered from the interviews, and generated ideas for a 3-year vision and
organizational priorities. Following the retreat, the planning committee identified six
organizational priorities that guided the remainder of the planning process.

The task to develop written 3-year goals and objectives on the basis of these priorities
was assigned to board committees or joint board–SPC work groups. These work groups
were staffed by members of the AFC management team. The drafts were brought back to
the strategic planning committee for review, discussion, revision, and, finally, adoption.
In this fashion, the strategic planning committee developed its entire 3-year written plan.
The plan included eight sections—Grant Making, Service Coordination, Advocacy/
Policy, Governance/Board Development, Financial Development/Fundraising, Diversity,
Marketing/Public Relations, and Management—each section had goals and objectives
stated in a form to describe general directions for the 3-year period covered by the plan.
Specific work plans were to be developed annually by the specific board committee or
other AFC group responsible for overseeing implementation. This plan was reviewed,
revised, and adopted by the AFC board of directors 10 months after the process was
initiated (AFC, 1995).

As associate director, the advanced practice public/community health nurse had both
general and specific responsibilities in the strategic-planning process. He was an active
participant in both the strategic-planning committee and all its meetings, as well as the
two half-day retreats. The nurse's organizational responsibilities had largely to do with
the foundation's service coordination work, so he took responsibility for coordinating the
work of the SPC work groups around building the Council, furthering its leadership in
the development of a comprehensive system of care and prevention for people with HIV/
AIDS in the Chicago metropolitan area, and building the integration of the Council and the
board. This meant that the nurse facilitated and provided staff support at committee meetings for creating goals and objectives related to organizational priorities, either directly or
through supervision of other staff. He wrote or oversaw the writing of the draft goals and
objectives for the service coordination-related section of the strategic plan and made necessary revisions per committee and strategic-planning committee input. Finally, once the
strategic plan was adopted by the board, the nurse directed and supervised the program
department staff in development of quarterly work plans for staff and committee activities
that guided the implementation of the strategic plan.

Community-Wide Planning

It was the implementation of one of the strategic plan's goals (" Work to ensure the further
development of a comprehensive integrated system of HIV/AIDS services" [AFC, 1995, p. 10])
that led to another set of planning activities: creating a 5-year housing plan for people
living with HIV/AIDS in the nine-county Chicago metropolitan area. This population-
focused planning effort was centered on service system planning for a specific population

and based on both the Community Organization Model and a modification of the McLaughlin (1982) health program planning model. This planning effort was titled the "HIV Service Needs Matrix," and is illustrated in Figure 9.5. This model is based on an understanding of the multiple factors that influence each HIV-affected individual's service needs and the changing nature of needs over time. For the person with HIV, service needs are the product of both a person's progression on the continuum of HIV disease and the adequacy of each person's own social support system in meeting his or her goals (Kuehnert, 1993).

Chicago, like other major U.S. cities in the early 1990s, was home to a growing population of HIV-infected and -affected individuals and families who faced a complex set of medical and social needs with very limited personal/family economic and social support resources. This created a rapidly escalating demand for services, such as housing, that had already outstripped the supply of such services. Long-lasting institutional inequities resulting from racial discrimination and segregation further exacerbated the problems, because the HIV epidemic was disproportionately affecting Chicago's ethnic minority communities. Limited resources in an area of burgeoning demand for services created a severe ethical dilemma for the community that needed to be directly addressed. This central fact created the demand for both a planning process that would be inclusive and a plan that would be equitable and just.

The goal of the planning process was twofold: to identify strategies to expand the availability of comprehensive HIV/AIDS housing services in the Chicago area and to gain community buy-in of those strategies. The 8-month planning process included quantitative and qualitative housing needs assessment, identification and discussion of strategic issues facing HIV/AIDS housing consumers and service providers, and the development of consensus on priorities for the further development of HIV/AIDS housing resources in the Chicago metropolitan area. More than 90 people, including 15 self-identified HIV/AIDS housing consumers, representatives from 60 HIV/AIDS service provider agencies, and 18 governmental agencies, participated in what became the ad hoc housing planning committee.

The full committee met four times, and a smaller group of 12 to 15 volunteers from the larger group met an additional three times. Staff from the AFC and its consultant organization, AIDS Housing of Washington, surveyed case managers and conducted site visits and semistructured interviews with management staff from all identified HIV/AIDS housing

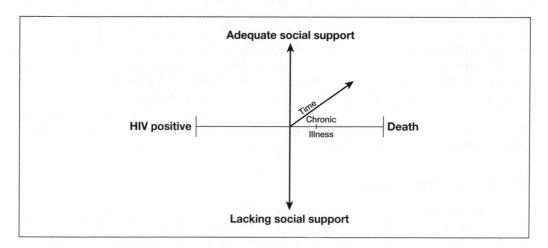

FIGURE 9.5 HIV Service Needs Matrix.

programs in the area. More than 800 individuals living with HIV/AIDS in the Chicago area responded to a survey developed by the AFC and the consultants regarding their housing needs and preferences (AIDS Housing of Washington, 1995).

This process led to the development of a planning document that identified the need for HIV/AIDS housing in the Chicago metropolitan area. Also identified in the document were four key system-level barriers to HIV housing service delivery. In addition, the planning document contained recommendations for improvements to the system of HIV housing services in the Chicago metropolitan area and for the allocation of HIV/AIDS housing funding from public sources to be implemented over the same 5-year period (AIDS Housing of Washington, 1995).

In this planning effort, the advanced practice nurse had management and leadership responsibilities for the entire AIDS housing planning effort. He selected and supervised the consulting firm that staffed the plan. Along with the consultants, the nurse attended all meetings with governmental funders. He identified and invited ad hoc planning committee participants and assisted in designing the consumer survey and the approaches used to distribute it. He chaired all meetings of the planning committee and its work group and facilitated many of the discussions within these meetings. In addition, the advanced practice nurse supervised the drafting and revising of the plan document. Following the adoption of the plan, he also had responsibility of planning follow-up activities by AFC staff and committees to monitor and respond to issues arising from the implementation of the recommendations.

Program Planning

As a direct result of the *Chicago EMA Five-Year HIV/AIDS Housing Plan* (AIDS Housing of Washington, 1995), the Chicago Department of Health released a request for proposals to develop and implement a centralized rent-subsidy program for low-income persons with HIV/AIDS in the Chicago metropolitan area. In responding to this proposal, the AFC developed a program plan that was initially written as a grant proposal. This program plan involved the development of a consortium of agencies to deliver the rent subsidies, so it was based on both the Community Organization Model and the HIV Service Needs Matrix model.

The program plan envisioned a centrally coordinated rent-subsidy program, providing partial rent payments for low-income individuals disabled by HIV infection who would become homeless or institutionalized without the rent subsidy. The program was to serve residents of the nine-county Chicago area. It was designed to have multiple points of access for the client and provide long-term, individualized rent subsidies. The program in consistence with the service priorities determined by the *Chicago EMA Five-Year HIV/AIDS Housing Plan* (AIDS Housing of Washington, 1995) would target those with very low incomes who were homeless or at risk of homelessness and disabled by HIV/AIDS. The program was to be integrated into three existing AFC programs, centrally coordinated case management, emergency financial assistance, and transportation, resulting in an efficient, comprehensive, client-centered array of social support services.

After receiving the grant award, some planning steps were necessary to ensure the development of an equitable, centrally coordinated system that would replace the existing fragmented arrangement. AFC developed a budget and a detailed, time-related program plan that set quarterly service targets (numbers of clients receiving subsidies) by region of the metropolitan area. The targets were related to reported prevalence of AIDS in each of the regions. Program policies and procedures that governed all aspects of program administration were developed. After a little more than a year of implementation, the new centrally coordinated rent-subsidy program was providing ongoing rent subsidies to nearly 500 households throughout the metropolitan area. This was accomplished with the same funding level that had earlier provided fewer than 200 households with rent subsidies.

The advanced practice public/community health nurse, as program planner for this AFC initiative, was responsible for all aspects of program design, writing the grant proposal, developing a staffing and budget plan, and establishing an implementation strategy and timetable. The new program initiative involved developing a consortium of service providers, so it was necessary to develop much of the program plan with the input of management staff from the four subcontracting agencies. This required the use of good communication and negotiations skills to develop program policies and procedures that each agency found acceptable and workable.

■ SUMMARY

Planning is a key component of advanced public/community health nursing practice, providing a vital link between assessment and diagnosis, on the one hand, and intervention and evaluation on the other. Planning is a process involving a series of intentional, time-related actions taken by a group or an individual that are designed to move an idea from vision into reality. The core of the planning process itself is generic and consists of four interdependent steps: defining, analyzing, choosing, and mapping.

Planning encompasses a set of skills and competencies that are vital to the successful implementation of advanced public/community health nursing practice. The remaining chapters in this section provide a detailed, in-depth examination of these vitally important skills.

■ SUGGESTED CLINICAL OR PRACTICUM ACTIVITIES

1. Meet with the director or manager of a nonprofit agency in the geographical area of your clinical placement to discuss how the agency uses the planning process to provide direction for its services.
2. Discuss with your nurse preceptor or nurse manager in the local health department how the health department collaborates with other agencies when planning programs and/or services.
3. Review program plans from both nonprofit agencies and the local health department.

■ ACKNOWLEDGMENT

The author acknowledges the staff and board of directors of the AIDS Foundation of Chicago, particularly former Executive Director Karen Fishman, for their support and encouragement of the planning activities detailed in the case study presented in this chapter.

REFERENCES

AIDS Foundation of Chicago. (1995). *AIDS Foundation of Chicago: Strategic plan, March 1, 1995-June 30, 1998*. Chicago, IL: Author.

AIDS Housing of Washington. (1995). *Chicago EMA five-year HIV/AIDS housing plan*. Seattle, WA: Author.

American Nurses Association. (2013). *Public health nursing: Scope and standards of practice* (2nd ed.). Silver Spring, MD: Author.

Beauchamp, D. E. (1985). Community: The neglected tradition of public health. *Hastings Center Report, 15*(6), 28–36.

Bekemeier, B., Walker Linderman, T., Kneipp, S., & Zahner, S. J. (2015). Updating the definition and role of public health nursing to advance and guide the specialty. *Public Health Nursing, 32*(1), 50–57.

Bellah, R. N., Madsen, R., Sullivan, W. M., Swidler, A., & Tipton, S. M. (1985). *Habits of the heart*. New York, NY: Harper & Row.

Bellah, R. N., Madsen, R., Sullivan, W. M., Swidler, A., & Tipton, S. M. (1991). *The good society*. New York, NY: Alfred A. Knopf.

Bigbee, J. L., & Issel, L. M. (2012). Conceptual models for population-focused public health nursing interventions and outcomes: The state of the art. *Public Health Nursing, 29*(4), 370–379.

Centers for Disease Control and Prevention. (2014). *The public health system and the 10 essential public health services*. Retrieved from https://www.cdc.gov/nphpsp/essentialservices.html

Chalmers, K., & Kristajanson, L. (1989). The theoretical basis for nursing at the community level: A comparison of three models. *Journal of Advanced Nursing, 14*, 569–574.

Finnegan, L., & Ervin, N. E. (1989). An epidemiological approach to community assessment. *Public Health Nursing, 6*(3), 147–151.

Gebbie, K. M., & Turnock, B. J. (2006). The public health workforce, 2006: New challenges. *Health Affairs, 25*(4), 923–933.

Hamilton, P. (1983). Community nursing diagnosis. *Advances in Nursing Science, 5*(3), 21–36.

Hamilton, P. A., & Bush, H. A. (1988). Theory development in community health nursing: Issues and recommendations. *Scholarly Inquiry for Nursing Practice: An International Journal, 2*(2), 145–159.

Hanchett, E. S. (1988). *Nursing frameworks and community as client*. Norwalk, CT: Appleton & Lange.

Hanchett, E. S. (1990). Applications of systems theory in community health nursing. In S. J. Wold (Ed.), *Community health nursing: Issues and topics* (pp. 1–11) Norwalk, CT: Appleton & Lange.

Higgs, Z. R., & Gustafson, D. D. (1985). *Community as client: Assessment and diagnosis*. Philadelphia, PA: F. A. Davis.

Institute of Medicine. (1988). *The future of public health*. Washington, DC: National Academies Press.

Kuehnert, P. L. (1991). Community health nursing and the AIDS pandemic: Case report of one community's response. *Journal of Community Health Nursing, 8*(3), 137–146.

Kuehnert, P. L. (1993, February). *Assessing community HIV/AIDS service needs*. Paper presented at the Illinois Ryan White CARE Act Title II Consortia Conference, Starved Rock, IL.

Kuehnert, P. L. (1995). The interactive and organizational model of community as client: A model for public health nursing practice. *Public Health Nursing, 12*(1), 9–17.

Maurer, F. A., & Smith, C. (2013). *Community/public health nursing practice: Health for families and populations*. St. Louis, MO: Elsevier.

McLaughlin, J. S. (1982). Toward a theoretical model for community health programs. *Advances in Nursing Science, 5*(1), 7–28.

Minkler, M. (1990). Improving health through community organization. In K. Glanz, F. Lewis., & B. Rimer (Eds.), *Health education and health behavior*. San Francisco, CA: Jossey-Bass.

Moccia, P. (1988). At the faultline: Social activism and caring. *Nursing Outlook, 36*(1), 30–33.

Nutt, P. C. (1984). *Planning methods for health and related organizations*. New York, NY: John Wiley.

Piercy, D. (1996). *Day's strategic planning manual for non-profit organizations*. Chicago, IL: CreateNet.

Public Health Accreditation Board. (2011). *Guide to national public health department accreditation. Version 1.0*. Washington, DC: Author.

Public Health Functions Steering Committee, American Public Health Association. (1995). *Public health in America*. Washington, DC: Author.

Rodgers, S. S. (1984). Community as client—A multivariate model for analysis of community and aggregate health risk. In B. W. Spradley (Ed.), *Readings in community health nursing* (3rd ed., pp. 146–156). Boston, MA: Little, Brown.

Ross, M. G. (1967). *Community organization: Theory, principles and practice* (2nd ed.). New York, NY: Harper & Row.

Rothman, J., & Tropman, J. E. (1987). Models of community organization and macro practice perspectives: Their mixing and phasing. In F. Cox, J. L. Erlich, J. Rothman., & J. E. Tropman (Eds.), *Strategies of community organization* (4th ed., pp. 3–26). Itasca, IL: Peacock.

Stanhope, M., & Lancaster, J. (2016). *Public health nursing: Population-centered health care in the community* (9th ed.). St. Louis, MO: Elsevier.

Schultz, P. R. (1987). When client means more than one: Extending the foundational concept of person. *Advances in Nursing Science, 10*(1), 71–86.

Sills, G. M., & Goeppinger, J. (1985). The community as a field of inquiry in nursing. In H. H. Werley & J. J. Fitzpatrick (Eds.), *Annual review of nursing research* (Vol. 3, pp. 3–23). New York, NY: Springer Publishing.

Smith, K., & Bazini-Barakat, N. (2003). A public health nursing practice model: Melding public health principles with the nursing process. *Public Health Nursing, 20*(1), 42–48.

Storfjell, J. L., & Cruise, P. A. (1984). A model of community-focused nursing. *Public Health Nursing, 1*(2), 85–96.

Tilson, H., & Gebbie, K. M. (2004). The public health workforce. *Annual Review of Public Health, 25*, 341–356.

Walgren, D. J. (1984). Conceptual framework: A basis for community health nursing practice. In J. A. Sullivan (Ed.), *Directions in community health nursing* (pp. 45–68). Boston, MA: Blackwell.

Watson, N. M. (1984). Community as client. In J. A. Sullivan (Ed.), *Directions in community health nursing* (pp. 69–90). Boston, MA: Blackwell.

Weil, M. (Ed.). (2004). *The handbook of community practice*. Thousand Oaks, CA: Sage.

White, M. S. (1982). Construct for public health nursing. *Nursing Outlook, 20*, 527–530.

CHAPTER 10

Formulating Program Goals and Objectives

■ STUDY EXERCISES

1. How are goals and objectives related to program planning?
2. How do goals and objectives differ?
3. What approaches are used for developing program objectives?
4. What elements are required for complete objectives?
5. Write a set of goals and objectives for a program plan based on a community diagnosis.

One of the first steps in developing a sound program plan is to write the program goals and objectives, as indicated in Figure 10.1, which lists the steps in program planning. Goals are long-range specified states of accomplishment toward which programs are directed. Objectives are statements of what is to be achieved through the program activities or services (Timmreck, 1995). Each group of objectives is related to a specific goal and spells out steps that move toward achievement of the goal.

The process of writing goals and objectives is a valuable task for the program planner or planning committee. Forcing oneself to state precisely what is expected to be achieved in a program sets the stage for more successful outcomes. Objectives lead the way to precisely stated activities. Programs may claim outcomes that could never be achieved because the program activities are not aimed at achieving the outcomes. Program planners are often required to write outcomes or measurable objectives, so the objectives may be done as an exercise. When measuring the program achievements, the outcomes fall short of their intended mark because of the lack of coordination of the objectives, activities, and the program focus. A well-thought-through set of goals, objectives, and activities will make implementation easier and provide the basis for a useful evaluation plan. This chapter assists you in learning how to formulate goals and objectives that provide a sound foundation for program planning.

■ RELATIONSHIP OF GOALS AND OBJECTIVES TO PROGRAM PLANNING

Goals and objectives are important both to operationalize the priorities from the community assessment and to guide the program planning. Although goals provide the big picture, objectives tell the painter what colors to put where, when, and how on the canvas. Just as with a coherent picture in which shapes, colors, and images are conceived as a

Identify the priority community diagnosis.
Develop goals and objectives.
Develop activities to achieve the objectives.
Develop a plan to implement the activities.
Develop a budget to implement the activities.
Write the total program plan.

FIGURE 10.1   Steps of the planning process.

whole, a coherent program plan requires a conception of how the goals, objectives, and activities come together to make a whole.

Operationalizing Community Assessment Priorities

After completion of the community assessment, the advanced practice public/community health nurse will engage in activities to establish priorities among the various community diagnoses that have been identified. Approaches to validation of community diagnoses and setting priorities are discussed in Chapter 11. The planning process contains the initial efforts to address the priorities, as indicated in Chapter 9.

Objectives for community health programs often entail areas that lack a sound research or experience base, for example, how many home visits are needed to result in a positive pregnancy outcome? Although we have some knowledge, not enough is always known to make predictions about the outcomes that result from an intervention. The best we can do is to use the available knowledge and our professional expertise to come as close as possible to what we think is needed in terms of an intervention and how much of it is needed (White, Dudley-Brown, & Terhaar, 2016).

Regardless of the lack of a research base, advanced practice public/community health nurses often develop plans to address complex, long-term community problems. One way to do this is through outcome objectives that help programs to truly focus on what are the causes or probable causes and risk factors related to a problem identified as a community diagnosis. A program plan lacks direction without a search into the causes or probable causes of a problem. The linkage between the problem and the causes sets the stage for writing goals and objectives to address a community diagnosis as the basis of a program plan that may be effective.

Guiding Program Planning

The approaches that may be used to address a specific community diagnosis are perhaps endless. To move forward in planning a program, the potential areas for programming must be identified and then narrowed to one or perhaps two areas. The goals and objectives for one specific program area can then be written.

NARROWING THE AREA FOR PROGRAM PLANNING

In Chapter 8, community diagnoses were identified as the conclusions of the analysis and synthesis of data about the community. If a well-stated community diagnosis is a problem that requires intervention, there are potentially numerous ways to approach the intervention. Goals are used to narrow program planning from the broad area of a community assessment. Specifics about how to achieve the goal are identified in the objectives.

For example, infant mortality may be a topic of a community diagnosis: Risk of death among infants in Sullivan County (a hypothetical county) related to 6% of infants weighing less than 2,500 g at birth, 23% of infants born to females younger than 18 years, and 5% of pregnant women receiving late or no prenatal care, as demonstrated in an infant mortality rate of seven deaths per 1,000 live births in 2015. Discovering the causes or risk factors related to infant deaths in a specific community leads the program planner to areas for goal exploration.

After the causes are discovered, there are still various strategies that could be chosen to decrease infant mortality. If a major cause of many infant deaths was low birth weight, several approaches could be taken to decrease the number of low-birth-weight infants, thus decreasing the number of infant deaths. A potentially very successful program would be one planned to address the specific causes of or risk factors related to low birth weight in the specific target community. A goal for such a program could be to decrease infant mortality. Objectives would be related to the major cause of low birth weight, such as to decrease the level of low-birth-weight infants from 6% to 4% over the next 2 years.

A temptation for a program planner, especially one new to the activity, is to write many goals and objectives to accomplish as much as possible in one program. However tempting this approach may be, the advanced practice public/community health nurse is advised to avoid grand-scale thinking about what can be accomplished with a small amount of money and effort. Nurses tend to think that goodwill accomplishes much, which it does, but goodwill cannot make up for a shortfall in the resources required to produce change through a program intervention.

Health and social services are faced with problems that have persisted over many generations and resisted many interventions. Many problems are multidimensional and do not respond to quick fixes. For example, a onetime educational session is inadequate for most people who desire to make behavior changes toward better health. In addition, research has demonstrated that most people have better outcomes from healthcare and program interventions if they are involved in making decisions about their own health (Glanz, Rimer, & Viswanath, 2008).

If a program has more than one facet, for example, a program that includes exercise and dietary interventions to decrease deaths from cardiovascular disease, more than one set of goals and objectives is usually needed. To reiterate, one should not be overly ambitious when planning one program that is expected to address several aspects of one problem or several problems without adequate resources.

SETTING GOALS FOR THE PROGRAM FOCUS

Different goals may be needed for one program. Examples of categories of goals are program achievement, behavior change, change in health status, and maintenance of a level of health. One example of each goal category is given in Box 10.1. Other categories of goals may be needed for a specific program, for example, stability of a change, but all should be

---

BOX 10.1 EXAMPLES OF GOALS

Program achievement goal: Make primary care accessible to the total community.

Behavior change goal: Decrease the level of smoking among residents of the community.

Change in health status goal: Decrease deaths from cardiovascular disease.

Maintenance of health status goal: Maintain the infant mortality rate at the current level.

written so as to focus on the community and clients. The program planner and planning committee will need to discuss what should be the long-term focus of the specific program.

Goals that address the continuation of a program are usually not useful for directing activities for the improvement of the health of a community. An example of a goal for program continuation is to continue to screen adults for high blood pressure. Although a screening program may be beneficial at a point in time, screening alone does not address what will be done if high blood pressure is discovered. In addition, screening programs do not usually address problem prevention. The goal may be better stated as: Increase the number of adult residents of the county who have blood pressures within the normal range. The next sections address ways to state useful goals and objectives.

REVISING OBJECTIVES

Although writing objectives before developing the program plan is highly recommended, this does not mean that objectives are never changed during or after program planning has been completed. On the contrary, the planner may find that objectives written before identification of interventions and activities are unrealistic. For example, an objective to increase access to prenatal care by opening a clinic in an underserved area would have to be changed if the only potential location became unavailable.

Resources that were not known when objectives were written may become available, so expanded objectives would be needed. At times this occurs with the number of clients or communities that can be served by a program. Sometimes during program implementation, services cannot meet the demand, and objectives would need to be changed to reflect this situation. For instance, a program may be much more popular than the planners had anticipated. If an objective is for 100% of clients to have comprehensive education about sexually transmitted diseases, a demand that exceeded resources, for example, staff time or number of hours of operation, would result in not achieving the objective. A rewritten objective could modify the 100%, for example, 100% who present between 8 a.m. and 3 p.m. Information collected about the excess demand over capacity would be very valuable in requesting additional funds to expand the program.

■ GOALS AND OBJECTIVES

As indicated earlier, goals and objectives are one route to operationalize the priorities identified after the community assessment. Well-conceptualized and well-written goals and objectives provide the program-planning team with valuable direction for the rest of the planning process.

Goals

In healthcare, a goal is a statement of a long-term future situation, condition, or status. Goals are stated in terms that may not be measurable but are usually attainable, if not in the long run, then at some time in the distant future (Dignan & Carr, 1992; Timmreck, 1995). An example of a goal is to improve the quality of life of the community. Unlike an objective, this goal has no timeline and is not measurable the way it is written.

Quality of life is a multidimensional concept that has different interpretations for various individuals and groups. To achieve the goal of improving the quality of life of the community, many years and many projects may be required. Thus, the goal may never be achieved to the satisfaction of everyone in the community, but it could be achieved by the attainment of specific objectives written for specific programs.

STATING GOALS AS OUTCOMES

Goals are better stated as long-term outcomes rather than activities. Thus, it is better to avoid writing goals that begin with words such as *to provide, to establish,* and *to develop.* These statements are usually activities or methods but do not clearly identify what is to be changed as a result of a program. Even if the goal is reached, it is unlikely that the outcome of the goal is known. To provide services or interventions without the direction of an intended outcome is too costly for most organizations. Comparisons of ways to state goals are given in Box 10.2.

Objectives

Objectives are statements of expected outcomes that are measurable, time limited, and action oriented (Timmreck, 1995). Objectives and goals differ in the projected time frame for achievement, that is, short term versus long term, and in specificity. Although objectives are often stated as activities (e.g., to provide services to the elderly in the community), it is preferable to focus objectives on outcomes rather than on what will be done. That is, what will be the results of providing services to the elderly? Will their health status change? Will they have fewer hospitalizations? What clinical indicators will change, if any? What will happen with the rate of chronic illness?

RATIONALE FOR BEHAVIORAL OBJECTIVES

The purpose of a program may be to provide services, but the objectives should be focused on what is expected to change in the target population as a result of providing services. There are several reasons for writing objectives that meet the criteria just described. Probably, the most important reason is that the objectives will more likely be interpreted similarly by everyone. Another reason is that the program implementer does not have to guess the meaning of objectives that were written several months before program implementation. Furthermore, objectives that are measurable and describe behavior help to keep the program interventions focused to those very specific areas that may result in the desired changes. An example of this advantage is illustrated in the following paragraph.

An objective to reduce deaths from cardiovascular disease by 10% in 5 years may be approached from many methods and interventions. One tendency is to develop a program that approaches the situation from many directions, for example, reduction of dietary fat

---

BOX 10.2 COMPARISONS OF GOALS

Weak Goal Statements	Stronger Goal Statements
To give immunizations	To increase the immunization level among the 2-year-old population
To screen for hypertension	To increase the proportion of individuals who maintain normal blood pressure through screening and referral for diagnosis and treatment
To develop a respite program for caregivers	To improve the quality of life for caregivers of home-dwelling disabled individuals

intake, increasing exercise, controlling high blood pressure, smoking cessation, and weight reduction—in other words, to simultaneously attack all known risk factors for cardiovascular disease. This approach may result in no progress toward the objective because resources were spread too thin and not enough attention was paid to the areas that may be more effective. As mentioned earlier, identifying the causes or probable causes and risk factors for a specific community diagnosis is important for developing programs that may be more effective.

Following is another way to write the reduction-in-cardiovascular-disease objective: Increase the proportion of adults who engage in aerobic physical activity of at least moderate intensity for 150 minutes/week or 75 minutes/week of vigorous intensity or an equivalent combination (Office of Disease Prevention and Health Promotion [ODPHP], 2016b). After identifying baseline activity levels for specific segments of the community, high-risk groups with low levels of activity could be targeted, and a program developed to achieve the objective of increasing physical activity. Then, other objectives could be written to address additional risk factors in the specific community.

Additional advantages to writing clearly defined objectives are as follows:

- The evaluation of a program is much easier.
- Program implementers have clear directions.
- Potential funders and/or grant administrators have fewer questions about the direction of the program.
- Staff is able to carry out the specified activities in a better way.

RELATIONSHIP OF OBJECTIVES TO GOALS

Objectives are related to goals in that the objectives spell out precisely what outcomes are expected as means to achieve the goals. Furthermore, a group of objectives is written to be specifically related to each goal. As an example, Box 10.3 contains one goal and a list of related objectives.

Although it is not easy to write clear objectives, the program will be stronger and have better results if the hard work is put into writing measurable, outcome-oriented objectives. The following section presents in detail how to develop such objectives.

BOX 10.3 A PROGRAM GOAL AND RELATED OBJECTIVES

Program Goal

To decrease violence in the community

Objectives

1. To decrease the number of weapons carried to school by students and adults as measured by random searches of backpacks, briefcases, and other bags brought into schools by 50% in the next 6 months
2. To decrease the number of reported conflicts in schools and public places by mandatory attendance of offenders and voluntary attendance of all other community members at conflict-avoidance sessions by 20% in the next year
3. To improve the safety of residents and property through community policing, as demonstrated by a 5% decrease in reported crimes against residents and property, by increasing the number of police officers by 20% during the next 6 months

■ ELEMENTS REQUIRED FOR COMPLETE OBJECTIVES

Objectives need to contain specific elements to be considered complete. Objectives need to use action verbs that describe terminal behaviors. Furthermore, objectives need to state **who** will perform the behaviors under what conditions. Often, the quality and quantity of the behaviors will need to be stated as part of the objectives. Including **how** behaviors will be measured adds to the completeness of objectives. How objectives relate to the goal and a specified time frame are additional elements of complete objectives (Dignan & Carr, 1992; Kiritz, 1980; Mager, 1962). See Box 10.4 for a summary of the characteristics of complete objectives.

Behavioral Terms

An objective needs to be written in behavioral terms. This means using an action verb. Usually, a change in behavior is **what** can be observed as a result of an intervention (Dignan & Carr, 1992).

DESCRIBING TERMINAL BEHAVIORS

In healthcare, the behavior change may be a physical act, such as not smoking; a mental act, such as correctly listing the food groups; or a physiological state, such as blood pressure within normal range. For a community, similar behavior changes are possible. For example, a behavior change may be a decrease in the smoking level from 25% to 22% of the population in 1 year. Although smoking behavior would be changed by individuals as a result of class sessions, individual counseling, or self-initiation, the community decrease in smoking prevalence as a whole could be measured. Behavior changes for a community may also be related to status (e.g., income level), condition (e.g., free of toxic waste sites), trends (e.g., increasing employment levels), and strengths (e.g., building on community pride).

USING ACTION VERBS

To describe a measurable change, precise verbs need to be used to convey a meaning that can be interpreted by everyone in the same way. Table 10.1 contains lists of verbs that are useful and those to be avoided when writing measurable objectives.

BOX 10.4   CHARACTERISTICS OF COMPLETE OBJECTIVES

Stated in Behavioral Terms

- Uses action verbs
- Describes terminal behavior
- States who will perform the behavior under what conditions
- Describes the quality of performance
- Describes the quantity of performance
- Describes how performance will be measured
- Relates to goal
- Delineates the time frame

Sources: Adapted from Green, L. W., & Kreuter, M. W. (2005). *Health promotion planning: An educational and ecological approach* (4th ed.). St. Louis, MO: McGraw-Hill; Mager, R. F. (1962). *Preparing instructional objectives.* Palo Alto, CA: Fearon; Timmreck, T. C. (1995). *Planning, program development, and evaluation.* Boston, MA: Jones & Bartlett.

TABLE 10.1 Verbs for Writing Objectives

Useful Verbs for Writing Objectives	Verbs to Avoid	Useful Verbs for Writing Objectives	Verbs to Avoid
Decrease	Know	Select	Acknowledge
Increase	Understand	Apply	Experience
Identify	Appreciate	Complete	Enjoy
List	Believe	Develop	See
Demonstrate	Realize	Open	Grasp
State	Verbalize	Answer	Imagine
Define	Aware	Calculate	Learn
Diagram	Comprehend	Report	Perceive
Evaluate	Feel		

To locate an appropriate verb, the advanced practice public/community health nurse needs to identify the behavior expected at the end of the program or intervention by name (Green & Kreuter, 2005). This may be an act (e.g., walk), an intellectual behavior (e.g., recognize), a physiological response (e.g., normal blood pressure), or a changed state (e.g., decreased infant mortality). If a statement begins with words such as *to provide, to create,* or *to establish,* the statement is a method and not an objective.

Suggested verbs for objectives in the cognitive, motor, and affective domains are shown in Table 10.2. The organization and content of Table 10.2 are selected on the basis of the work of Bloom et al. (Bloom, 1956; Krathwohl, Bloom, & Masia, 1964) and Mager (1962). Other verbs may be discovered through brainstorming, in dictionaries, and in a thesaurus. Books on writing educational objectives may be good sources of verbs for outcome objectives. Nursing textbooks contain examples that usually refer to individuals but may be useful for generating ideas about outcomes for communities and groups.

At times, it is difficult to find just the right verb to match what the planner has in mind. Then a temptation is to state an objective in a negative form, such as: Parents will not abuse their children. Stating objectives as negatives or behaviors not performed is not a desired format because you are then collecting data about the absence of some behavior. In rare instances when only negative wording comes to mind, identify the behavior that is desired. If the negative behavior is, for example, not to abuse children, the desired behavior may be for parents to describe their feelings when they have an urge to abuse their children. A clear description of the desired behavior may require more than a verb and phrase. Writing a complete description of the behavior may be needed before an outcome objective is written.

After writing an objective, ask yourself: "Can I answer yes or no that this objective has been met when the program is completed?" If you are unable to give an unequivocal answer, rewrite the objective because it is not clearly measurable. Moreover, if an objective is not clear to you, it will not be clear to anyone else.

DESCRIBING BEHAVIORS UNDER SPECIFIC CONDITIONS

For some objectives, the behavior of program participants will need to occur under specific conditions or circumstances. The description of the behavior within the context of the conditions is important for having a measurable objective. For example, if smoking cessation

TABLE 10.2 Verbs in the Cognitive, Motor, and Affective Domains

Cognitive Domain Verbs

Knowledge	Comprehension	Application	Analysis	Synthesis	Evaluation
Cite	Associate	Apply	Analyze	Arrange	Appraise
Count	Classify	Calculate	Categorize	Assemble	Assess
Define	Compare	Correlate	Contrast	Collect	Choose
Identify	Contrast	Demonstrate	Criticize	Compose	Critique
Indicate	Describe	Operate	Diagram	Construct	Debate
Label	Differentiate	Practice	Examine	Diagnose	Determine
List	Discuss	Relate	Infer	Formulate	Evaluate
Name	Explain	Schedule	Inspect	Generalize	Grade
Order	Illustrate	Solve	Inventory	Integrate	Judge
Outline	Interpret	Use	Question	Manage	Justify
Recognize	Predict	Utilize	Separate	Organize	Measure
Relate	Review	Write	Solve	Produce	Prescribe
Repent	Translate		Summarize	Synthesize	Rank
Select					Rate
Tell					Recommend
Write					Revise
					Score
					Test

Motor Domain Verbs

Add	Do	Handle	Meet	Set
Be present	Drop	Hold	Move	Take
Call	Give	Keep	Place	Turn
Contaminate	Give care	Make	Position	

Affective Domain Verbs

Receiving	Responding	Valuing	Conceptualization	Characterization
Realize	Willing to	Assume responsibility	Admire	Develop consistency about
Accept	Contribute to	Adopt	Find pleasure in	Relate beliefs to the problem
Listen to	Obey	Challenge		
Be alert to	Practice	Prefer		

Sources: Adapted from Bloom, B. S. (Ed.). (1956). *Taxonomy of educational objectives. Handbook 1: Cognitive domain.* New York, NY: David McKay; Krathwohl, D. R., Bloom, B. S., & Masia, B. B. (1964). *Taxonomy of educational objectives. Handbook II: Affective domain.* New York, NY: David McKay; Mager, R. F. (1962). *Preparing instructional objectives.* Palo Alto, CA: Fearon.

is to occur after attending five sessions of the program, then the objective will be better stated including that caveat, such as: After attending five smoking-cessation sessions, 40% of participants will stop smoking.

Contrast this objective with one that does not contain behavioral terms for the program participants: to conduct smoking-cessation sessions every month for a year. This describes an activity but does not describe the effectiveness of the sessions or the behavior change of the program participants.

WRITING REALISTIC OUTCOMES

A word of caution is also needed in objective writing. Often, program planners are enthusiastic about how much a program will potentially accomplish and want to promise great outcomes, often well beyond what could be expected. For example, expecting that 70% of program participants will stop smoking is probably not realistic. If continued funding is based on achievement of objectives, funding is in jeopardy when those objectives are not achieved. It may be helpful to use national objectives as benchmarks. For example, there are 42 health-related topic areas and 1,200 objectives in *Healthy People 2020* (ODPHP, 2016b).

Thus, keeping objectives realistic, yet optimistic, is a matter of skill and having others provide critique before the program plan is finalized. Asking others what they think could be accomplished by knowing the target population. You could ask the target population what they want to accomplish. Objectives need to be realistic in relation to other factors, for example, availability of qualified staff, an accessible target population, and adequate funding.

Specifying Who

After finding a verb that describes the terminal behavior, the next step is to describe the behavior in more detail by stating who will perform the behavior under what conditions. Objectives should describe the population or aggregate served or targeted for the program (Green & Kreuter, 2005).

Without specification of the target population and the conditions under which the behavior is to occur, the grant funding source and the program implementer will have difficulty relating the pieces of the proposal and outcomes together. For example, if the objective is smoking cessation, must the smoker attend three of four smoking-cessation classes? Or is it necessary for the smoker to attend all four sessions? Is the program intended for pregnant women, adults, or adolescents?

SPECIFYING QUALITY AND QUANTITY OF PERFORMANCE

If quality of performance, or how well the behavior is performed, is important for the achievement of an objective, describe how well the aggregate or population must perform to meet an acceptable level (Dignan & Carr, 1992). For example, must participants get eight of 10 questions correct on a posttest? How will the program evaluator know whether the program participants are performing a behavior correctly?

Closely related to quality of performance is quantity of performance. The objective should include how much of the behavior is acceptable. Quantifying behavior in an objective is preferable because of the greater ease of collecting and analyzing data. Does achievement of the objective require that the population perform all of the behavior or 50% of the behavior? Must the smoker have no cigarettes? Or is it okay for the smoker to have had one or two cigarettes after stopping smoking? Will infant mortality be decreased by 10% or 20%? Objectives that are aimed at increases or decreases in behavior must be related to the baseline behavior or state of the participants.

Measuring the Behavior

How the behavior will be measured is another important component of the objective. Often, measurement of a behavior is stated through a phrase at the end of the objective that starts with *by*. For example: To make a 40% decrease in smoking among adult participants who attend five smoking-cessation sessions as measured *by* self-report.

When writing objectives, it is sometimes necessary to include the baseline behavior in order to measure an increase or decrease. For example, a decrease of 10% in infant mortality would require that we know what the infant mortality rate was when the objective was written. This objective will be measured by a change in the infant mortality rate. Thus, if the baseline infant mortality rate was 14 deaths per 1,000 live births, a 10% decrease would be 0.10×14 or 1.4 deaths. Usually, for events such as infant deaths, a 3-year or longer time period is specified in the objective.

The *Healthy People 2020* document incorporates baseline information for each objective as follows: Reduce cigarette smoking by adults. Baseline: 20.6% of adults aged 18 years and older were current cigarette smokers in 2008. Target: 12% (ODPHP, 2016a).

The baseline statistic or behavior could also be incorporated into the objective by stating: Reduce cigarette smoking from 20.6% to 12% of the adult population aged 18 years and older. If subpopulations are different targets of the program, a different objective may need to be written for each subpopulation; for example, 19.5% of adolescents in grades 9 to 12 smoked cigarettes in the past 30 days in 2009; the target is 16% (ODPHP, 2016a).

COST OF OBTAINING DATA TO MEASURE BEHAVIORS

Careful thought needs to go into the measures to be used because of the potential cost and effort required to obtain data for measuring achievement of the objectives. As much as possible, data collected for objective achievement should be the same as that required by external funding sources, part of ongoing record systems, and not time-consuming to compile. For example, if attendance at three of four smoking-cessation sessions is part of the measurement for objective achievement, attendance records should be built into the program routine.

If an objective requires an inordinate amount of data collection at great cost, such as extensive surveys or record reviews, the advanced practice public/community health nurse's time would be better spent rewriting the objective for more efficient time use. Planning for data collection before program implementation is also very important because often baseline data are needed to measure improvement. If data collection is not started as the program is implemented, it may be impossible to recover useful data for objective measurement.

Relating Objectives to the Goal

Not only must the verb be appropriate but also the content must be related to the goal for an objective to be considered complete. This is an area in which objective writers often go astray. To focus the objectives, write several that you decide are related to the goal. Then ask yourself: If this objective is met, will achievement of the goal be closer? If you can answer yes, then perhaps the objective is on track. If you answer no, delete or rewrite the objective. At times, you may not know whether the answer is yes or no. Then ask others the same questions about the objectives. In this way, you may come closer to having objectives that truly relate to the goal.

In his seminal work, Kiritz (1980) provided the following example of a well-defined objective: "At the conclusion of the five-day workshop, at least 20 to 25 participants will demonstrate a pre-/posttest gain of at least 25 percent on the Evaluator's Competency Test, covering the areas of (1) introductory statistical terminology,

(2) measurable objectives, and (3) educational program evaluation concepts" (p. 20). Kiritz's work has been updated and more information may be found at the website (www.tgci.com/grantsmanship-program-planning-proposal-writing).

Another test of having appropriate content that is related to the goal is to analyze how much the objectives are related to each other. A diagram of how the goal and objectives relate to each other is one approach to analyzing the relationships of the statements.

Delineating the Time Frame

Another component of complete objectives is delineating the time frame for accomplishment of the specified outcome. Often this time frame is at the termination of the program, for example, after 1 or 2 years of funding. At times when it is awkward to insert the time frame into each objective, an alternative approach is to have a stem that introduces a set of objectives. A stem such as "By the end of the program, participants will be able to . . ." may be used for the objectives that follow.

A second approach to set the time frame for accomplishment of objectives is to use results of research studies. A review of the literature will provide information and justification for specific points in time. With this approach, a word of caution is also in order. Results obtained in research studies cannot always be replicated in the real world because of the myriad differences between controlled research designs and the community setting (Green & Kreuter, 2005).

Determining the time frame is not always a scientific endeavor but requires a thoughtful discussion among the people who will implement the program. In addition, lead time is often needed to acquire equipment, hire staff, and accomplish tasks requisite to implementation of the program. One approach for determining the time frame for accomplishment of objectives is to use a Gantt chart to plan the total project timeline (White et al., 2016). Then this information can be used to set time frames for the objectives. Other methods used to determine time frames for accomplishment of objectives include basing them on the past year's performance, using what other similar programs have achieved, and using a consensus process with experienced individuals (Green & Kreuter, 2005).

Objectives are an important component of program planning and offer a good beginning for conceptualizing what is intended to occur as a result of the program. Complete and measurable objectives take time to develop but are well worth the time and effort expended. The characteristics of complete objectives are summarized in Box 10.4.

■ APPROACHES FOR SPECIFYING PROGRAM OBJECTIVES

Various approaches for specifying program objectives may be used to gain more precision and detail. The three approaches explained in this section are levels of objectives, process objectives, and outcome objectives.

Levels of Objectives

One approach to write objectives is to break them down into levels. Levels of objectives are usually needed more often in a complex or large program because greater detail may be needed to guide the implementation. In addition, levels of objectives may be used in a specific organization because formats for goals and objectives differ among organizations. Although the development of the detail required in levels of objectives may be tedious, full implementation of a program may be dependent on this level of detail.

Often after program implementation is started, the staff responsible for implementation finds that they do not understand what is to be done and must write or figure out what those other unwritten objectives or activities would have been. Unfortunately, they often guess what was intended and may be wrong or change the original intention of the program. The approach of levels of objectives may prevent unintentional changes being made during program implementation or with change of staff.

Greater detail may be achieved by developing two or three levels of objectives. A two-level approach will have "higher than low-level" and "low-level" objectives. The three-level approach includes high-, intermediate-, and low-level objectives. The lower level objectives in both approaches are more detailed and more specific than the higher level ones. Other terms for the lower level objectives are *action objectives, subobjectives, short-term objectives,* and *activity-directed objectives* (Timmreck, 1995).

The terminology is not as important as the clarity and consistency with which a specific approach is applied. For example, if a program planner has used high-, intermediate-, and low-level objectives, switching to objectives and activities in the middle of a program plan would be inconsistent. Examples of the two approaches to objective development are given in Box 10.5.

Although levels of objectives may be appropriate for a specific project, other approaches may be needed for other projects. Process and outcome objectives may be used together or in combination with levels of objectives.

Process Objectives

Although this chapter has concentrated on encouraging you to write behavioral objectives in terms of program participant behaviors, there is a place for process objectives that are measurable and behavioral in terms of employee behaviors. Process objectives spell out

---

BOX 10.5   EXAMPLES OF LEVELS OF OBJECTIVES

Example of Three-Level Objectives

Goal 1: To improve the quality of life of community residents

Objective 1.1: To increase the number of families living in housing units that meet the city housing code (high-level objective) by 10% in 1 year

Objective 1.2: To complete applications for relocation by at least 75 families who have filed complaints about housing-code violations in their current housing units within the past 3 months (intermediate-level objective)

Objective 1.3: To identify with owners and families all housing units that cannot be repaired (low-level objectives)

Example of Two-Level Objectives

Goal 2: To decrease deaths due to smoking among community residents

Objective 2.1: To decrease the number of smokers in the working population from 25% to 22% in 2 years by providing smoking-cessation programs for all worksites in the county (higher than low-level objective)

Objective 2.2: To gain commitment from half of the worksites in the county to sponsor smoking-cessation programs within 1 year (low-level objective)

the actions of staff or others involved in the program. Process refers to what the individuals or groups will do. Although some process objectives may be written as activities, it should be clear what will be the outcome of the activities, and it is the outcome that is stated in an objective.

Process objectives allow the program implementer to know that the program is being put into place as intended by the planners. For example, the objective, "Staff will implement the intervention according to the protocol," is critical for staff to achieve so that a program component will be successful. Although some modifications may be necessary as a program plan is implemented, a program implemented as intended can be evaluated better than one that is changed without documentation of the changes.

In the previous example ("Staff will implement the intervention as specified in the protocol"), many activities are required for the staff to implement the intervention. The intervention will be based on research results, so it will be more effective if the fidelity (i.e., correspondence with the protocol) of the intervention is maintained during the program.

A group of process objectives would be helpful when staff training, new procedures, or other system changes are needed. Such changes may be a new computer software package, new forms to be completed by staff, a new appointment system, teaching protocols for clients, a new client record system, or a new treatment protocol. Staff training is needed for many of these changes.

Often implementation of new programs is begun only for administrators to discover that some vital pieces are missing, for example, training new staff or obtaining new equipment. These situations slow or stop implementation and result in more cost. Process objectives that are carefully thought through will make these oversights less likely.

Outcome Objectives

Outcome objectives are statements of what the program participants will achieve at the end of the program. These statements are measurable, behavioral, concise, time-limited, expected end points for the individuals, groups, aggregates, or communities who participated in the program at the specified level (Dignan & Carr, 1992). *Outcome objectives* may seem a redundant term, but because many sources give examples of process objectives or even objectives that sound like activities, differentiation has been made of the types of objectives used in this book.

PARTICIPANT AND COMMUNITY OUTCOMES

The meat and potatoes, so to speak, of program objectives are the outcomes that participants or communities are expected to reach as a result of the program. Advanced practice public/community health nurses are often confused when writing outcome objectives because the nursing approach to writing care plans has centered around nursing actions. This process approach is often carried over into program planning as demonstrated in the following example from the literature.

The authors described a program designed "to promote intergenerational exchange between community-based seniors and elementary school children." The specific objectives to reach this goal were listed as "(a) establishing positive, ongoing relationships between the students and seniors; (b) facilitating communication between the two intergenerational groups; and (c) providing a supportive environment for this exchange to occur" (Poole & Gooding, 1993, p. 78).

To write behavioral objectives for this example, we would need to know the intended outcome of the intergenerational exchange. Was it to improve the quality of life for both generations? Was it to improve the health status of the adults? Was it to delay dependency or institutionalization of the adults? For the children, was the intention to improve school performance, enhance their socialization, or to increase their appreciation of older adults? Perhaps, it was an opportunity to have students exposed to grandparent figures.

The objectives from this intergenerational study described what the program activities would be, not the outcomes. Outcomes may be behaviors such as enhanced quality of life for the senior adults by improved scores on a quality-of-life measure, communication between the groups as measured by number and length of contacts, and an adequate level of satisfaction with the environment as specified by survey results. Contacts between generations may also result in better mental and physical functioning of the older generation. Without more information, we are at a loss to develop objectives that describe the intended outcomes of the program as described in Poole and Gooding (1993).

While writing outcome objectives, developers should ask themselves what will the participants of this program look like, act like, or sound like at the end of their participation? Will they be healthier? What will be the specific description of that healthier state? For example, will their blood pressures be within recommended limits? Will their weight be more or less than when they started the program? What will they purchase when they shop for food? What will be the birth weights of their infants? What skills will the participants be able to perform? The time spent in developing outcome objectives, especially in a small group, should provide a realistic set of objectives that is more likely to be addressed in the program interventions.

INVOLVING COMMUNITY MEMBERS

How do we know whether the program participants want to achieve the outcomes developed for the program? We do not know unless we ask the participants or potential participants. This means that we must involve the community in program-planning activities in several ongoing ways (Anderson & McFarlane, 2015). Community involvement in community assessment and program planning has been emphasized throughout previous chapters and is addressed more specifically for program planning in Chapter 12.

WEIGHING COSTS AGAINST OUTCOMES

An additional focus of outcome objectives is that they address areas that will have the greatest effect on the problem at a reasonable cost. For example, we know that smoking by pregnant women often results in infants of low birth weight (Zhang et al., 2017). An intervention to reduce smoking by pregnant women will probably have a greater cost-benefit than, for example, screening every pregnant woman for HIV infection.

■ SUMMARY

One of the first steps to begin program planning is to write the goals and objectives. In healthcare, goals are statements of long-term future situations, conditions, or status. Objectives are statements of what is to be achieved through the program activities or services (Timmreck, 1995).

As statements of what is to be achieved through program activities, objectives provide the road map for where the program is headed. In an unfamiliar area, a road map shows the driver what roads to take and lets the driver know that the destination has been reached. Clearly written objectives give this kind of guidance to the people implementing the program plan. Without clear objectives, program staff will neither know what route to take nor when the destination has been reached.

Complete objectives are written in behavioral terms using action verbs to describe terminal behaviors. Objectives need to contain qualifying phrases about who will perform the behaviors under what conditions. Quantity and quality of performance, as well as how the behavior will be measured, adds to the completeness of objectives. Approaches for specifying program objectives included in this chapter are levels of objectives, process objectives, and outcome objectives.

■ SUGGESTED CLINICAL OR PRACTICUM ACTIVITIES

1. Locate a written program plan in a local health department or nonprofit agency. Compare the goals and objectives to the characteristics described in this chapter.
2. Meet with a program planner at a nonprofit agency to discuss how the agency approaches the process of program planning.
3. Interview a public health nurse about how new programs are implemented from written plans, if they are. If written plans are not used, how does the nurse know how to implement the program?

REFERENCES

Anderson, E. T., & McFarlane, J. (2015). *Community as partner: Theory and practice in nursing* (7th ed.). Philadelphia, PA: Wolters Kluwer.

Bloom, B. S. (Ed.). (1956). *Taxonomy of educational objectives. Handbook 1: Cognitive domain*. New York, NY: David McKay.

Dignan, M. B., & Carr, P. A. (1992). *Program planning for health education and promotion* (2nd ed.). Philadelphia, PA: Lea & Febiger.

Glanz, K., Rimer, B. K., & Viswanath, K. (Eds.). (2008). *Health behavior and health education: Theory, research, and practice* (4th ed.). San Francisco, CA: Jossey-Bass.

Green, L. W., & Kreuter, M. W. (2005). *Health promotion planning: An educational and ecological approach* (4th ed.). St. Louis, MO: McGraw-Hill.

Kiritz, N. J. (1980). *Program planning & proposal writing*. Los Angeles, CA: The Grantsmanship Center.

Krathwohl, D. R., Bloom, B. S., & Masia, B. B. (1964). *Taxonomy of educational objectives. Handbook II: Affective domain*. New York, NY: David McKay.

Mager, R. F. (1962). *Preparing instructional objectives*. Palo Alto, CA: Fearon.

Office of Disease Prevention and Health Promotion. (2016a). Physical activity. In *Healthy people 2020*. Washington, DC: U.S. Department of Health and Human Services. Retrieved from https://www .healthypeople.gov/2020/topics-objectives/topic/physical-activity

Office of Disease Prevention and Health Promotion. (2016b). 2020 topics and objectives – Objectives A–Z. In *Healthy people 2020*. Washington, DC: U.S. Department of Health and Human Services. Retrieved from https://www.healthypeople.gov/2020/topics-objectives

Poole, G. G., & Gooding, B. A. (1993). Developing and implementing a community intergenerational program. *Journal of Community Health Nursing, 10*(2), 77–85.

Timmreck, T. C. (1995). *Planning, program development, and evaluation*. Boston, MA: Jones & Bartlett.

White, K. M., Dudley-Brown, S., & Terhaar, M. F. (Eds.). (2016). *Translation of evidence into nursing and health care* (2nd ed.). New York, NY: Springer Publishing.

Zhang, X., Devasia, R., Czarnecki, G., Frechette, J., Russell, S., & Behringer, B. (2017). Effects of incentive-based smoking cessation programs for pregnant women on birth outcomes. *Maternal and Child Health, 21*(4), 745–751. doi:10.1007/s10995-016-2166-y

CHAPTER 11

Focusing Evidence-Based Program Planning

■ STUDY EXERCISES

1. What steps are taken to focus program planning after completion of the community assessment?
2. What methods may be used to identify causes of adverse situations identified in community diagnoses? Evaluate each method in terms of efficiency, effectiveness, and appropriateness for working with a community.
3. What factors are considered in selecting the appropriate level of program focus: individual, group, or community?
4. How would you go about identifying, critiquing, and selecting a research-based or evidence-based intervention to address an adverse situation specified in a community diagnosis?
5. How may theory be used to develop an intervention to address a community diagnosis?

After completion of a community assessment, the advanced practice public/community health nurse may be involved in the development of a program plan to address a community diagnosis. If program planning is the next step, additional work is needed to expand upon the community diagnosis and to narrow the areas to be addressed in the program and specific intervention. This chapter presents details about focusing program planning on the areas that require intervention.

■ STEPS TO FOCUS PROGRAM PLANNING

As discussed in Chapter 8, community diagnoses provide a picture of the community health status, but not specific answers to what is needed to address identified adverse situations. Thus, several steps need to be completed before beginning the development of a written program plan: validating the community diagnoses; prioritizing the community diagnoses; identifying the causes or possible causes of adverse situations addressed in the community diagnoses; selecting the level of program focus; and identifying alternative, research-based interventions to address the community diagnoses. The next sections address these steps.

Validating Community Diagnoses

Validation is a process of verification or substantiation of the community diagnoses. Validation of community diagnoses by community members is an important step for focusing the program plan. As emphasized earlier, communities must be involved in the solutions to their own problems. The advanced practice public/community health nurse has a specific job to carry out, but cannot do all the work required to make or keep communities healthy. The involvement of community residents is imperative to long-term, sustained improvement of all communities.

Stakeholders for each community diagnosis may be involved in validation, or all diagnoses may be validated through wide community representation. In an ideal world, the validation would be part of the continuing involvement of the community that had input into the community assessment. Thus, the concerns, observations, and opinions of community residents would already be captured in the community diagnoses.

The wording of the diagnoses is important for clear communication. In some instances, the professionally oriented wording of diagnoses, such as the approaches presented in Chapter 8, need to be modified to convey meaning in terms used by the community. For example, a diagnosis that includes the phrase "as demonstrated in" could be worded "as shown by the following." Community diagnoses may need to be translated to languages other than English. Graphics, pictures, slides, videotapes, or other visuals may be helpful in displaying the results of the community assessment.

METHODS FOR VALIDATING COMMUNITY DIAGNOSES

Many methods may be used to validate community diagnoses. Some methods that are also used for data collection are described in Chapter 6, such as focus groups, the Delphi technique, and surveys. Two additional methods described in this section are the nominal group process and rating tools.

Nominal Group Process. The nominal group process is a technique used to obtain a great deal of information from participants in a brief period. The process consists of a series of very specific steps that are facilitated by a leader who is an objective implementer of the steps. Specific training for leading a group helps to make the process proceed smoothly and on time.

Steps of the nominal group process are to compose groups of not more than 10 participants, pose a question to the group, ask group members to write down their answers to the question without discussion, conduct a round-robin procedure (i.e., ask each person around the table to state one item from her or his list), record all items as given, clarify each response, conduct a preliminary vote on ranking each item, discuss the preliminary vote, conduct a final vote, and tally the total vote (Delbecq, Van de Ven, & Gustafson, 1975).

Following is the question that may be posed to the group: What do you think are the most important health and social issues facing our community? If the same areas are identified as found in the community assessment, then validation is determined. If different areas are identified, the assessment team or the advanced practice public/community health nurse may have to reanalyze the assessment data, collect additional data, or link existing data to the identified community issues.

Ranking Tools. A second method for validation of community diagnoses is the use of ranking tools. These may be developed by the nurse or adapted from tools in the literature (Anderson & McFarlane, 2015; Helvie, 1998). The tool should ask community members to specify to what extent they believe the community diagnoses exist in the community and

TABLE 11.1 Priority Ranking Tool for Community Diagnoses

Community Diagnoses (Problems)	How Important to Solve: 1 = Low 2 = Medium 3 = High	Positive Change for Community if Solved: 0 = None 1 = Low 2 = Medium 3 = High	Improvement in Quality of Life if Solved: 0 = None 1 = Low 2 = Medium 3 = High	Rank All Problems From 1 to 6: 1 = Least Important 6 = Most Important

to what extent they are correctly identified. These rankings are then used to compare with the diagnoses developed by the advanced practice public/community health nurse or assessment team. An example of a tool that combines validation and ranking is presented in Table 11.1.

Prioritizing Community Diagnoses

Usually, several community diagnoses are identified in one community assessment. Not all can be addressed at the same time for program planning, so some system of placing them in order of importance, or prioritization, is needed. Prioritization should follow validation because not all diagnoses may be validated.

METHODS FOR PRIORITIZING DIAGNOSES

Methods of placing community diagnoses in order of importance are neither totally objective nor do all who may participate accept all methods equally. It is best to use a method that is most compatible with the characteristics of the group or groups that will do the prioritizing. Different methods may be used with different groups. For example, a method that requires little reading and writing, such as one using graphs and pictures, is best to use with a low-literacy group.

Paper-and-Pencil Tools. A tool that places all community diagnoses in random order using a scale to rate their importance to the community may be easily constructed. Other indicators of importance may be added, such as the number of people affected, potential magnitude of change for the community if the adverse situation is addressed, and potential effect on the quality of community life if the adverse situation is solved. An example of a tool is shown in Table 11.1. Another example is found in the section on causal analysis that follows in this chapter.

Such a tool for prioritizing diagnoses may be used during group meetings of citizens, professionals, political officials, church congregations, volunteers, and business owners. A survey tool could be mailed to a random sample of registered voters or parents of schoolchildren. Children could be asked for their opinions in a variety of settings. The use of several groups will decrease the chance of getting a bias toward one or two diagnoses.

All approaches to using tools for prioritizing will require resources for their implementation; therefore, the use will depend on the availability of time, money, personnel, and other resources.

Verbal Group Priority-Setting Methods. Some of the methods explained in Chapter 6 that are used for data collection may also be applied to the task of priority setting. For example, surveys could be conducted face to face. Ranking diagnoses by asking people what is more important for the future of the community is one such survey approach.

Identifying Causes or Possible Causes of Diagnoses

As discussed in Chapter 8, causes or possible causes of diagnoses are not necessarily discovered during the community assessment process. To plan a program that will specifically target the causes of a diagnosis, causes or possible causes must be identified to the extent possible after the diagnoses are formulated. Also, as pointed out earlier, not all adverse situations have known causes. In those instances, risk factors or other characteristics of the situation are used to focus the program intervention.

METHODS FOR CAUSAL ANALYSIS

Causal analysis can be used to identify unidentified needs or to analyze factors contributing to known problems or adverse situations. "Without causal analysis, it is all too easy to settle for solutions or programs that do not really meet the need" (Witkin & Altschuld, 1995, p. 269). Three methods for conducting causal analysis are presented next: literature searches, fishboning, and cause-and-consequence analysis.

Literature Searches. A first approach for all community diagnoses that will be the basis for a program plan is to complete a literature search. This may have already been done during the data-collection phase of the community assessment to assist with identification of risk factors and other clues to needed data. In any case, additional literature may need to be explored to assist with identification of causes. Coupled with local data, the literature search will provide the advanced practice public/community health nurse enough information to proceed with the use of an additional method of causal analysis or to work with the planning team. More detail about literature searches is provided later in this chapter under techniques for identifying an intervention.

At times, the use of an additional causal analysis method will be needed or desired to obtain local ideas about causes of adverse situations. For example, several explanations may be found in the literature for intergenerational conflict. However, without including the opinions of community residents, a program may not be successful because it fails to account for local variations on what was found in the literature.

Fishboning. As a technique for identifying causes of an existing adverse situation or problem, fishboning is a quick and easy method to use. This technique could be used to identify causes of community diagnoses that do not have clear scientific explanations, for example, failure of parents to obtain immunizations for their children when no-cost services are available. Combined with data from the community assessment and a literature search, the results from a fishboning session may be very useful to focus and tailor a program to meet a local specific situation.

In a fishboning exercise, groups of 10 to 12 people who are familiar with the problem are assembled, with each group having a facilitator. As many groups as are needed may be assembled to represent various viewpoints or expertise. Each group is presented with a fishbone diagram of the problem, as shown in Figure 11.1. The problem is indicated on the head of the fishbone and the major categories of the problem are listed on the ribs,

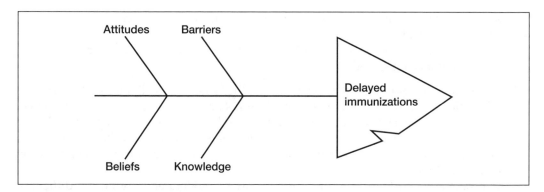

FIGURE 11.1   Fishbone diagram of delayed immunizations.

Source: Adapted from Ishikawa, K. (1992). *Guide to quality control.* Tokyo, Japan: Asian Productivity Organization.

extending to the left. The ribs may be filled in with ideas generated from the group or the facilitator may fill in the ribs while the group is generating ideas. Generally, the number of ribs is kept to fewer than 10 and usually four or five ribs are used, as indicated in Figure 11.1.

The facilitator begins the session by describing the reason for the meeting and the problem to be addressed. The next step is to have each person write down without discussion as many causes of the problem as can be thought of in about 10 minutes. Each person is then asked by the facilitator to name one cause and indicate where it should be placed on the fishbone diagram as a line radiating from the appropriate rib. This process is continued until all ideas are exhausted.

After review of the diagram and restructuring as needed, the facilitator asks the group to indicate whether each cause is important by a show of hands. Those causes receiving no votes are deleted. Group members then individually assign a number from 1 (most likely) to 5 (least likely) to each item, indicating the likelihood of each as a cause of the problem. After the votes are tallied and displayed on the diagram, there is general discussion of the diagram (Witkin & Altschuld, 1995).

The results may be displayed for all interested parties to review, or distributed via various means such as newsletters or websites. For program planning, the advanced practice public/community health nurse will have a good beginning template of causes to begin the planning process.

Cause-and-Consequence Analysis.   Cause-and-consequence analysis encourages the uncovering of both causes and effects of current problems or situations as well as potential future effects. This method works best with small groups of key informants who have various perspectives on the problem.

In cause-and-consequence analysis sessions, groups of five to eight individuals work separately to develop ideas to address areas displayed in five columns on a large chart. The five columns are as follows:

Column 1: List the problems or adverse situations identified in the community assessment.
Column 2: List all possible causes of each problem.
Column 3: List all consequences if the causes are not removed and the problems are not solved.

Column 4: Enter a rating (low, medium, or high) of the difficulty of correcting the problem after it has occurred.

Column 5: Enter a rating on a scale of 1 (least critical) to 5 (most critical) for the problem if it is not solved.

Each group member rates each problem individually, and the facilitator tallies the votes for all members to derive a group score for columns 4 and 5. The scores for all groups may also be tallied to reach a total rating for columns 4 and 5. Although each problem may have many causes and consequences, the problem is evaluated only for its difficulty to correct and the degree of criticality. An example of the results of a cause-and-consequence session is displayed in Table 11.2.

The problems rated high on criticality and low or moderately low on the difficulty-to-correct scale may be best to address for short-term planning. Long-term planning will be needed for the problems that are both difficult to correct and high in criticality (Witkin & Altschuld, 1995).

TABLE 11.2 Cause-and-Consequence Analysis of Community-Assessment Findings

Problems	Causes	Consequences	Difficulty to Correct (Low, Medium, High)	Criticality (1 = Low; 5 = High)
Violence	• Drug use • Available guns • Alcoholism • Influence of media • Lack of parental supervision	• More violence • Decrease in quality of life • More victims • Fear • Families move away from high-crime areas • Businesses move • Tax base decreases • Taxes increase	High	5
Teen pregnancy	• Unprotected sex • Desire for someone to love • Sexual assault/rape • Rebellion	• School dropout • Low educational level • Underemployment/unemployment • Adverse pregnancy outcomes	Medium	4
Smoking	• Peer pressure • Rebellion • Role models • Advertisement	• Addiction • Diseases in self and others • Death • Low–birth-weight infants • Loss of productivity in jobs	Medium	4
Unintentional injuries	• Vehicle crashes • Farm mishaps • Falls	• Deaths • Permanent disabilities • Loss of ability to work • Pain and suffering • High healthcare costs	High	4

Selecting the Level of Program Focus: Individual, Group, or Community

The community diagnosis and cause of the adverse situation will provide initial guidance on selecting the level of the program focus as individual, group, or community. The levels may be combined or they may be addressed in stages. For example, a community level may be used to raise awareness of a specific problem followed by group and individual interventions to assist with behavior change. This section provides information about selecting the level for the program plan. After the level of the plan is selected, the research-based intervention or theory is matched with the behaviors, level, and community characteristics. These areas are addressed in this section.

IDENTIFYING BEHAVIORS

A program focus at the individual, group, or community level requires a careful identification of the behaviors of the target group. In addition, identifying those who experience the behaviors and the mechanisms that maintain the behaviors are important. The ethnic and cultural components of all behaviors must be examined as part of the community characteristics and may have been identified as part of community diagnoses.

Most behaviors do not exist as singular acts but constitute a chain of behaviors that lead to adverse or unwanted outcomes. For example, overeating leads to weight gain, which leads to decreased activity and obesity and eventually to weight-related illnesses. The feelings or circumstances that trigger the overeating may be unrelated to the need or desire for food, but eating may be used to compensate for something missing from an individual's life.

Other behaviors are not at the individual-client level but may be those of healthcare providers. For example, the use of emergency rooms for primary care may be a result of physicians in the community not accepting new patients or because an ill person is unable to get an appointment with a physician for several weeks. If the advanced public/community health nurse attempts to change the behavior of individuals who use emergency rooms without looking at other factors, the intervention is unlikely to succeed.

Behaviors may also occur at more than one level. For example, failure of single mothers to obtain immunizations for their young children may be a result of lack of transportation to get to the county health department, whereas the lack of transportation is a result of the county government's not acting to address a serious situation for the total county. Interventions at the individual, group, and community levels may be needed to improve the immunization rate for the total group of young children.

METHODS USED TO IDENTIFY BEHAVIORS

Systematic methods may be used to collect data about behaviors and outcomes. Direct observation and self-report are two methods that would require a few additional resources, especially the time of the advanced practice public/community health nurse. Another method is the PRECEDE Model (Green & Kreuter, 2005). This model comes from the field of health education and has been applied by nurses while working with communities. The model is described in more detail in Chapter 16.

The PRECEDE Model is an acronym for predisposing, reinforcing, and enabling causes in educational diagnosis and evaluation. The first parts of the model provide a guide for identifying the behaviors to be targeted in an intervention. From the community diagnosis, an understanding of the adverse situation and its extent are identified. The reason for the adverse situation is derived from the causal analysis, but the behaviors are not always clear with causal analysis.

Phase 1 of the PRECEDE Model is the social diagnosis; phase 2 is the epidemiologic diagnosis. These steps should usually be achieved in the community assessment process. The third phase of the PRECEDE Model is the behavioral and environmental diagnosis. If behaviors have not been identified in previous steps, the PRECEDE Model may be useful.

The following five steps are suggested for diagnosing behavior:

1. Separate behavioral and nonbehavioral causes of the health problem. The differentiation may begin by examining the risk factors for the disease, condition, or situation. Risk factors related to behavior, either directly (e.g., smoking) or indirectly (e.g., high serum cholesterol), may be separated from nonbehavioral risk factors (e.g., gender).
2. Develop a classification of behaviors. The behavioral factors may be divided into preventive behaviors and treatments. The aim of this step is to identify a list of very specific actions to be used in writing the behavioral objectives for the program.
3. Rate behaviors in terms of importance. Behaviors that occur more frequently (e.g., smoking) and are clearly linked to health problems (e.g., smoking and cancer) are more important.
4. Rate behaviors in terms of changeability. Behaviors that are more susceptible to change make better targets for health promotion and prevention programs.
5. Choose behavioral targets. After the behaviors have been ranked by importance and susceptibility to change, the program planner may select the focus of the program.

Identification of behaviors is crucial for program planning because behaviors are used to develop measurable objectives and lay the basis for an effective evaluation plan (Green & Kreuter, 2005).

Identifying Research-Based Interventions

After determining the level of the program, the next step in focusing program planning is to identify an intervention or interventions to address the adverse situation or problem. All interventions should be research based and, if possible, based on programs that have been shown to be effective. This step will require a thorough literature search to discover programs about which something has been written. Unfortunately, information about many effective programs will not appear in print. Other sources for material on programs are colleagues, university faculty, unpublished master's and doctoral theses, state health departments, federal agencies, *Healthy People 2020 Evidence-Based Resources* (Office of Disease Prevention and Health Promotion, 2017), and voluntary organizations, for example, the American Lung Association and the March of Dimes.

Literature Search

A literature search begins with the identification of key words to be explored in the literature databases. Identifying accurate key words may take some time, but the starting point could be important words in the community diagnosis (e.g., tuberculosis), causes of the adverse situation (e.g., smoking), or the target group (e.g., adolescents). As the search continues, refinement of key words becomes possible.

The other area for a literature search is the theory base on which a successful program was developed. Often, the initial sources for this search will be found in the reference lists of the studies about the intervention or program. If no theory is mentioned in the literature about an intervention, the advanced practice public/community health nurse will want to explore the theory base as a separate literature search to relate the program with a theory.

For some topics, a review of literature might have been published. Literature reviews are very useful tools and should be located if they exist. Also for some areas of research, reviews or systematic syntheses have been conducted. These syntheses may be in the form of narratives or statistical summaries such as meta-analyses (Cooper, 1998; Cooper, Hedges, & Valentine, 2009). Research summaries are very useful but should be scrutinized for accuracy and bias.

In the next sections, some examples of theories with related research are presented. These are examples of theories to guide intervention development or to use as a base for a literature search of interventions.

FOCUS AT THE INDIVIDUAL LEVEL

Numerous theories and interventions at the individual level of health behavior have been tested. Three theories that have volumes of research based on them are the Health Belief Model (HBM), social support theory, and the Transtheoretical Model. Nurses and other disciplines have tested these theories with various populations and various conditions.

The Health Belief Model. This model was developed to predict health-related behaviors and compliance with treatment regimens (Becker, 1974). The HBM is based on the work of Kurt Lewin (1951) in field theory. Two assumptions form the basis of the HBM: (a) people behave on the basis of their perceptions and (b) people are attracted to areas of positive value (health) and repelled by areas of negative value (illness) in their lives. The HBM postulates that the value associated with the desire of the individual to avoid illness and achieve health, coupled with an estimate that a particular course of action will bring about the desired value, will result in a reduction in the threat of illness.

Five major variables or concepts make up the HBM and are considered important in explaining and predicting health-related behaviors: perceived susceptibility, perceived severity, perceived benefits, perceived barriers, and cues to action. Self-efficacy was added to the HBM as the sixth concept to increase its explanatory power (Rosenstock, Strecher, & Becker, 1988).

The HBM has been used in research about many conditions and situations of interest to advanced practice public/community health nurses (Janz & Becker, 1984). Some of these are AIDS, smoking, immunizations, breast cancer screening, and compliance (Champion & Skinner, 2008; Champion et al., 2002; Dawkins, Ervin, Weissfeld, & Yan, 1988; VanDyke & Shell, 2017).

Social Support Theory. Cumulative research evidence demonstrates that social support has beneficial effects on both psychological and physical well-being (Heaney & Israel, 2008). Social support appears to have not only direct effects but also stress-buffering effects on well-being (Glanz & Schwartz, 2008). Numerous studies have demonstrated that social support can influence how people adapt psychologically to a stressful event such as an illness or pregnancy.

Some examples of studies of interest to advanced practice public/community health nurses are as follows: those demonstrating effectiveness in improving pregnancy outcomes (Elsenbruch et al., 2007; Norbeck, DeJoseph, & Smith, 1996), adherence to medical regimens (DiMatteo, 2004), and the influence on health outcomes (Reifman, 1995).

The Transtheoretical Model. This theory integrates processes and principles of change from major theories of intervention. Five stages of change are conceptualized as a process through which people progress: precontemplation, contemplation, preparation, action, and maintenance. Termination is a sixth stage in which individuals do not return to their old habits. This stage applies to some behaviors, such as addictions, but is achieved by few.

The processes of change are the overt and covert activities that individuals use to progress through the six stages of change. The Transtheoretical Model is also composed of 15 core constructs that have been tested in about 48 studies. These constructs of change provide important guidelines for interventions. The Transtheoretical Model has been used in studies of smoking cessation, alcohol and substance abuse, delinquency, eating disorders and obesity, high-fat diets, HIV prevention, mammograms, cervical cancer screening, compliance, unplanned pregnancy prevention, and other behaviors. The one area that has not shown to be effective is in primary prevention of substance abuse in children (Prochaska, Redding, & Evers, 2008).

FOCUS AT THE GROUP LEVEL

At the group level, theories that may be useful are found in several disciplines, including nursing. The social support literature contains research about group interventions as well as individual interventions (Heaney & Israel, 2008; Norbeck et al., 1996). Other theories explored here for group interventions are diffusion of innovations theory and stage theory of organizational change.

Diffusion of Innovations Theory. An innovation is any idea, practice, or object that is seen as new by someone or a group. Diffusion is the process used to spread the use of an innovation over time among members of a group or social system (Rogers, 2003). Five adopter categories have been identified as innovators, early adopters, early majority adopters, late adopters, and laggards. These categories form the basis for designing and implementing intervention strategies targeted at specific groups of people.

In addition, five characteristics most likely to affect the speed and extent of the diffusion process have been identified through research as relative advantage, compatibility, complexity, trialability, and observability (Rogers, 2003; Zaltman & Duncan, 1977). These characteristics need to be addressed during the development stage of an intervention and communicated to the potential users (Oldenburg, Hardcastle, & Kok, 1997).

Diffusion of innovations theory has been used for many interventions. Some examples are an intervention to decrease alcohol consumption through a program of primary care physicians and office receptionists (Oldenburg et al., 1997), diffusion of AIDS education in schools (Paulussen, Kok, Schaalma, & Parcel, 1995), a program to reduce risk of cardiovascular disease (Graham-Clarke & Oldenburg, 1994; Oldenburg, Graham-Clarke, Shaw, & Walker, 1996), and programs to increase physical activity (Glowacki, Centeio, Van Dongen, Carson, & Castelli, 2016) and fruit and vegetable intake (Oldenburg & Glanz, 2008).

Stage Theory. Stage theory of organizational change provides an explanation of how organizations put innovations into place (Butterfoss, Kegler, & Francisco, 2008; Hernandez & Kaluzny, 1997). The relevance of this theory for advanced practice public/community health nurses lies in the fact that organizations (e.g., schools, worksites, voluntary groups, and healthcare agencies) are often required to change in order to implement an intervention or the intervention is a change in the organization. Any organizational change requires a great deal of effort and planning. Some models for organizational change may be found in Cameron and Green (2015).

One model of stage theory has seven stages (Beyer & Trice, 1978): sensing unsatisfied demands on the system, a search for possible responses, evaluation of various alternatives, decision to adopt a course of action, initiation of action within the system, implementation of the change, and institutionalization of the change. An example of the use of stage theory is shown in a study about disseminating health curricula to schools (Goodman, Tenney, Smith, & Steckler, 1992).

FOCUS AT THE COMMUNITY LEVEL

Theories to develop interventions at the community level are not as numerous or as well developed as at the individual level. However, some theories presented earlier are also used at the community level. Examples of community-level programs that incorporate social support may be found in the literature, such as the de Madres a Madres program (Mahon, McFarlane, & Golden, 1991), the Friends Can Be Good Medicine campaign in California (Hersey, Klibanoff, Lam, & Taylor, 1984), and social support for migrant populations (Hernández-Plaza, Alonso-Morillejo, & Pozo-Muñoz, 2006). The two additional theories discussed in this section are social change theory and community organization theory.

Social Change Theory. Change at the community level recognizes that behavior is greatly influenced by the environment in which people live. Social change theory advocates for changing the standards of acceptable behavior in a community, and, thus, by changing community norms about health-related behavior, individual behavior will change (Institute of Medicine, 2012; Thompson & Kinne, 1990). Most major health-promotion interventions at the community level over the past several years have used public education through mass media, schools, and other organizations. Many studies have addressed reduction of multiple risk factors for cardiovascular disease (Carlaw, Mittlemark, Bracht, & Luepker, 1984; Cohen, Stunkard, & Felix, 1986; Elder et al., 1986; Tarlov et al., 1987). Others have been aimed at reduction of smoking (Syme & Alcalay, 1982), reduction in preterm births (Shapiro-Mendoza et al., 2016), and cancer prevention (Van Parijs & Eckhardt, 1984). Other examples of community-level interventions are found in the literature.

Community Organization Theory. *Community organizing* has been defined as "the process by which community groups are helped to identify common problems or goals, mobilize resources, and develop and implement strategies to reach goals they have set collectively" (Minkler, Wallerstein, & Wilson, 2008, pp. 287–288). In the strict definition of community organization, communities themselves must have identified the problem or situation to address. In addition, for community organization to take place, community problem-solving ability must have increased (Ross, 1955).

Community organization has a long history of application in the United States and around the world. Various phases of application of the concepts may be found in the literature (Rothman, Erlich, & Tropman, 1995). One international project is the World Health

Organization (1986) Healthy Cities movement, which aims to create healthy public policies, achieve high-level participation in community-directed projects, and eventually reduce inequities and disparities among groups. In the United States, the Healthy Cities concept has been applied in several states and facilitated by nurses (Flynn, 1992).

Another community organization project incorporated social support and social action among elderly residents in a San Francisco district. The Tenderloin Senior Organizing Project was aimed at facilitating a process that encouraged residents to work together to solve shared problems, for example, poverty, social isolation, malnutrition, and depression (Minkler, 1985).

■ USING RESEARCH IN PRACTICE

When attempting to translate research into practice, several steps should be taken to ensure that an intervention is based on sound research results. A complete literature search is needed to identify all studies about interventions that have addressed the problem or adverse situation of interest. The following steps are recommended as minimum criteria for identifying appropriate research to put into practice:

1. Review the scientific merit of each study. Table 6.3 (in Chapter 6) is a useful data-collection tool when reviewing studies. Summarize each study on a grid as displayed in Table 11.3.
2. Use research results that have been replicated in more than one study. Always use more than one study as a basis for a change in practice.
3. Identify the degree of potential client risk associated with the implementation of findings. Also identify risks of maintaining current practice.
4. Determine the feasibility of implementing the change. Include resources needed as well as the clinical merit, clinical significance, and the amount of control and influence nursing has over the practice to be changed.
5. Complete a cost–benefit analysis (Beaudry, VandenBosch, & Anderson, 1996; Horsely, Crane, Crabtree, & Wood, 1983; White, Dudley-Brown, & Terhaar, 2016).

Detailed criteria to use for critiquing studies for scientific merit may be found in research books and will provide guidance for most studies. However, some study results may require the use of a consultant for appropriate interpretation. Often, university faculty are available to provide such consultation.

If the evaluation of the research demonstrates that an intervention was successful, it may be used as described in the literature or adapted to meet local conditions. It is important to keep in mind that interventions under more controlled situations, such as in research studies, will usually be more effective than the same activities implemented in clinical practice. We do not often see the results of tested interventions used in advanced

TABLE 11.3 Data-Collection Tool for Reviewing Research Studies

Author(s) and Year	Theory	Design	Setting	Sample	Variables	Statistical Methods	Findings

Sources: Adapted from Cooper, H. (1998). *Integrating research: A guide for literature reviews* (3rd ed.). Thousand Oaks, CA: Sage; Ganong, L. H. (1987). Integrative reviews of nursing research. *Research in Nursing & Health, 10*(1), 1–11.

public/community health nursing practice; therefore, the differences between research results and practice results are not always known.

If no studies can be located that directly address the community diagnosis, a search should be attempted to locate studies of similar areas. For example, if the identified community situation is a low immunization rate of children younger than 2 years, studies to increase immunization rates in all children may be helpful.

Guidance for conducting a cost–benefit analysis may be found in finance textbooks and articles about the topic (e.g., Issel, 2013; Tomey, 2000). Assistance may also be sought from the fiscal office of the agency. One suggested approach is to document all costs for the innovation as planning is done. The planning team will not have all information about costs; therefore, requests will need to be made to the fiscal officer and others in the agency.

■ USING THEORY IN PRACTICE

At times, the advanced practice public/community health nurse will be unable to locate studies that directly or indirectly address the community diagnosis for which an intervention is to be developed. Then the choice of action is to explore the use of theory to fashion an intervention. This is not an exact process and may require the use of a consultant and/ or a group of nurses with some background in the critique and use of theory as well as clinical expertise in the intervention area.

Ideally, nursing theory would be used in the construction of interventions to be implemented by nurses, but nursing theories are not yet available for all areas. If a nursing theory cannot be located, the use of a related or borrowed theory may be helpful. If the intervention is to be interdisciplinary, theories from various disciplines should be explored. In addition, theories that are classified as middle range or practice theories are more appropriate to use as a basis for practice interventions.

The following criteria have been proposed for use in selecting a behavior theory for practice use. The criteria are also useful for selecting any theory for use in developing an intervention (Thomas, 1984).

> *Content relevance:* Does the content embrace the appropriate target persons, behaviors, and related behavioral and social conditions?
> *Content inclusiveness:* Does the behavior theory embrace the relevant independent and dependent variables pertaining to the behavioral domain of the intervention?
> *Knowledge validity:* Have the propositions of the behavioral theory been corroborated in appropriate research?
> *Knowledge power:* Are the variables of the theory capable of accounting for a large portion of the behavior to be explained or predicted?
> *Knowledge engineerability:* Are the real-world referents of the knowledge capable of being successfully implemented because the indicators are identifiable, accessible, potent, economically feasible, and ethically suitable to manipulate?

Constructing an Intervention From Theory

A theory is a statement or explanation about the relationship among phenomena or the prediction about the effects of one phenomenon on another (Fawcett, 1995; Wood & Ross-Kerr, 2011). The advanced practice public/community health nurse uses the relational statements in a theory to develop a protocol that puts into place the hypothesized relationships and expected outcomes. These steps are illustrated in Figure 11.2.

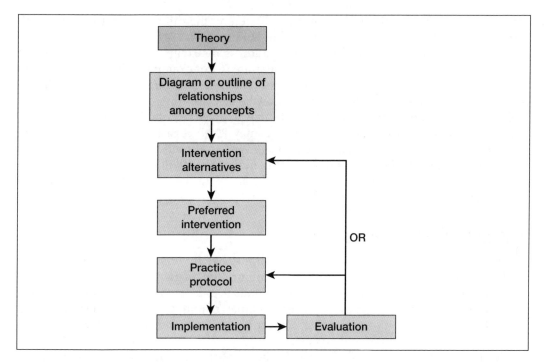

FIGURE 11.2   Steps in using theory to develop an intervention.

Analysis of the theory should proceed with a thorough reading of the original publication followed by reading all publications that further illuminate the details of the theory. The next step is to develop a diagram or narrative picture of the relationships among the concepts explicated in the theory. The diagram provides guidance for the advanced practice public/community health nurse in the design of the actual intervention. A simplistic example of a diagram is shown in Figure 11.3.

The structure of the theory may take any form (e.g., overlapping circles, branching circles, triangles) but may not always be clear from the written information. If a structure cannot be developed, an outline of the concepts in the order presented will assist with the analysis process (Chinn & Jacobs, 1991).

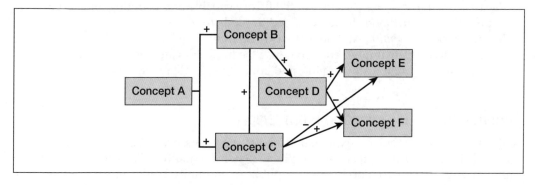

FIGURE 11.3   Relationships among theory concepts.

Several approaches may be used to design an intervention, for example, brainstorming, group exercises, committee work, or a written paper that is reviewed by several people. Individuals who are representative of the intervention recipient group should be involved in providing information for the development of the intervention. Involvement of groups and/or individuals may be obtained in numerous ways as indicated in Chapter 6 for community assessment methods.

Focus groups and individual interviews are especially fruitful for gathering in-depth information from the recipient group. One example of the use of both techniques to develop a social support intervention for African American women is given in a study by DeJoseph, Norbeck, Smith, and Miller (1996). Focus group information was used to develop semi-structured, individual interviews, which were used to confirm and/or amplify the themes about social support, stress, and pregnancy identified in focus groups. This information was used to develop the intervention.

The intervention developed by DeJoseph et al. (1996) consisted of two parts: skill building by African American women to develop self-esteem and to access support, and acknowledgment of the women's lives and experiences.

A group developing several alternative intervention strategies will allow for consideration of a broader range of ideas than could be imagined by just one person working alone. Creative ideas that build on the theory, yet incorporate aspects of known effective interventions, should be encouraged. For example, from research findings, it is known that structured teaching approaches, such as planned teaching, independent study, and multiple strategies, are more effective than informal teaching (Theis & Johnson, 1995).

The intervention should also, of course, incorporate the behaviors identified earlier in the program-planning process. Keeping the intervention development focused on the identified behaviors will allow for a quicker realization of the objectives.

Although the intervention is not being developed for testing per se, a protocol based on a theory is a test of the relationships posited in the theory. As with any intervention that is part of a program, evaluation is needed to determine the effectiveness, cost, and conditions under which the intervention works or does not work. Instead of conducting a research study, the advanced practice public/community health nurse will conduct a well-designed evaluation to make determinations about the effectiveness of an intervention. Evaluation also provides data to allow for adjustments in the intervention if warranted by the results of the evaluation. Program evaluation is covered in depth in Section V.

■ SUMMARY

This chapter has continued the content on program planning by providing information for focusing the program at the individual, group, or community level. Validation and prioritization of community diagnoses are necessary steps before causes of the adverse situations and behaviors are identified. With these steps accomplished, the advanced practice public/community health nurse is ready to develop or identify the interventions needed to address the adverse situation.

Interventions based on research are potentially much more effective than those that have no basis in evidence. If research cannot be located to use to fashion an intervention, theory is preferred over atheoretical planning. The development of an intervention based on a theory is not an exact process but requires creativity as well as knowledge of research about the factors or variables to be included in the intervention.

■ SUGGESTED CLINICAL OR PRACTICUM ACTIVITIES

1. Select one community diagnosis from your community assessment. Review the literature for a cause or causes of the diagnosis.
2. Locate an evidence-based intervention that addresses the diagnosis and specific cause of the problem. Compare the intervention with a program that was implemented to address the diagnosis.
3. Interview an advanced practice public/community health nurse about how evidence is used in programs and services.

REFERENCES

Anderson, E. T., & McFarlane, J. (2015). *Community as partner: Theory and practice in nursing* (7th ed.). Philadelphia, PA: Wolters Kluwer.

Beaudry, M., VandenBosch, T., & Anderson, J. (1996). Research utilization: Once-a-day temperatures for afebrile patients. *Clinical Nurse Specialist, 10*(1), 21–24.

Becker, M. H. (Ed.). (1974). The health belief model and personal health behavior. *Health Education Monographs, 2*, 324–473.

Beyer, J. M., & Trice, H. M. (1978). *Implementing change: Alcoholism policies in work organizations.* New York, NY: Free Press.

Butterfoss, F. D., Kegler, M. C., & Francisco, V. T. (2008). Mobilizing organizations for health promotion: Theories of organizational change. In K. Glanz, B. K. Rimer, & K. Viswanath (Eds.), *Health behavior and health education: Theory, research, and practice* (4th ed., pp. 336–361). San Francisco, CA: Jossey-Bass.

Cameron, E., & Green, M. (2015). *Making sense of change management: A complete guide to the models, tools and techniques of organizational change* (4th ed.). London, UK: Kogan Page.

Carlaw, R. W., Mittlemark, M. B., Bracht, N., & Luepker, R. (1984). Organization for a community cardiovascular health program: Experiences from the Minnesota heart health program. *Health Education Quarterly, 11*, 243–252.

Champion, V. L., & Skinner, C. S. (2008). The health belief model. In K. Glanz, B. K., Rimer, & K. Viswanath (Eds.), *Health behavior and health education: Theory, research, and practice* (4th ed., pp. 45–65). San Francisco, CA: Jossey-Bass.

Champion, V. L., Skinner, C. S., Menon, U., Seshadri, R., Anzalone, D. C., & Rawl, S. M. (2002). Comparisons of tailored mammography interventions at two months postintervention. *Annals of Behavioral Medicine, 24*(3), 211–218.

Chinn, P. L., & Jacobs, M. K. (1991). *Theory and nursing: A systematic approach* (3rd ed.). St. Louis, MO: Mosby.

Cohen, R. Y., Stunkard, A., & Felix, M. R. (1986). Measuring community change in disease prevention and health promotion. *Preventive Medicine, 15*, 411–421.

Cooper, H. (1998). *Integrating research: A guide for literature reviews* (3rd ed.). Thousand Oaks, CA: Sage.

Cooper, H., Hedges, L. V., & Valentine, J. C. (Eds.). (2009). *The handbook of research synthesis and meta-analysis* (2nd ed.). New York, NY: Russell Sage Foundation.

Dawkins, C. E., Ervin, N. E., Weissfeld, L., & Yan, A. (1988). Health orientation, beliefs, and use of health services among minority, high-risk expectant mothers. *Public Health Nursing, 5*(1), 7–11.

DeJoseph, J. F., Norbeck, J. S., Smith, R. T., & Miller, S. (1996). The development of a social support intervention among African American women. *Qualitative Health Research, 6*(2), 283–297.

Delbecq, A. L., Van de Ven, A. H., & Gustafson, D. H. (1975). *Group techniques for program planning.* Glenview, IL: Scott, Foresman.

DiMatteo, M. R. (2004). Social support and patient adherence to medical treatment: A meta-analysis. *Health Psychology, 23*(2), 207–218. doi.org/10.1037/0278-6133.23.2.207

Elder, J. P., McGraw, S. A., Abrams, D. B., Ferreira, A., Lasater, T. M., Longpre, H., … Carleton, R. A. (1986). Organizational and community approaches to community-wide prevention of heart disease: The first 2 years of the Pawtucket Heart Health Program. *Preventive Medicine, 15,* 107–117.

Elsenbruch, S., Benson, S., Rücke, M., Rose, M., Dudenhausen, J., Pincus-Knackstedt, M. K., … Arck, P. C. (2007). Social support during pregnancy: Effects on maternal depressive symptoms, smoking and pregnancy outcome. *Human Reproduction, 22*(3), 869–877. doi:10.1093/humrep/del432

Fawcett, J. (1995). *Analysis and evaluation of conceptual models of nursing* (3rd ed.). Newbury Park, CA: Sage.

Flynn, B. C. (1992). Healthy cities: A model of community change. *Family & Community Health, 15*(1), 13–23.

Ganong, L. H. (1987). Integrative review of nursing research. *Research in Nursing and Health, 10*(1), 1–11.

Glanz, K., & Schwartz, M. D. (2008). Stress, cooping, and health behavior. In K. Glanz, B. K. Rimer, & K. Viswanath (Eds.), *Health behavior and health education: Theory, research, and practice* (4th ed., pp. 211–236). San Francisco, CA: Jossey-Bass.

Glowacki, E. M., Centeio, E. E., Van Dongen, D. J., Carson, R. L., & Castelli, D. M. (2016). Health promotion efforts as predictors of physical activity in schools: An application of the diffusion of innovations model. *Journal of School Health, 86*(6), 399–406. doi:10.1111/josh.12390

Goodman, R. M., Tenney, M., Smith, D. W., & Steckler, A. (1992). The adoption process for health curriculum innovations in schools: A case study. *Journal of Health Education, 23*(4), 215–220.

Graham-Clarke, P., & Oldenburg, B. F. (1994). The effectiveness of a general practice based physical activity intervention on patient physical activity status. *Behavior Change, 11*(3), 132–143.

Green, L. W., & Kreuter, M. W. (2005). *Health promotion planning: An educational and ecological approach* (4th ed.). San Francisco, CA: Jossey-Bass.

Heaney, C. A., & Israel, B. A. (2008). Social networks and social support. In K. Glanz, B. K. Rimer, & K. Viswanath (Eds.), *Health behavior and health education: Theory, research, and practice* (4th ed., pp. 190–210). San Francisco, CA: Jossey-Bass.

Helvie, C. O. (1998). *Advanced practice nursing in the community.* Thousand Oaks, CA: Sage.

Hernandez, R., & Kaluzny, A. (1997). Organizational innovation and change. In S. Shortell & A. Kaluzny (Eds.), *Essentials of health care management* (pp. 355–380). Albany, NY: Delmar.

Hernández-Plaza, S., Alonso-Morillejo, E., & Pozo-Muñoz, C. (2006). Social support interventions in migrant populations. *British Journal of Social Work, 36*(7), 1151–1169.

Hersey, J. C., Klibanoff, L. S., Lam, D. J., & Taylor, R. L. (1984). Promoting social support: The impact of California's "Friends Can Be Good Medicine" campaign. *Health Education Quarterly, 11,* 293–311.

Horsely, J., Crane, J., Crabtree, M. K., & Wood, D. J. (1983). *Using research to improve nursing practice: A guide (CURN project).* Philadelphia, PA: Saunders.

Institute of Medicine. (2012). *Accelerating progress in obesity prevention: Solving the weight of the nation.* Washington, DC: National Academies Press.

Ishikawa, K. (1992). *Guide to quality control.* Tokyo, Japan: Asian Productivity Organization.

Issel, L. M. (2013). *Health program planning and evaluation: A practical, systematic approach for community health* (3rd ed.). Sudbury, MA: Jones & Bartlett.

Janz, N. K., & Becker, M. H. (1984). The health belief model: A decade later. *Health Education Quarterly, 11,* 1–47.

Lewin, K. (1951). The nature of field theory. In M. H. Marx (Ed.), *Psychological theory.* New York, NY: Macmillan.

Mahon, J., McFarlane, J., & Golden, K. (1991). De Madres a Madres: A community partnership for health. *Public Health Nursing, 8*(1), 15–19.

Minkler, M. (1985). Building supportive ties and sense of community among the inner-city elderly: The Tenderloin Senior Outreach Project. *Health Education Quarterly, 12*(4), 303–314.

Minkler, M., Wallerstein, N., & Wilson, N. (2008). Improving health through community organization and community building. In K. Glanz, B. K. Rimer, & K. Viswanath (Eds.), *Health behavior and health education: Theory, research and practice* (4th ed., pp. 287–312). San Francisco, CA: Jossey-Bass.

Norbeck, J. S., DeJoseph, J. F., & Smith, R. T. (1996). A randomized trial of an empirically-derived social support intervention to prevent low birthweight. *Social Science & Medicine, 43*(6), 947–954. doi:10.1016/0277-9536(96)00003-2

Office of Disease Prevention and Health Promotion. (2017). *Healthy people 2020 evidence-based resources.* Washington, DC: U.S. Department of Health and Human Services. Retrieved from https://www .healthypeople.gov/2020/tools-resources/Evidence-Based-Resources

Oldenburg, B., & Glanz, K. (2008). Diffusion of innovations. In K. Glanz, B. K. Rimer, & K. Viswanath (Eds.), *Health behavior and health education: Theory, research, and practice* (4th ed., pp. 312–333*). San Francisco, CA: Jossey-Bass.

Oldenburg, B., Hardcastle, D. M., & Kok, G. (1997). *Diffusion of innovation*. In K. Glanz, B. K. Rimer, & F. M. Lewis (Eds.), Health behavior and health education: Theory, research and practice (2nd ed., pp. 270–286). San Francisco, CA: Jossey-Bass.

Oldenburg, B. F., Graham-Clarke, P., Shaw, J., & Walker, S. (1996). Modification of health behavior and lifestyle mediated by physicians. In K. Orth-Gomér & N. Schneiderman (Eds.), *Behavioral medicine approaches to cardiovascular disease prevention* (pp. 205–226). Mahwah, NJ: Lawrence Erlbaum.

Paulussen, T. G., Kok, G., Schaalma, H. P., & Parcel, G. S. (1995). Diffusion of AIDS curricula among Dutch secondary school teachers. *Health Education Quarterly, 22*, 227–243.

Prochaska, J. O., Redding, C. A., & Evers, K. E. (2008). The transtheoretical model and stages of change. In K. Glanz, B. K. Rimer, & K. Viswanath (Eds.), *Health behavior and health education: Theory, research, and practice* (4th ed., pp. 97–121). San Francisco, CA: Jossey-Bass.

Reifman, A. (1995). Social relationships, recovery from illness, and survival: A literature review. *Annals of Behavioral Medicine, 17*(2), 124–131.

Rogers, E. M. (2003). *Diffusion of innovations* (5th ed.). New York, NY: Simon & Schuster.

Rosenstock, I. M., Strecher, V. J., & Becker, M. H. (1988). Social learning theory and the health belief model. *Health Education Quarterly, 15*(2), 175–183.

Ross, M. G. (1955). *Community organization: Theory and principles.* New York, NY: HarperCollins.

Rothman, J., Erlich, J. L., & Tropman, J. E. (Eds.). (1995). *Strategies of community organization* (5th ed.). Itasca, IL: Peacock.

Shapiro-Mendoza, C. K., Barfield, W. D., Henderson, Z., James, A., Howse, J. L., Iskander, J., & Thorpe, P. G. (2016). CDC grand rounds: Public health strategies to prevent preterm birth. *Morbidity and Mortality Weekly Report, 65*(32), 826–830.

Syme, S. L., & Alcalay, R. (1982). Control of cigarette smoking from a social perspective. *Annual Review of Public Health, 3*, 179–199.

Tarlov, A. R., Kehrer, B. H., Hall, D. P., Samuels, S. E., Brown, G. S., Felix, M. R., & Ross, J. A. (1987). Foundation work: The health promotion program of the Henry J. Kaiser Family Foundation. *American Journal of Health Promotion, 2*(2), 74–80.

Theis, S. L., & Johnson, J. H. (1995). Strategies for teaching patients: A meta-analysis. *Clinical Nurse Specialist, 9*(2), 100–105, 120.

Thomas, E. J. (1984). *Designing interventions for the helping professions.* Beverly Hills, CA: Sage.

Thompson, B., & Kinne, S. (1990). Social change theory: Applications to community health. In N. Bracht (Ed.), *Health promotion at the community level* (pp. 45–65). Newbury Park, CA: Sage.

Tomey, A. M. (2000). *Guide to nursing management and leadership* (6th ed.). St Louis, MO: Mosby.

Van Parijs, L. G., & Eckhardt, S. (1984). Public education in primary and secondary cancer prevention. *Hygie, 3*(3), 16–28.

VanDyke, S. D., & Shell, M. D. (2017). Health beliefs and breast cancer screening in rural Appalachia: An evaluation of the health belief model. *Journal of Rural Health, 33*(4), 350–360. doi:10.1111/jrh.12204

White, K. M., Dudley-Brown, S., & Terhaar, M. F. (Eds.). (2016). *Translation of evidence into nursing and health care* (2nd ed.). New York, NY: Springer Publishing.

Witkin, B. R., & Altschuld, J. W. (1995). *Planning and conducting needs assessments: A practical guide.* Thousand Oaks, CA: Sage.

Wood, M. J., & Ross-Kerr, J. C. (2011). *Basic steps in planning nursing research: From question to proposal* (7th ed.). Sudbury, MA: Jones & Bartlett.

World Health Organization. (1986). *Ottawa charter for health promotion.* Copenhagen, DK: Author.

Zaltman, G., & Duncan, R. (1977). *Strategies for planned change.* New York, NY: John Wiley.

CHAPTER 12

Developing a Program Plan

■ STUDY EXERCISES

1. How are the components of a program plan used to develop a specific plan?
2. What resources should be considered in program planning?
3. Use a specific planning model to guide you in the development of a program plan.
4. What relationship do interventions have with program plans?
5. How is research used to develop an intervention?
6. How are program plan components used at each level of intervention: individual, group, and community?

The development of a program plan usually begins long before the formal development. Advanced practice public/community health nurses are often familiar with the communities with which they work and are thus aware of many factors that may make a program successful. *Nevertheless, it is very important that premature conclusions not be drawn about the design of a program before the steps discussed in previous chapters are completed.* This chapter continues the explanation of program planning and incorporates previous content to assist you in developing a comprehensive program plan.

■ COMPONENTS OF A PROGRAM PLAN

As introduced in Chapter 9, planning is a process of the four interdependent steps of defining, analyzing, choosing, and mapping. In this chapter, program planning is examined as a subset of planning and is defined as a series of detailed steps carried out to address a problem or adverse situation that requires a solution through a structured intervention.

Steps of the Planning Process

The specific steps of program planning are to formulate a planning group, develop goals, develop objectives, explore resources and constraints, and select methods and activities to reach the goals (Dignan & Carr, 1992).

FORMULATE A PLANNING GROUP

Program planning is directly linked to community assessment. Without a community assessment, or a targeted assessment of one segment of a community, planning is a futile exercise. Therefore, members of a program-planning group should be chosen on the basis of the community assessment, the topic of the priority community diagnosis, and the focus of the intervention. At times, the advanced practice public/community health nurse may develop a program plan alone, but this would be a rare event. The program-planning group needs to include members of the target group for the program. As mentioned earlier, community member involvement should be part of the total community assessment process, so the continued involvement of a specific group or community will be a natural extension of the earlier activities.

The composition of the planning group should reflect the expertise needed to accomplish the tasks for program planning while remaining small enough to move the work forward. The outcomes of a small working group may be taken to others for preliminary critique during the planning process. Other mechanisms may be used to obtain feedback on the developing plan, for example, focus groups, community forums, or questionnaires.

If possible, those who have more than one area of expertise should be chosen as group members. For example, a program-planning effort on control and prevention of lead poisoning would need members with backgrounds in environmental health, budget expertise, child health, and building codes. One person may have knowledge in two or three of the needed content areas. Also, experts may be consulted during the development process. Much information is available on the Internet, so someone with computer skills may be a valuable resource on several topics.

DEVELOP GOALS

Development of goals for the program plan is also very much related to the community diagnosis. As indicated in Chapter 10, goals are broad statements of what is to be accomplished. Using the focus of the intervention, some goals should be written to encompass the general aims of the program. Depending on the size of the program, one to three goals will often be adequate.

DEVELOP OBJECTIVES

The development of objectives is closely related to the goals. Each goal should be accompanied by few objectives so that the direction is set for making progress toward the goal. Objectives should meet criteria as set forth in Chapter 10.

EXPLORE RESOURCES AND CONSTRAINTS

The potential availability of resources needs to be explored for successful program planning. The political environment is one area that will have been explored all along during the community assessment. At the point of program planning, the exploration needs to center on the support for change, which may be found in the political environment. Ways to increase or stabilize that support should be built into the plan. For example, if key informants indicated interest in the outcome of the community assessment, they should be kept informed and, perhaps, involved in other steps along the way in program planning. If new individuals hold key positions in political bodies, they should be informed and consulted about the developing plan.

Other types of resources that need to be explored are possible services and supplies to be donated or given in kind to the project. Often community businesses and organizations will support an effort that directly benefits the community. Examples of donations include space for clinics or centers, office supplies, food for special events, volunteer time, and money (Ervin & Young, 1996).

Constraints are forces likely to interfere with or inhibit the attainment of goals and objectives (Dignan & Carr, 1992). Analysis of potential and real constraints is very important because modifications in the program plan may be made on the basis of thorough identification of constraints. The identification of constraints allows opportunity to convert some of them to resources. For example, if inadequate funds are available for equipment, a donor may be located before the program is due to begin.

IDENTIFYING METHODS AND ACTIVITIES

The intervention used to address a specific behavior and behaviors was discussed earlier. In this next step of program planning, the exact activities will be delineated for implementing the intervention (method). Activities are linked to each objective and spell out how each objective will be achieved. For example, an objective to decrease the percentage of employees who smoke could use the intervention of group support for a smoking-cessation program. The activities to implement the group-support method need to be clearly stated. How often will the group be held? Where? Who will lead? What will be the content of each session? These kinds of activities and many others need to be detailed for the program to be implemented.

It is better to write out all the details of the program activities even though the planning group may believe that the directions are clear. Often, there are many possible interpretations of simple activities. In addition, the intervention chosen from the literature was carried out in a specific way and needs to be replicated or appropriately modified if projected outcomes are to be achieved. If the intervention is not described in adequate detail in the literature, the researchers will need to be contacted to obtain a copy of the protocol used in the studies.

The Budget

Another area for development in the program plan is the budget. Identifying the resources needed, including staff, time, and space, is the first step in developing a useful budget. In Chapter 13, budget development is covered in detail.

■ RESOURCES TO CONSIDER IN PROGRAM PLANNING

The incentive for planning a program may be the potential availability of funds. Many agencies submit program plans or proposals to an external organization to obtain funds to meet an identified problem. At times, agencies submit proposals for unclear reasons. Therefore, the true problem has not been identified, but the temptation of possible funding is too great, so a proposal is submitted without a truly good idea being developed.

In addition to money, resources needed to develop and carry out a program plan are qualified staff, equipment, supplies, space, protocols, instructions, forms, and baseline data. This section discusses these resources and how to deal with obtaining them or finding alternatives. Program planning will be enhanced if these resources are identified during the planning period rather than waiting until the program is funded. The success of a program is closely related to adequate and appropriate resources, so these items should not be left to chance or last-minute efforts.

Qualified Staff

A program planner is often required to stipulate details about the qualifications and sources of staffing for a project (Hale, Arnold, & Travis, 1994). The success of a program often depends on the efforts of personnel who implement the program and conduct the intervention. Depending on several factors, qualified staff may be difficult to locate and hire. A shortage of baccalaureate and master's-prepared nurses has been a situation whose solution requires creativity. Recruitment for a nurse with a needed specialty (e.g., public health nursing or a family nurse practitioner) should start well before program implementation is anticipated. If funding is pending, recruitment could start before the funds arrive in the agency with advertising using the phrase *anticipated opening.*

Another approach is reassigning and training current staff to implement a new program. Advantages to this approach are that these individuals are familiar with the agency, know the community, and may be motivated to try something new. There are, of course, disadvantages to having current staff take on a new program. Foremost among the disadvantages is the resistance to change. As discussed earlier, almost all changes will be met with resistance from some staff members. This is far less likely to happen if individuals who will implement the program have been part of the planning.

Without newly hired qualified staff, a program may often be started with temporary reassignment of current staff, but care needs to be taken to have adequate coverage for all assignments. A program may be unsuccessful if adequate time is not allowed for trial and error in the early weeks of implementation. Also, new program start-ups will often take more time than expected because of unanticipated events.

Equipment, Supplies, and Space

A new program may suffer when equipment and supplies were not ordered far enough in advance or, if ordered, were not delivered when expected. Starting a new program without the necessary equipment and supplies can range from frustrating to impossible. If the start of the program can be delayed, this should be done until all necessary items are in place and staff has been oriented to their use.

The details about obtaining equipment and supplies may be incorporated into the program plan, which will also assist in the development of the budget. Actual ordering or procurement of equipment and supplies may be done during planning for implementation of the program if funding is secured.

Another component of program requirements is space. At times, additional space must be procured to implement a new program. Alterations or renovations of existing space may be needed. These activities require lead time for contracts to be signed and the work to be completed. These details should be specified in the program plan, if possible.

In one instance of starting a community nursing center, the renovations of the donated space were delayed for several months. The staff was able to begin minimal services in the space used by the collaborating community organization so as not to lose momentum and to use funding. This arrangement allowed the staff and the organization to develop working relationships and give credibility to the new program (Ervin & Young, 1996).

If space and equipment are acquired before the program is due to start, a trial run of the program and use of equipment will be possible. For example, a run-through of all components with a few clients or role-playing staff members would be a valuable exercise, 2 or 3 weeks before the program is scheduled to premiere. If this is not possible, a walk-through of the program on site by the assigned staff and the advanced practice public/community health nurse would be an acceptable substitute.

Protocols and Instructions

Most new programs will require the development of research-based protocols. As discussed in Chapter 11, the work required to do literature searches, to critique research studies, and to decide on an appropriate intervention is time-consuming. This work should be done before program- plan writing is begun, but the protocols based on the research may not have been developed. Although this phase could wait until the program is funded, often the program plan must include enough detail to let the funding source know what activities are proposed. If not a detailed protocol, the program plan must be clear about the intervention or focus of the program.

Orientation of personnel to the new protocols must also be planned but not be carried out until the program implementation is begun. If the program plan includes an outline of the orientation and training for staff, implementation of the intervention will be facilitated.

Another required need for new programs is the development of written instructions about how to perform specific tasks. This process is sometimes done verbally, with one staff member instructing another about the way to carry out some task. The difficulty with this is the loss of precision that is possible in verbal translation. How many of us have heard someone instructing another person say, "This is how it is supposed to be done, but this is how I do it"? Although the staff member's shortcut may be acceptable, it is this kind of change that may contribute to the lack of success in a program. Written instructions provide documentation for program orientation, staff development, implementation, and evaluation. If changes are made in a program, written instructions should be updated and used as the basis of in-service education for the personnel who deliver the program.

Forms

The forms required for new programs may be extensive or minimal. Most organizations require that one or more committees and/or individuals approve new forms. Also, forms must be printed or made available on the computer system used in the agency. All these steps take more time than often anticipated.

During the planning phase, the advanced practice public/community health nurse will want to think through and document any need for new forms. A draft document may be included in the program plan or perhaps only a narrative description of what will be developed is included, depending on the requirements of the funding source. At times, a program will be required to use forms supplied by the funding source. This is more common with state- and federally funded projects. Many reports are submitted through the computer, so staff members may need to have training to comply with the computer-submission protocols.

Baseline Data for Program Evaluation

The need for specific data to evaluate a program is often discovered after the program has begun. At that point, it is usually too late to collect baseline data so that change in the target population or community can be measured. The advanced practice public/community health nurse will need to think ahead of the program evaluation to avoid this unfortunate situation. This is not to say that the evaluation plan must be written before the program plan is completed, but the evaluation design and the data needed to measure change will be required for incorporation into the data-collection aspects of the program plan.

If a change in knowledge of program participants, for example, is one program objective, the program plan should include the tool, test, or other instrument that will be used for pre- and posttests. The pretest and posttest scores will become part of the evaluation.

A specific literature search to locate an appropriate instrument or the development of a reliable tool will require more time and thus will be accomplished best if adequate time is allotted and adequate efforts are made.

Many programs partially evaluate effectiveness by obtaining a count of the number of people served. Procedures for collecting basic demographic data, services provided, expenditures of resources, and evidence of program effectiveness are other areas for baseline data collection to be included in the program plan. If forms are designed with these items in mind, data collection for program evaluation will be facilitated.

■ USING A MODEL FOR PROGRAM-PLAN DEVELOPMENT

Use of a model for program-plan development provides the advanced practice public/community health nurse with a conceptual focus for guiding the planning team. Although not always apparent in the written program plan, a planning model serves to keep the team on target. In this section, three planning models are introduced. Advantages and disadvantages of each model are discussed.

Planning Models

Planning is not an exact science, but several planning models have been developed to provide more guidance for the planning process. The three models introduced in this section are McLaughlin's (1982) Model for community health programs, Timmreck's (2003) 10-step planning model, and the PRECEDE–PROCEED Model (Green & Kreuter, 2005). Examples of the use of these models are found in the literature.

McLAUGHLIN'S MODEL FOR COMMUNITY HEALTH PROGRAMS

McLaughlin's Model is based on the Health Belief Model and the concept of intentionality, which includes both belief strength and referent group attitudes (see Chapter 9). This model clusters populations into groups according to where individuals would fall in one of four quadrants formed by the intersection of two axes. The horizontal axis is the continuum of perceived wellness, ranging from a perception of illness to that of high-level wellness. The vertical axis is a continuum of perceived psychological readiness to act on health benefits, ranging from little readiness to a high intention to act.

Furthermore, McLaughlin views cues to action as central to both the Health Belief Model and intentionality. Thus, "program development in community health nursing is an effort to organize services for the provision of appropriate and meaningful cues" (McLaughlin, 1982, p. 14). The three levels of prevention—primary, secondary, and tertiary—provide the basis for the sections of the model termed *health promotion* (primary), *health supervision and early detection* (secondary), *disease avoidance and heath protection* (secondary), and *disease control and monitoring* (tertiary).

On the basis of a community assessment, the advanced practice public/community health nurse could develop goals, objectives, and activities to address each of the four quadrants described. An example of application of McLaughlin's Model to lead poisoning has a goal of "elimination of lead hazards from the community's environment" with sample activities of inspections prior to home or apartment occupancy and enforcement of housing codes (Ervin & Kuehnert, 1993, p. 27).

One advantage of McLaughlin's Model is that it is based on theory with which nurses are familiar. It was specifically developed for use with a variety of community health programs, so it provides a guide for many different types of program plans. In addition, the guidance provided is applied to aggregates across the two important continua of psychological readiness and health. This conceptualization encourages the development of programs that apply to diverse groups of people-provided services in a community, for example, elderly and middle-aged adults.

Although very useful for program planning, the McLaughlin Model does not provide as much direction as some other models. The nurse planner must have a good grasp of the theoretical foundation and behaviors of the population to effectively apply this model.

TIMMRECK'S 10-STEP PLANNING MODEL

Timmreck's model provides a straightforward approach to the process of planning. The 10 steps are as follows: (1) review or develop the mission statement; (2) complete assessment and evaluation of organization, inventory resources, and review regulations and policies; (3) write goals and objectives; (4) conduct need assessments; (5) determine and set priorities; (6) write goals and objectives; (7) determine the step-by-step activities and procedures; (8) develop timeline charts; (9) implement the project; and (10) evaluate and provide feedback (Timmreck, 2003).

This book has so far led the reader through much of the first six steps of Timmreck's 10-step process. The next step would be to determine the step-by-step activities and procedures. Timmreck pointed out several items addressed earlier in the section on resources. Other questions to answer in this step of the planning process are, "What needs to be done first? What needs to be done before other activities can take place? What items or processes need to be in place before others can start?" (Timmreck, 2003, p. 138).

Advantages of the 10-step model are its straightforward approach, easy-to-follow format, and the detail provided to complete each step. This general model would be useful for many types of program-planning efforts. One disadvantage is that it has little theoretical basis.

PRECEDE–PROCEED MODEL

This health-promotion planning and evaluation model consists of two components, PRECEDE and PROCEED, which have six basic phases that can be extended to eight phases with the addition of evaluation of program impact and outcomes. The PRECEDE component was introduced in Chapter 11. "The Precede–Proceed model takes into account the multiple factors that determine health and quality of life. It helps the planner arrive at a highly focused subset of those factors as targets for intervention" (Green & Kreuter, 1999, p. 34). The five phases of the PRECEDE component are social assessment, epidemiologic assessment, behavioral and environmental assessment, educational and ecological assessment, and administrative and policy assessment.

In phase 1, the social assessment considers the quality of life by subjectively defined hopes, problems, and priorities of individuals and communities. Involving the people in a self-study is recommended as an approach to complete this phase.

The purpose of phase 2 is to identify the specific health goals or problems that may contribute to the social goals identified in phase 1. Health and illness data are gathered and analyzed to complete this step. The end point of phase 2 is the selection of the problem of the highest priority, considering educational and promotional resources.

Phase 3 involves techniques to identify the specific health-related behavioral and environmental factors that could be linked to the health problem chosen in phase 2.

In phase 4, the factors that have potential to influence a specific health behavior are organized into predisposing, enabling, and reinforcing factors. The program planner then studies the factors to determine which have the highest priority as the focus of the intervention.

Phase 5 of the PRECEDE component is administrative and policy diagnosis. In this phase, an assessment of the resources needed and those available to carry out the methods and strategies is completed. Time, personnel, and the budget are major items to be addressed. An assessment of barriers to implementation completes the administrative assessment. The policy assessment consists of an assessment of policies, regulations, and organizations followed by an assessment of political forces. Implementation and evaluation complete this phase and are addressed in detail later in Sections IV and V of this book.

PROCEED stands for policy, regulatory, and organizational constructs in educational environmental development. The PROCEED component of the model provides a guide for a thorough examination of factors for program planning and implementation. This level of examination would be especially important for planning controversial programs, for example, a needle exchange program or programs in a highly polarized community. This advantage of the model may also be viewed as a disadvantage. The detail of assessment required to apply the model correctly would require a great deal of time, especially the first time it is used.

Phase 6 is implementation of the program and builds on a good program plan, an adequate budget, good organizational and policy support, good training and supervision of staff, and good monitoring in the process-evaluation stage. Program implementation is covered in detail in Chapters 14 and 15. Although evaluation phases 7 and 8 of the PROCEED components are last, they are a continuous part of working with the entire PRECEDE–PROCEED model and are discussed in Section V.

Example Application of a Planning Model

For purposes of illustrating application of a model, McLaughlin's Model of community health program planning is used in this section. The community diagnosis for this application is risk of death from cardiovascular disease among adults in the county. Cardiovascular disease has several risk factors, including smoking, high-fat diet (elevated serum cholesterol), hypertension, lack of exercise, diabetes, stress, family history, and obesity (Valanis, 1999), so using a multifaceted program to address cardiovascular disease is appropriate.

A specific behavior inventory would have been conducted during earlier stages of the planning process to identify the exact behaviors and their quantity in the county adult population. For example, the percentage of smoking adults, the percentage of adults with elevated blood cholesterol levels, the level of exercise, obesity levels, and other pertinent levels would be known to target those behaviors that have the greatest potential for decreasing the risk factors for cardiovascular disease for the population as a whole. For this program plan, the risk factors of smoking and lack of physical activity will be addressed.

One study demonstrated that cardiovascular risk factors for U.S. adults, ages 20 to 49 years, have become worse over the past 40 years (Casagrande, Menke, & Cowie, 2016). In 2015, 15.3% of U.S. adults aged 18 and older were cigarette smokers (Office of Disease Prevention and Health Promotion, 2018). Smoking was higher among adults aged 25 and over for those with no high school diploma or general equivalency diploma (GED) (25.6%) than among adults aged 25 and over with a bachelor's degree or higher (5.9%). Smoking levels also varied widely by age, poverty status, and race/ethnicity. The *Healthy People 2020* objective is to reduce cigarette smoking by adults from the 2008 baseline of 20.6% to 12.0% (Office of Disease Prevention and Health Promotion [ODPHP], 2016a). These data provide content for objectives for the program plan.

Many people are at risk for cardiovascular disease due to lack of physical activity. In 2014, data showed that 23.7% of adults are engaged in no leisure-time physical activity. The levels of no physical activity ranged from 16.4% in Colorado to 31.6% in Mississippi (CDC, 2014). The *Healthy People 2020* objective is to reduce the proportion of adults who engage in no leisure-time physical activity (ODPHP, 2016b). Both areas, a decrease in smoking and an increase in physical activity, will contribute to a decrease in obesity in the community as well as to improve other indicators of health.

Each quadrant of the McLaughlin Model provides guidance for directing program activities to a different segment of the community. The health-promotion quadrant of McLaughlin's (1982) Model is defined as the area of interventions used to prevent illness and is aimed at people who are healthy. Measures under health promotion are designed to help individuals develop lifestyles to maintain health. General cues are needed to encourage health behavior.

The disease-avoidance and health-protection services are designed to use cues about specific illness conditions. Thus, this program area is aimed primarily at illness behavior to limit adverse effects of health problems. Health supervision and early detection, the other areas of secondary prevention, are aimed at people who believe themselves to be at risk. The cues for action rely primarily on education and support directed at influencing attitudes and beliefs.

Disease control and monitoring services are related to cues that limit behaviors in conflict with health. These tertiary services are aimed at sick-role behavior to contain the effects of disease or restore individuals to an optimal state of function.

Box 12.1 shows examples of goals, objectives, and activities for each quadrant aimed at the community diagnosis of risk of death from cardiovascular disease. A comprehensive program to reduce the risk of death from cardiovascular disease may encompass some or all these activities. In addition to the goals, objectives, and activities for each quadrant of the McLaughlin (1982) Model, a research-based protocol for each intervention is needed for successful program implementation.

■ RELATIONSHIP OF INTERVENTIONS TO PROGRAM PLANS

A *nursing intervention* is defined as any treatment based on clinical judgment and knowledge performed by a nurse to enhance client outcomes (McCloskey & Bulechek, 1996). An intervention in advanced public/community health nursing practice differs in several ways from this definition of a nursing intervention. Advanced public/community health nursing practice focuses on improving the health of the total community, though interventions may be aimed at the individual, group, or community. A nurse may perform interventions at the community level on behalf of the community, but it is much more likely that the intervention would be implemented in partnership with the community.

Moreover, an intervention at the community level is direct care but often appears very different than an intervention at the individual or group level. For example, working with a community to develop areas for exercise and family recreation to promote health looks very different than individually instructing people about getting adequate exercise to promote cardiovascular health. Nonetheless, both interventions are examples of direct care to promote health of communities.

Nurses in advanced public/community health nursing practice are involved with developing interventions at the group and community levels, but often these are delivered to the individual or family unit to reach people with appropriate care. Thus, an intervention in advanced public/community health nursing practice is a direct-care treatment in terms of a very broad definition of *treatment*, which is the application of a remedy to effect a cure.

BOX 12.1   APPLICATION OF McLAUGHLIN'S MODEL TO CARDIOVASCULAR DISEASE

Health-Promotion Services

Goal: To increase positive attitudes of the population toward exercise

Objective 1: To increase knowledge level in the county population about the positive benefits of exercise

Activities

1.1. Hold community-wide monthly programs to promote positive attitudes and outcomes of family exercise activities.
1.2. Work with community organizations and worksites for promotion of exercise as a positive benefit to quality of life.

Objective 2: To reduce from 30% to 25% the percentage of adults 18 years and older in the county who do not engage regularly in light to moderate physical activity for at least 150 minutes per week

Activities

2.1. Organize walking clubs for all county worksites with 10 or more employees.
2.2. Work with sponsors to develop community walking trails, bike paths, outdoor fitness courses, and worksite fitness centers.
2.3. Provide incentives for walking instead of driving to events (e.g., free parking away from events).

Disease Avoidance and Health Protection

Goal: To reduce the proportion of adults in the county who smoke cigarettes

Objective 1: To reduce from 20.8% to 15.0% the percentage of adults in the county who smoke cigarettes

Activities

1.1. Enforce nonsmoking regulations in all locations.
1.2. Increase the number of workplaces with nonsmoking policies from 50% to 80% of local work settings.
1.3. Offer smoking-cessation programs at factories and other locations with a high proportion of employees with high school diplomas and/or GEDs.

Objective 2: To increase the local tax on a pack of cigarettes from $0.50 to $0.80

Activities

2.1. Work with local organizations to form a coalition to support the effort for a tax increase.
2.2. Provide the coalition with information and expertise about the need for a tax increase.

Early Detection and Health-Supervision Services

Goal: To detect risk factors for cardiovascular disease
Objective: To maintain serum cholesterol levels in the adult population of the county to no more than 200 mg/dL

(continued)

BOX 12.1 APPLICATION OF McLAUGHLIN'S MODEL TO CARDIOVASCULAR DISEASE *(continued)*

Activities

1. Provide cholesterol testing sites at regularly scheduled times and locations for easy access for adult population (e.g., shopping malls, worksites, community events, churches).
2. Provide dietary counseling for all adults with cholesterol levels over 200 mg/dL and who desire it; provide counseling for all others who request a consultation.
3. Promote monthly community activities to highlight fat content in food and methods to decrease fat intake (e.g., public service announcements on television and radio, food store displays).

Disease Control and Monitoring Services

Goal: To decrease barriers to regular medical care for people with cardiovascular disease

Objective 1: To increase access to regular medical care for 80% (currently 60%) of the county population

Activities

1.1. Provide information to employers about need for insurance coverage for cardiac follow-up after hospitalization for cardiac events.
1.2. Organize, in cooperation with the local medical society, programs about the benefits of regular medical follow-up for all cardiac patients.

Objective 2: To decrease the number of hospitalizations for cardiac events

Activities

2.1. Provide case management services to all patients discharged from the local hospital with cardiac diagnoses.
2.2. Conduct education and support groups for patients with cardiac diagnoses.

In health promotion and disease prevention, which are keystones of public/community health nursing practice, a cure is not needed, but efforts to prevent the need of a cure are targeted for action in programs.

Multidisciplinary Interventions

In advanced public/community health nursing practice, the nurse is often engaged in multidisciplinary program planning, which may include more than nursing interventions. Thus, the nurse is called upon to work with others to develop interventions that may be delivered by a variety of health and social service workers.

This type of program planning requires that the interventions be coordinated as well as compatible. For example, instructions given by the nurse and the housing inspector to a family about control of lead hazards in the home must be the same or at least compatible to avoid confusing the family. Although the nurse and the other team members may not implement interventions at the same time, the planning requires a coordinated and synchronized effort for a cohesive program that is aimed at accomplishing the same ends.

Delivery Method and Intervention

A program includes both the delivery method for the intervention and the intervention itself, so details about both are needed for a successful program. The delivery method must be detailed enough for planning a budget and for delineating the activities to be carried out by the staff who will deliver the intervention to the targeted individuals, groups, and/or communities. For example, in a program to increase the immunization level among children ages 2 years or younger, the immunizations themselves are the intervention. Details about where, by whom, and how the immunizations will be given are also needed, in addition to a marketing plan for reaching the target population, which is explained in Chapter 14.

At times, the intervention and delivery method are not separate but are interwoven. For example, the intervention of group support for weight loss includes both the intervention (which must be detailed) as group support and the delivery method as group sessions. However, the details about where and when the groups will be held, who will be targeted for attending, who will conduct the groups, and other details of the delivery method need to be thought through and documented. Less off-the-cuff planning and more preplanning are better for program success.

Documentation of Activities in the Program Plan

As indicated earlier, activities will take two forms in the actual program-plan document. One form includes the activities that spell out the methods and approaches for objective attainment. The second form of activities is the details about the intervention that is delivered by the program. For example, home visiting has been demonstrated through numerous research projects to be effective in improving outcomes for young mothers and their infants (Olds & Kitzman, 1990; Olds et al., 2014). How many home visits to make to which clients is not entirely clear in the research reports. A structured program is needed to provide guidance to the program staff about how many home visits to make, how far apart they should be scheduled, when to terminate home visits, and various other details about effectively scheduling visits.

The other major component of the program plan about home visits is what to do during each one. What assessment tools are used? How often is assessment done? What educational content does the nurse provide and how? What skills are taught? The level of detail will vary with the purpose and objectives of the program, but consideration of key questions is crucial so that important details are not inadvertently omitted. Programs have failed or have not achieved the projected objectives because some needed details were left undocumented during the planning phase.

In the preceding example of home visits to young mothers and infants, the content of each visit could be unspecified and tailored by each nurse to the mother's perception of need at each home visit. If a pilot study was conducted to determine the effectiveness of the two approaches, then evaluation would provide some data for choosing an approach for future programs of home visiting. For example, a review of randomized trials of parenting interventions to improve health outcomes and development of infants and children found that home visitation by nurses showed more positive outcome behaviors (Olds, Sadler, & Kitzman, 2007); interventions based on research do work. The content to be included in each home visit has been documented by Olds and colleagues. Information to become a site for the program, the Nurse–Family Partnership program, may be obtained by contacting the organization. Information can be obtained at www.nursefamilypartnership.org. The home visiting program is a good example of a research-based intervention.

Content of a Program Plan Document

The basic components of a program plan are outlined in Box 12.2. Greater detail may be added to the outline as indicated by the complexity of the program. The outline may be provided with page numbers as an index on the front of a written program plan, or it may be used only to guide the final writing of the plan.

Providing the rationale for the goals and objectives makes it clear why the specific goals and objectives were chosen. Recall that in earlier chapters, discussion included focusing the program plan to one or more levels and numerous factors to consider in choosing goals and objectives. No one approach to solve a problem is ever obvious, so the program planner needs to be explicit about the choices made. In addition, if the rationale is clear to the program planner, it is more likely to be clear to potential funding sources and others who will read the program plan.

Often, a funding source will specify the page limit for the program plan to be submitted for funding consideration. This often poses a challenge for the writer of a program plan. The detail needed to implement a program need not be included in a plan for funding consideration unless it is the focus of the RFA (request for applications) from the

---

BOX 12.2   OUTLINE FOR A WRITTEN PROGRAM PLAN

I. Executive summary
    Table of contents (optional)

II. Introduction
    A. Summary of community assessment
    B. Community diagnosis
    C. Target population description
    D. Program-planning model

III. Goals
    A. Goals and rationale
    B. Relationship of goals to community diagnosis

IV. Objectives
    A. Objectives and rationale
    B. How objectives relate to the goals
    C. Relationship of objectives to target population

V. Program
    A. Description of program
    B. Expected outcomes of program
    C. Activities related to program delivery

VI. Intervention
    A. Description of intervention
    B. Expected outcomes of intervention
    C. Activities related to intervention delivery

VII. Resources and constraints
    A. Available and potential resources
    B. Current and anticipated constraints

VIII. Budget

IX. Appendices

funding source. Often, the detail may be included in an appendix or referred to in the body of the program plan as "available upon request." A brief summary of the intervention may be adequate to reassure the funding source that the planners have thought through what is needed to successfully implement the program.

An executive summary of usually no more than two pages may be provided at the beginning of a written program plan. Writing the summary last is important so that the total program plan is presented. An executive summary includes the major points of the program plan, including community diagnosis or problem, target population, goals, objectives, intervention, delivery system, and evaluation. Program evaluation is addressed in Section V.

■ USE OF A RESEARCH BASE FOR INTERVENTION DEVELOPMENT

In Chapter 11, the use of research for intervention development was discussed. In the actual program-plan document, the details of the intervention need to be stated. This statement could take the form of the protocol or procedure developed during the previous phase of the planning process. A trial of the intervention should be completed before the full program is implemented to have a more successful program. A consultant may be contacted for details about the actual intervention during program planning. A consultant may be conferred with in person, on a telephone or video conference call, in written form, in a computer email exchange, or other form of computer program. If funding is required for the use of a consultant, a request should be made after determining the actual fees with the consultant.

Research Utilization

Research-based interventions are developed and implemented using the research utilization process, which consists of the following steps:

- Systematically identify patient care problems or community diagnoses.
- Identify and assess the research-based knowledge to solve the identified problems.
- Adapt and design the nursing practice innovation.
- Conduct a clinical trial and evaluation of the innovation.
- Decide whether to adopt, alter, or reject the innovation.
- Develop the means to extend (or diffuse) the new practice beyond the trial phase.
- Develop mechanisms to maintain the innovation over time (Horsley, Crane, Crabtree, & Wood, 1983; White, Dudley-Brown, & Terhaar, 2016).

For advanced public/community health nursing practice, this process begins with the community assessment followed by the validation and prioritization of the community diagnoses. A clinical trial may not be needed if the innovation (intervention) is well established and has generally been implemented by other agencies or organizations as accepted practice. However, if the intervention has not been implemented and evaluated with the target population, a trial project is more likely to be needed. If there is doubt or disagreement about the implementation of an intervention, a clinical trial or pilot project is the preferred approach used to settle the disagreement.

If the intervention is on a community-wide basis, a trial may be difficult to conduct. In instances such as these, materials or techniques may be introduced to groups of the target population to evaluate before the intervention is implemented across the total community. At the point of pilot testing, changes could still be made.

■ PROGRAM-PLAN COMPONENTS AT INDIVIDUAL, GROUP, AND COMMUNITY LEVELS

In Chapter 11, theory and research were presented as bases for the development of interventions at the individual, group, and community levels. In some instances, intervention components will be used at all three levels to achieve program objectives. For example, social support may be provided at the individual and/or group level, but involvement of the community may be an integral part of the intervention. A study examined community and organizational support needed to improve women's rural health in Ontario, Canada. Findings indicated that factors at multiple levels, including community, governmental, institutional, professional, and persona, l contributed to public/community health nursing practice for more effective promotion of rural women's health (Leipert, Regan, & Plunkett, 2015).

From diffusion theory, we know that people adopt innovations at different rates (Rogers, 2003). Thus, different intervention strategies are needed to reach various groups. "For example, mass media are most efficient with innovators and early adopters, but outreach methods such as home visits are necessary with late adopters" (Green & Kreuter, 1999, pp. 179–180).

Irrespective of whether one, two, or three levels of intervention are planned, all must be documented in the program plan with an explanation of how they fit together. In addition, different people may be involved with implementation of various aspects of the program at various levels. For example, public health nurses may deliver the intervention at the individual level, and health educators work at the community level in an immunization program. Also, community members may be more involved at the community level than at the individual level, such as with a campaign to increase the rate of women screened for breast cancer.

Individual-Level Program-Plan Components

Individual-level programs are based on the premise that individuals have the ability and resources to initiate and maintain the behavioral changes on their own (Dignan & Carr, 1992). This is not always true and should be addressed in the program plan. For example, many behavior changes require coaching and reinforcement before the change becomes a permanent part of the individual's life. Therefore, a one-time educational program is not an appropriate intervention for all topics with all individuals. In addition, some behaviors are difficult to maintain because of factors outside the control of the individual, for example, diet when the individual does not purchase and prepare the food.

The intervention protocol may specify what the exact intervention is, but not who carries it out. For example, in a program to prevent falls among elderly living at home, both the home healthcare nurse and the home health aide could be involved. The program plan should specify what the nurse will do and what the activities of the home health aide will be in the program.

An example of a program plan aimed at the individual level with involvement of a family (group level) is presented at the end of this chapter.

Group-Level Program-Plan Components

Groups may be specified as small (e.g., eight to 10 individuals) or large (e.g., community aggregates of several thousand). Programs delivered to groups of various size require different types of plans, with interventions tailored to address the characteristics of the various groups. More than one model of an intervention may also be needed.

Groups may include families, peer groups, worksite groups, and small organizations that often influence behavior change. The use of group-dynamics principles is needed with small groups. In groups of this size for face-to-face sessions, individuals must feel part of the group to have a successful outcome (Dignan & Carr, 1987).

A program to increase the number of pregnant women who start prenatal care in the first trimester is an example of a group-level program that is aimed at an aggregate. Although prenatal care is provided at the individual level, the outreach to encourage prenatal-care initiation in the first trimester could be accomplished through group networking.

There may be more than one aggregate also. The aggregates may be defined as females in the reproductive age groups who have been seen to delay the start of prenatal care. Characteristics associated with late or no prenatal care include women who are less educated, have no health insurance, abuse tobacco and other drugs, are multiparous, and are living with at least one child (Maupin et al., 2004).

Interventions to reach pregnant women with these various characteristics would require different techniques. For example, reaching women who abuse drugs would require an approach to involve significant others who are in close contact with the women. Many women who abuse drugs do not come forward because of concern of being arrested, so programs would need to stress the nonpunitive aspects.

A potentially successful program should be tailored to fit the characteristics of the groups targeted in the specific community. The community assessment and subsequent steps for program planning will assist the advanced practice public/community health nurse to fold these into the program plan.

Community-Level Program Plan Components

Identifying characteristics of a community for program planning is difficult because most communities are diverse. So, a program tailored to fit one community segment may be inappropriate for another segment of the community. There are, however, some guidelines that may be helpful.

Consideration needs to be given to what is acceptable to the community, including literacy, degree of auditory or visual stimulation in the lives of the community, customary ways of gaining information, cost of the intervention, feasibility, and anticipated effectiveness (Dignan & Carr, 1992). More than one method may be needed for an intervention at the community level depending on the community profile.

Asking members of the various community aggregates what they would like to see in an intervention will assist greatly with the design and implementation of the specifications for a program plan. Techniques outlined earlier may be helpful in the process of asking community members, for example, focus groups, surveys, and community meetings.

For purposes of program planning, large organizations may be considered communities. Appropriate interventions must also be used with organizations to bring about changes to meet goals and objectives. Chapter 9 provides more guidance about planning at the organizational level.

The following example of a program plan incorporates the points made in this chapter as well as in other chapters of Section III.

◼ PLAN FOR THE SAFETY-FIRST AT HOME PROGRAM

Executive Summary

The Safety-First at Home program is designed to decrease the number of deaths or complications from a fall among elderly who experience a fall in their homes. Falling in the home is the third leading cause of death among elderly in Alexander County. In addition, the program is expected to decrease the number of elderly who require emergency care and hospitalization due to falls in the home.

At the end of 2 years of the program, a decrease in deaths by 30% is projected as one outcome of this program. Emergency visits and hospitalizations are projected to decrease by 20% by the end of the first program year.

Two approaches to reach the objectives are proposed: enhancing safety at home and increasing the strength and ambulation ability of the program participants. Using assessments of the home and the individual, a public health nurse, a physical therapist, and a safety engineer will recommend changes needed in the home and a program of exercise to each program participant and the family. Physician approval will be obtained for participation in the exercise program component. The public health nurse will do follow-up in the home.

The effectiveness of the program will be measured by a decrease in the number of deaths and by a decrease in the number of emergency visits and hospitalizations due to falls or complications from falls. Long-term support for the program, if effective, will be obtained through a combination of funding from donations, agency in-kind contributions, grants, and reimbursement.

Introduction

A community assessment conducted in Alexander County, in 2015, discovered that the third leading cause of death among residents aged 65 years or more was a fall or complications following a fall in the home. The following community diagnosis was developed on the basis of data collected in the community assessment:

> Risk of death due to falls *among* Alexander County residents aged 65 years or older *related to* side effects or interactions of medications, impaired balance and ambulation, hazards inside the home, and unsafe use of tools or devices as *demonstrated in* 10 deaths reported in 2014, due to falls or complications after falls in the home, and 110 calls and visits to emergency departments related to falls in the home.

Goals

The following goals are the aims of the program:

1. To decrease the number of deaths due to falls among the home-dwelling elderly in Alexander County
2. To decrease the number of injuries from falls requiring emergency treatment among the home-dwelling elderly in Alexander County

These goals were formulated to focus the program intervention on areas that will have concrete outcomes for the elderly residing in Alexander County. On the basis of data collected in the community assessment, it is projected that 10 deaths, 30 hospital admissions, 110 emergency department visits, and 10 nursing home admissions could be avoided with use of preventive methods in the home. The annual cost savings is conservatively estimated at $265,000. Moreover, the cost in terms of loss of quality of life and pain would be reduced.

Objectives

1. To reduce the number of deaths related to falls in the home by 30%, by the end of the second year of the program (baseline 10 deaths annually)
2. To reduce the number of hospital admissions and emergency visits by 20% in the first year (baseline 30 hospital admissions and 110 emergency department visits in 2014)

Two years are needed for the program to reach an adequate number of people to have an impact. By the end of the first year, no decrease in deaths may be expected, but some reduction in injuries should be apparent. The interventions and processes will be examined and altered as needed, if the objectives are not achieved.

Data indicate that deaths and injuries due to falls in the home are leading causes of mortality, morbidity, and loss of quality of life for older residents of Alexander County. As the proportion of the older-than-65 population continues to increase, an increase in deaths and injuries due to falls can be expected. A program, such as the one proposed in this plan, if effective, will decrease this burden on the elderly as well as on their families.

Program

The focus of the Safety-First at Home program is twofold: (a) enhancing the safety of homes of elderly, and (b) improving balance and ambulation ability of elderly living at home through exercise. A public health nurse, a physical therapist, and a safety engineer for residential property will assess the physical conditions of all participants and their homes. A component of the physical condition assessment will be the balance and ambulation status of the program participant.

Following the assessments, recommendations will be made to the participant and the family for alterations in factors related to the physical condition of the program participant and correction of safety hazards. Family members and the participant will decide what changes they want to make and the assessment team will make referrals. The public health nurse will continue follow-up until all corrections are made.

If the program participant has deficits in balance and/or ambulation, the second component of the program will be offered. The program participant's primary care provider must approve in writing the participation in the exercise part of the program. An individualized program of exercise to improve balance and strength of the program participant will be devised by the physical therapist, who will work with the public health nurse, client, and family for 1 week to teach the exercises and evaluate their effectiveness.

During the second week of program participation, the public health nurse will visit the family three times to continue teaching and assisting with the exercises. Following this, once-a-week home visits will be made for a month by the public health nurse to evaluate progress, to reinforce teaching, and to encourage continuation of exercise. Home visits will be made once a month for 1 year by the public health nurse to assess progress and to encourage continued participation. After 1 year of participation, the physical therapist will evaluate each participant for balance and ambulation status.

It is expected that safety hazards will be eliminated in the homes of 50% of the program participants. If it is impossible to eliminate hazards (e.g., structural faults), a plan will be devised to decrease risk of the adverse situation. It is expected that of the program participants who enroll in the exercise part of the program, 30% will complete 1 year. They will have improved balance and ambulation status, thus decreasing their risk of falling.

Intervention

HOME SAFETY ASSESSMENT

This program component will consist of a physical inspection of the inside of the home. All identified hazards will be noted and recommendations will be made in writing for the family. For example, if throw rugs are used, the recommendations will be to remove them or secure them with appropriate methods.

INDIVIDUAL HEALTH AND PHYSICAL ASSESSMENT

The public health nurse will assess the program participant's physical and mental status, including medical diagnoses and medications. If drug side effects or drug interactions are indicated in the assessment, the primary care provider and/or pharmacist will be consulted about changes. The physical therapist will assess the participant's balance and ability to ambulate inside the home. All recommendations will be written and discussed with the participant and/or family members.

On the basis of research findings, it is expected that participants in the exercise component of the program will have improved balance and ambulation because of increased strength and improved cardiovascular conditioning. In addition, safety will be improved with instruction about proper use of aids for ambulation (e.g., canes, walkers, and wheelchairs). Other recommendations will be made as appropriate about safety in ambulation.

Resources and Constraints

The program will be funded by a grant for the first 3 years. If the program is effective, continued funding will be phased into all agencies in the county that provide services to the elderly population. A potential fund will be explored from the savings experienced by all agencies and managed care plans through avoidance of injuries from falls to clients. Future funding may also be secured from grant writing. Donations will be accepted from families, program participants, and other community members and organizations.

Personnel from the participating agencies will be assigned and trained to participate in the program through recruitment of participants and referral. All participating agencies will contribute secretarial time, office supplies, telephone, fax, and other day-to-day needs.

Anticipated constraints include resistance by some agencies to participate, especially if the program is not one of their current priorities. Funding may not be adequate to implement the program as outlined. Also, some personnel may be in short supply (e.g., physical therapists).

Budget

The total budget is estimated at $148,750 for the first year of the program. Details of the budget are as follows:

Personnel	$115,000
Benefits (25%)	$28,750
Equipment	$2,000
Mileage	$3,000
Total	$148,750

■ SUMMARY

This chapter addresses some of the nuts and bolts of developing a program plan. An example of a basic program plan was presented with goals, objectives, resources, constraints, methods, and activities for a program to decrease deaths due to falls among elderly living in their homes. On the basis of a community diagnosis of risk of death related to falls in the home, this program is intended to decrease the risk of falls and, thus, decrease the risk of death due to falls.

■ SUGGESTED CLINICAL OR PRACTICUM ACTIVITIES

1. Review a program plan at your clinical placement setting or a local health department.
2. Identify the strengths and areas for improvement in the written plan using the content of this chapter.
3. If possible, discuss the plan with a staff member who was involved in writing the plan. Ask about the process that was used to develop the plan.

REFERENCES

Casagrande, S. S., Menke, A., & Cowie, C. C. (2016). Cardiovascular risk factors of adults age 20–49 years in the United States, 1971–2012: A series of cross-sectional studies. *Public Library of Science, 11*(8), e0161770. doi:10.1371/journal.pone.0161770

Centers for Disease Control and Health Promotion. (2014). *State indicator report on physical activity, 2014.* Atlanta, GA: U.S. Department of Health and Human Services.

Dignan, M. B., & Carr, P. A. (1987). *Program planning for health education and promotion.* Philadelphia, PA: Lea & Febiger.

Dignan, M. B., & Carr, P. A. (1992). *Program planning for health education and promotion* (2nd ed.). Philadelphia, PA: Lea & Febiger.

Ervin, N. E., & Kuehnert, P. L. (1993). Application of a model for public health nursing program planning. *Public Health Nursing, 10*(1), 25–30.

Ervin, N. E., & Young, W. B. (1996). Model for a nursing center: Spanning boundaries. *Journal of Nursing Care Quality, 11*(2), 16–24.

Green, L. W., & Kreuter, M. W. (1999). *Health promotion planning: An educational and ecological approach* (3rd ed.). Mountain View, CA: Mayfield.

Green, L. W., & Kreuter, M. W. (2005). *Health promotion planning: An educational and ecological approach* (4th ed.). San Francisco, CA: Jossey-Bass.

Hale, C. D., Arnold, F., & Travis, M. T. (1994). *Planning and evaluating health programs: A primer.* Albany, NY: Delmar.

Horsley, J. A., Crane, J., Crabtree, M. K., & Wood, D. J. (1983). *Using research to improve nursing practice: A guide (CURN project).* New York, NY: Grune & Stratton.

Leipert, B. D., Regan, S., & Plunkett, R. (2015). Working through and around: Exploring rural public health nursing practices and policies to promote rural women's health. *Online Journal of Rural Nursing & Health Care, 15*(1), 74–99.

Maupin, R., Jr, Lyman, R., Fatsis, J., Prystowiski, E., Nguyen, A., Wright, C., … Miller, J., Jr. (2004). Characteristics of women who deliver with no prenatal care. *Journal of Maternal-Fetal & Neonatal Medicine, 16,* 45–50.

McCloskey, J. C., & Bulechek, G. M. (Eds.). (1996). *Nursing interventions classification (NIC)* (2nd ed.). St. Louis, MO: Mosby.

McLaughlin, J. S. (1982). Toward a theoretical model for community health programs. *Advances in Nursing Science, 5*(1), 7–28.

Office of Disease Prevention and Health Promotion. (2016a). Tobacco use. *Healthy people 2020.* Retrieved from https://www.healthypeople.gov/2020/topics-objectives/topic/tobacco-use

Office of Disease Prevention and Health Promotion. (2016b). Physical activity. *Healthy people 2020.* Retrieved from https://www.healthypeople.gov/2020/topics-objectives/topic/physical-activity

Office of Disease Prevention and Health Promotion. (2018). Tobacco use. *Healthy people 2020.* Retrieved from https://www.healthypeople.gov/2020/data-search/Search-the-Data#topic-areas-3510

Olds, D. L., & Kitzman, H. (1990). Can home visitation improve the health of women and children at environmental risk? *Pediatrics, 86*(1), 108–116.

Olds, D. L., Kitzman, H., Knudtson, M., Anson, E., Smith, J., & Cole, R. (2014). Effect of home visiting by nurses on maternal and child mortality: Results of a two-decade follow-up of a randomized, clinical trial. *JAMA Pediatrics, 168*(9), 800–806. doi:10.1001/jamapediatrics.2014.472

Olds, D. L., Sadler, L., & Kitzman, H. (2007). Programs for parents of infants and toddlers: Recent evidence from randomized trials. *Journal of Child Psychology and Psychiatry, 48*(3-4), 355–391. doi:10.1111/j.1469-7610.2006.01702.x

Rogers, E. M. (2003). *Diffusion of innovations* (5th ed.). New York, NY: Simon & Schuster.

Timmreck, T. C. (2003). *Planning, program development, and evaluation: A handbook for health promotion, aging, and health services* (2nd ed.). Sudbury, MA: Jones & Bartlett.

U.S. Department of Health and Human Services. Centers for Disease Control and Health Promotion. National Center for Health Statistics. (2017). *Health, United States, 2016.* DHHS Publication 2017–1232. Retrieved from https://www.cdc.gov/nchs/hus/hus16.pdf

Valanis, B. (1999). *Epidemiology in health care* (3rd ed.). Stamford, CT: Appleton & Lange.

White, K. M., Dudley-Brown, S., & Terhaar, M. F. (2016). *Translation of evidence into nursing and health care* (2nd ed.). New York, NY: Springer Publishing.

CHAPTER 13

Developing Budgets for Program Plans

STUDY EXERCISES

1. What is the relationship of budgets to program plans?
2. How do the types of budgets relate to parts of a program plan?
3. What are the advantages and disadvantages of the various budgeting approaches?
4. Describe the factors to be considered in planning budgets.
5. What approaches may be used to secure funding for community health programs?

After developing a program plan, the advanced practice public/community health nurse is faced with the challenge of putting the objectives and activities into numerical terms, specifically budgets. If the components of a program plan follow the guidelines in Chapter 12, a budget or budgets will be easier to construct because the resources required for the program will be clearly stated. For example, details in the program plan about implementation of the intervention provide the information needed to develop staffing plans, which can then be translated into the money amount needed to hire staff. Other parts of the program plan provide details about needed supplies, space, communications, and other resources for a successful program.

The planning process is not a linear one that proceeds smoothly from step 1 through step 10. As indicated in earlier chapters, planning needs to be flexible and allow time for going back and forth between and among steps of the process. Budgeting is a similar process in that the planner is often determining resources needed throughout the planning stages and may even begin to attach numerical amounts to items as the planning process goes along. This tentative list of resources should not be interpreted as true budget planning. A systematic approach to budgeting for a new program is required. This chapter concentrates on the nuts and bolts of budget development for program plans and also provides basic knowledge about budgets and the budgeting process. As with any new major topic, you will want to refer to other materials for other areas of budgeting with which you are not familiar.

RELATIONSHIP OF BUDGETS TO PROGRAM PLANS

Budgets are numerical expressions of program plans (Murray, 2014). In other words, budgets are translations of program-plan words into numbers. Budgets also serve as standards for comparing results with projections. These two relationships of budgets to program plans are addressed in this section.

Numerical Expressions of Program Plans

Planning a sound budget is an important step for ensuring program success. Programs often fail to reach their intended objectives for lack of adequate resources. In addition, budgets frequently do not allow for leeway in the expenditure of funds if emergencies, crises, or large changes occur during the program funding period. Different approaches to budgeting will be addressed later to deal with some of these contingencies. At times, the budget for a program plan is the last part to be written and is thus given less time than the actual plan. This lack of attention may result in a less-than-satisfactory document for implementing the plan.

More than anything else, budgets should reflect the resources truly needed to carry out the work to achieve the objectives. Setting words down on paper is much easier than accomplishing the task. For one thing, there are many unknowns in the program-planning process. Often the planner is making best educated guesses about the number of people who will use the program, the amount of time needed to hire and train staff, and how much effort will be required to bring about the changes projected in the objectives.

Box 13.1 gives examples of how objectives may or may not assist with planning a budget. If the objectives do not contain adequate detail, the activities from the implementation plan will be useful for connecting money amounts with what will be done in the program. Box 13.2 gives examples of using objectives with the associated activities. Examples are provided later in this chapter about how to build budgets from program objectives.

Although planners use their own and others' experiences, the literature, and other sources of information to make best guesses, there are always unknown experiences in the planning process. The skill of the planner is often a key factor in developing a sound plan for which an uncertain budget must be developed. If a planner omits a key component, the fiscal resources needed for that component will likely be omitted. Using a team to develop a program plan or asking others to review draft program plans will assist you in avoiding pitfalls of inadequate plans.

BOX 13.1   RELATING OBJECTIVES TO BUDGET PLANNING

Objective	Budget Items
To increase the immunization level from 75% to 95% of 2-year-olds in the county	(a) Staff to administer immunizations (b) Vaccines and supplies (c) Space and furniture
To reduce cardiovascular disease deaths from 125 per 100,000 to 100 per 100,000	Without more detail, budget items are almost impossible to list. A program aimed at changing dietary habits of a town would require different budget items than one to increase exercise among adults.
To increase the proportion of school-age children who engage in regular physical activity from 55% to 95%	More detail is needed to know what activities are to be implemented, for example, instituting physical education programs in all schools 5 days a week and during summers.

BOX 13.2 RELATIONSHIP OF OBJECTIVES AND ACTIVITIES TO BUDGET	
Objective and Activities	**Budget Items**
To increase the immunization level from 75% to 95% of 2-year-olds in the county (a) Hold four immunization clinics per month for 1 year in locations close to concentrations of 2-year-old children. (b) Staff with one RN and one volunteer per site.	(a) Vaccines and supplies for 48 clinics for 1 year (b) Four hours of one staff member and one volunteer needed per week
To reduce cardiovascular disease deaths from 125 per 100,000 to 100 per 100,000 in 5 years by decreasing dietary fat intake among the adult county population (a) Institute low-fat menus in all local restaurants and workplace cafeterias. (b) Provide a school-to-home educational program via Internet and brochures monthly for grades K–12.	(a) Hold a series of meetings with restaurant owners and cafeteria supervisors to distribute and discuss the process for implementing low-fat menus and/or low-fat substitutes for favorite menu items. Provide nutritional consultation on request during the planning and implementing of new menus. (b) Half-time project coordinator will develop the website and brochures during the first year of the program.
To increase the proportion of school-age children who engage in regular physical activity from 55% to 95% (a) Provide consultation to schools that do not have physical education programs during the school year. (b) Assist schools to obtain funding for physical education programs. (c) Assist schools to gain community support for summer physical education programs.	(a) Project coordinator to provide consultation to five schools 2 hours per week for a year. (b) Four hours per week per school for 1 year for project coordinator to assist with grant writing and funding (c) Ten hours per week for project coordinator to develop public awareness campaign for support for summer physical education programs

EXTERNAL FACTORS THAT INFLUENCE BUDGETS

Translating the plan into numbers is not as straightforward as using the objectives and activities to develop the dollar amounts needed to operate the program. In addition to the factors within the program itself, factors in the outside environment may influence how the program will proceed. Numerous changes and trends may not have been anticipated when a program was planned.

Economic Factors. Adverse changes in the economy of the United States may hinder a program by turning people's attention from health to basic needs of housing and food.

When a program was planned, the planners may not have had information to prepare for this type of situation. During difficult economic times when workers lose their jobs, often health insurance is lost and use of services decreases. On the other hand, in prosperous economic times, people often spend more money on health services and demand may be greater for a program than anticipated.

Political Factors. Becoming aware of factors in the political environment that may affect programs is a key skill for the advanced practice public/community health nurse to develop. Potentially successful programs have been scuttled because of adverse publicity even before the program was implemented. An example of this opposition is the opening of a halfway house for discharged mental health patients or released prisoners. A common response is "not in my backyard."

Any kind of program may have political ramifications. The advanced practice public/community health nurse needs to be tuned into community sentiment, values, beliefs, misconceptions, and norms while planning a program and the corresponding budgets. If opposition to a new program is anticipated, money should be allocated in the budget for an informational campaign or a positive public relations effort.

Community support for funding a program must be built from the early planning stages. Having the involvement and endorsement of community leaders and politically connected people may make the difference in a program's being accepted or rejected by the broader community.

Funding Factors. The reality of the funding world is that it is changeable. Often, funding sources target very specific areas that change each year. The most important source of priorities for federal government funding is *Healthy People 2020* (Office of Disease Prevention and Health Promotion, 2016). This document should be consulted for a match of priorities when writing any health-related grant proposal. If your program does not fit within the current guidelines or priorities of a funding agency, it is preferable to look elsewhere or refocus the program plan to fit the potential funding source. Alternative funding sources may be located, but relationships with the foundation or government agency need to be established in order to have a better chance of making a good match with the priorities of the funding source.

A second reality of funding is the difficulty securing funds for sustaining programs that have "soft" funds for a given number of years. For example, many innovative programs are started with 2 or 3 years of nonrenewable funds from a foundation or a government agency, for example, the Health Care Financing Administration or a state health department. After the initial period of funding is ended, additional funding is not always available or is available at a much reduced level. Planning for a 5-year or more funding cycle would provide more time to financially stabilize a new program.

Standards for Comparing Results With Projections

Once a budget is developed and determined to be sound, it can serve the purpose of standards for monitoring expenditures and revenues for the program. For example, if the expenditures for salaries meet the projections, then the program manager has confidence that funds will meet future needs. On the other hand, if salary expenditures are exceeding allocated amounts for more than 1 month, adjustments in the staffing patterns may save the program from running into more serious fiscal problems later in the fiscal year (FY).

Budgets that provide for variance in spending and revenue are often easier for the advanced practice public/community health nurse to monitor because specified spending and income levels do not have to be met each month but can be averaged over the year. The drawback, of course, is that variances may be allowed to go on too long before corrections are made. It is much more difficult to correct a 10% above budget expenditure in the ninth month than the third month of a budget year. Standards provided in the budget must be used within reasonably consistent parameters in order to be useful. For example, 5% variances from the budgeted amounts are carefully monitored each month and corrections are made to bring expenditures and expenses in line with the budgeted amounts.

■ FINANCIAL TERMS AND THE BUDGETING PROCESS

Usually, preparation for becoming a professional nurse does not include the background for developing budgets for operating programs and agencies. Terms used in financing and budgeting are often foreign to nurses, just as nursing jargon makes little sense to those in other professions. This section provides a brief primer for the novice budget preparer. General background such as that supplied here should be supplemented by reading about the budget process within a specific organization. Most organizations have documents that describe the internal budget process and the timeline for budget preparation and approval. Additional information about budgets and fiscal management may be obtained from textbooks (e.g., Finkler, Jones, & Kovner, 2013; Finkler & McHugh, 2008).

Fiscal Terms

The definitions of some basic fiscal terms are helpful for preparing budgets, working with others to prepare budgets, and monitoring budgets during a FY. The following terms are used in various aspects of financial management.

Cost center: Organizational unit, such as a department, for which costs can be calculated

Profit center: Organizational unit for which costs can be calculated and revenue produced

Fixed cost: Expense that is a function of time and not related to changes in volume (e.g., administrators' salaries)

Variable cost: Expenses that change in relation to volume changes (e.g., client supplies)

Direct cost: Expense that can be linked directly to a cost objective (e.g., salaries)

Indirect cost: Expense that cannot be linked to a cost objective (e.g., equipment depreciation)

Full-time equivalent (FTE): A unit of staffing measurement related to the time worked by a full-time employee in 1 year. This is usually 2,080 hours per year (40 hours per week) but may be any number of hours designated as *full time* by an agency

Fiscal year: The 12-month budget year designated by an agency; may be any consecutive 12 months

Variance: Difference in dollars or percentages between budgeted amounts and actual expenses

Accounts receivable: Funds owed to a provider

Accounts payable: Funds owed to other institutions for goods, services, or interest on loans

Balance sheet: A numerical statement of the status of a business on a particular date that includes assets (what is owned by the company), liabilities (what is owed by the company), and the difference between assets and liabilities (equity)

Income statement: A summary report of financial activity during an accounting period such as a month, quarter, or year; also referred to as the statement of revenue and expenses or the profit and loss (Finkler & McHugh, 2008; Murray, 2014)

The Budgeting Process

The budgeting process is a series of steps taken to develop a budget or budgets for a specific FY. Each organization has its own process that takes into consideration the unique characteristics of the organization. For example, the federal government has a very long budget process that culminates in a very large document for review and approval by Congress. For most healthcare organizations, the budget process is much less involved but may take several weeks to several months to complete (Finkler, Smith, Calabrese, & Purtell, 2017).

In established organizations, budget history is important in developing new budgets. Budget analysis of previous FYs, along with projected activities, revenue, and needs for the new FY, are compiled as one of the first steps in the budgeting process. If no historical material exists, as with developing budgets for a new program, it is best to start with a worksheet that can be displayed as a computer spreadsheet. Listing all the personnel needs in words will provide an initial working document needed for calculating numbers of employees and then amounts for salaries, benefits, and other personnel costs.

A worksheet should also be developed for nonpersonnel budget items. Reading through the program plan a couple times may be necessary to glean all the items needed in the non-personnel part of the budget. If money for capital projects is also part of the program plan, a capital budget must be developed. A capital budget is a plan for acquiring and replacing major pieces of equipment over a number of years (Finkler et al., 2013). Money is usually set aside for those purposes each FY.

■ TYPES OF BUDGETS

Program plans may call for more than one type of budget, depending on the program objectives, scope of the program, and resources required to carry out the program activities. In addition, budgets must be planned to fit within the format and specifications of a specific agency. Operating, cash, and capital expenditure budgets are discussed in this section.

Operating Budgets

The operating budget, the most common type, is a plan of expenditures and revenue for a specified period, usually 1 year (Finkler et al., 2013). For a program plan, the operating budget should be planned for the length of the projected program, for example, 1 to 3 years. If the first year is planned in detail, the other years can be developed in more detail after some experience with program performance. In many agencies, the operating budget is divided into expenses and revenue, often as two separate parts of the budget or separate budgets.

EXPENSE BUDGETS

The details for determining projected program expenses are derived from the program plan, specifically from the goals, objectives, and program activities. The major activities are examined to allocate dollar amounts. For example, if five home visits are to be made to each pregnant woman who smokes during pregnancy, the number of pregnant women who smoke needs to be determined. Then an average length of time for each home visit, including preparation, travel, documentation, and follow-up, needs to be calculated. A national average is 1.5 hours for a home visit (Michalopoulos et al., 2015). If five home visits per client are to be completed, then each client will require 1.5 times 5, totaling 7.5 hours per client. If 200 clients will be visited during the first year of the program, the total number of hours is 1,500. To translate that number into the number of public health nurses, or FTEs needed to complete the home visits, divide 1,500 by 2,080. This result is 0.72, meaning that 0.72 of a full-time nurse position, or 28.8 hours per week, is needed for this particular part of the program.

If the agency has standardized numbers for any of the preceding calculations, they should be used instead. For example, many agencies have a 37-hour workweek, with 3 weeks per year vacation. Other amounts of release time should be deducted from the FTE in order to have a realistic number of work hours per FTE when calculating employees needed for program implementation. (See Box 13.3 for an example of time to be deducted from working hours to determine time available for program activities.) You can readily see that if each position is calculated as having 2,080 hours available for work, the number of hours actually available will fall far short for program activities. The other difficulty encountered is that vacations occur often at the same time, so programs fail to achieve their objectives because of dramatic slowdowns in program activities at peak vacation and holiday times. These variations in program activities may be planned for in the budget using variable budgets discussed later.

REVENUE BUDGETS

Revenue budgets project program income from charges for expected levels of service. For example, if a program is planned to deliver five home visits per year to 200 pregnant women and 80% are projected to be reimbursed from the Medicaid program, the revenue may be projected to be $32,000 per year on the basis of 800 home visits at $40 per visit.

Often programs delivered by public/community health nurses are not reimbursed directly but are part of the package of services funded through an agency's budget. If specific charges to clients are built into the program, the anticipated revenue should be placed into the budget even if the collected funds are not returned directly to the program. Small charges cannot generate adequate funds to keep a program viable but may be used in

BOX 13.3 EXAMPLE OF CALCULATIONS FOR FTEs	
Total available hours per year	2,080
Vacation (3 weeks/year)	−120
Sick time (6 days/year)	−48
Continuing education (2 days/year)	−16
Rest breaks (½ hour/day)	−118.5
Staff meetings (1 hour/week)	−47
Hours available for program	1,730.5

FTEs, full-time equivalents.

grant applications to demonstrate client support and value for the program as well as the potential for future income to support the program. Advanced practice public/community health nurses are aware of the need to justify services while demonstrating the cost-effectiveness of prevention and health-promotion programs.

If a program's charges are on a sliding fee scale, the revenue is more difficult to forecast. On the basis of experience in the agency and/or data about the income levels of the program target population, the number of services provided at various fees should be projected for the FY. For example, if 20% of the clients are anticipated to be able to pay full fees, 20% of the revenue is calculated for full fees for each service. Projections for the volume of services at each level of the fee scale need to be determined with the appropriate amount of revenue calculated for the budget.

Setting fees is another area of learning for most advanced public/community health nurses. Various techniques are used to determine what will be charged. In nonprofit organizations, fees may be set below a break-even level and additional income obtained to supplement client fees. To determine a simple fee structure, you would divide the total budget by the number of services. For example, a budget of $100,000 divided by 10,000 units of service results in a fee of $10 per unit of service. Then the number of units for each type of service is determined. As an example, a physical examination is four units of service and is priced at $40. An immunization is one unit of service, or $10. Although this method may be somewhat arbitrary, a stronger basis would be to link charges more closely with time required for each unit of service, the qualifications of personnel involved, supplies consumed, and equipment used. There are more elaborate techniques for setting charges that could be used in complex programs, such as cost-based pricing and competition-based pricing (Zelman, McCue, Glick, & Thomas, 2014).

Reimbursement for many health services is done primarily under physicians' names, so nursing programs must be creative to maintain fiscal viability. A revenue budget that reflects this creativity will contain various sources of revenue for many programs. For example, foundation funding may account for 40% of the revenue budget, but client fees may be only 10%, depending on the income levels of the target population. Donations to the program should be included in the budget as revenue. For example, if the program is operated in donated space, the amount of rent that would have had to be paid should be included as an item in the revenue budget, as well as an item in the expense budget. Other donations, such as volunteer time, advertising, and supplies for special events, should be included so that a complete picture is available about how much it costs to operate the program (Ervin, Chang, & White, 1998).

Cash Budgets

Cash budgets are forecasts of how much cash the program or organization will have on hand and how much it will need to meet expenses. This type of budget is very valuable for a small program because of the great variability that is likely to occur in client volume and program activities from day to day and month to month. Without a money surplus or a line of credit, small programs may experience difficulty meeting payrolls and paying suppliers. Even large organizations, such as city and state governments, have failed to pay their bills on time or at all. The cash budget can also provide the information needed to make decisions about short-term investments with cash surpluses.

Cash budgets are usually prepared for monthly intake and disbursement of cash for a total FY. The starting cash balance is the starting point for each monthly cash budget. The expected revenues for the month are added to the starting cash balance to arrive at the total cash balance. Expected expenses for the month are subtracted from the cash balance

TABLE 13.1 Capital Budget for a Program Plan: A Community Nursing Center

Description	FY 1	FY 2
Building renovation	$10,000	
Exam table		$2,000
Centrifuge	$800	
Microscope		$2,300
Refrigerator	$700	
Total	$11,500	$4,300

FY, fiscal year.

to obtain a tentative cash balance. If expected expenses exceed cash, funds may need to be borrowed if a reserve fund is not available. With new programs, cash reserves are rarely available. If expected revenues exceed expenses, the excess cash can be invested or left to begin the next month's cash budget (Finkler et al., 2013).

Capital Expenditure Budgets

A capital budget is a long-range financial plan for the acquisition of fixed assets. Budgets for capital expenditures contain items, such as buildings, property, and major equipment, that are both costly and last for a number of years. Commonly any item or acquisition that costs more than, for example, $500 and will be in use 5 years is part of a capital budget. To plan for such expensive acquisitions, an organization needs to develop budgets for several years to show how the items will be financed or acquired out of operating funds or by repaying long-term loans. For community health programs, the advanced practice public/community health nurse may be involved in acquiring buildings for programs, equipment for patient teaching purposes (e.g., large-screen television, video camera), office equipment (e.g., copy machine, facsimile machine, computers), or patient examination equipment (e.g., examination table, centrifuge). (See Table 13.1 for an example of a simple capital budget developed for a program plan for 2 FYs.) Some equipment does not qualify as capital expenditure but may need to be planned for in the operating budget, for example, scales, stethoscopes, and sphygmomanometers.

■ BUDGETING APPROACHES

Although each organization has its own approach to budgeting, budgets fall into a few major types. This section deals with five types of budgeting approaches, including traditional, variable, program, planning-programming-budgeting system (PPBS), and zero based. Some organizations may use variations of these types or a combination of them for specific purposes or for some areas of budgeting; for example, a new program or activities added during an FY may use a combination of traditional budgeting and program budgeting.

Traditional Budgeting Approach

The traditional budgeting approach is also referred to as *fixed* or *incremental budgeting*. In this approach, funds are allocated to organizational units for specific amounts and are maintained at those levels throughout the FY or other budget period. The units decide how much funding to allocate to specific activities. A traditional budgeting approach is to develop a new budget from the previous one. This could be used if a program was already in place and a second-year budget was needed. However, a program budget usually has amounts of funds allocated by activities and thus does not fit well within a true traditional budgeting approach.

Variable Budgeting

The budgets in the previous section are classified as fixed budgets based on a single specified volume. Variable or flexible budgets are based on the assumption that costs, such as labor, supplies, and some overhead expenses, vary with volume. Variable budgeting has been described as a series of fixed budgets based on forecasts of varying client activity levels (Finkler et al., 2017).

In client-care operations, variable budgeting may be very helpful because it is based on known variations in client volume. For example, ambulatory client visits and home visits typically decrease at major holiday and vacation times. Peak times are usually right before and after school begins in the fall. Other peak times may be at the beginning of a new year and during flu and cold seasons. If a variable budget is developed for a new program, projections for decreases and increases in client volume may not be known, but following general guidelines for the target program population will allow for general forecasting. In the second year of the program, budget adjustments can be made on the basis of program experience.

Variable budgets may be more difficult to develop, but give a program manager better information for monitoring a budget. For example, if expenditures are greater in the first 3 months of the budget, a variable budget will put more funds into the first quarter, where the money will be spent. The manager then has a better idea whether expenditures are on target or vary from the projections. If the same amount is budgeted each month, as in a fixed budget, the manager must make adjustments for the remainder of the FY so that one twelfth of the budgeted amount is not spent each month.

Program Budgeting

This type of budgeting is more likely the type you will use for a new program. Program budgeting allocates funds to groups of activities that are needed to achieve specific objectives. This type of budgeting addresses the disadvantage of traditional budgeting, which does not specify how funds will be spent within an organizational unit. Elaboration about how to develop program budgets is presented in the following sections.

Planning-Programming-Budgeting System

This approach to budgeting is an elaboration of the program budgeting approach. The PPBS was originally developed for the Air Force by the RAND Corporation and has been used extensively by departments and agencies of the federal government. The PPBS combines budgeting with management by objectives. Management by objectives is a variation on the traditional approach to the development of objectives and requires that employees set specific performance objectives with their supervisors. Progress toward the objectives is monitored, and rewards are disbursed according to progress made (Robbins & Coulter, 1999).

When using the PPBS approach to budgeting, programs are planned with multiyear objectives and alternative methods of achieving the objectives. Budgets are then built for the programs rather than departments or other organizational units. If a program cuts across departments, one person is put in charge to facilitate program operations. The PPBS is a complex approach to budgeting and may be difficult to use because of the multiyear projections.

Zero-Based Budgeting

Zero-based budgeting is a technique that requires managers to justify their budget requests as if the unit were newly established. Amounts of services are identified with incremental amounts of money, in increments above zero. A process of three steps is followed to determine the amount of funding for each organizational unit:

1. Each activity is broken down into a decision package.
2. The individual decision packages are ranked by benefit to the organization.
3. Resources are allocated to the individual packages according to preferential rank in the organization (Pyhrr, 1970).

A decision package describes a specific activity, including a statement of the expected result of the activity, its costs, personnel requirements, measures of performance, alternative courses of action, and an evaluation of the benefits from performance and consequences of nonperformance. Each package lists alternative methods of performing the activity, recommends one of the alternatives, and defines effort levels that are tied to spending targets. A large organization that uses zero-based budgeting will have thousands of decision packages (Zelman et al., 2014).

For a new program plan, zero-based budgeting may be a useful approach coupled with the program-planning process itself, because alternative approaches to reaching objectives need to be identified. Disadvantages to this technique are that it is time-consuming and requires a level of knowledge about program alternatives not always possessed by advanced practice public/community health nurses.

■ FACTORS TO CONSIDER IN PLANNING A BUDGET

The budget for a new program is an estimate of what the costs will be for the projected activities. The activities have not always been tested, so some will need to be modified during the program implementation. In addition, Murphy's laws may come into play: "If anything just cannot go wrong, it will anyway," and "everything takes longer than you think" (Peers, 1979, p. 36). Almost everyone has tales to tell about the foibles of starting a new program. Although all potential pitfalls cannot be predicted, you will want to include in the budgets all exigencies with high probability of occurring. For example, if the costs of any equipment, supplies, or services have a chance of increasing from the time the budget is planned until the program is implemented, the higher cost estimate should be placed in the budget rather than the current cost.

Rising Costs or the Inflation Factor

Increases in the prices of goods and services are not always predictable in the long run but may be planned for in the short run. Information from vendors and suppliers should be obtained during the budget preparation period. Any near future increases should be put into the budget. A contract should be signed to obtain goods and services at current charges for at least a year, if possible. The budget is then protected by unanticipated increases in those areas. If the suppliers are not willing to sign a contract for 1 year, you should attempt to extend the agreement for as many months as possible.

The same logic applies to capital projects. Often, the lead time for capital expenditures is very long, for example, 5 or 10 years. With such projects and even shorter time frames, the advanced practice nurse needs assurance that the cost of a capital project will not exceed the budget. A written and signed contract provides the legal documentation to keep the cost within the budgeted amount.

The most common mistake in budget planning is probably the failure to build in basic, planned increases in salaries, wages, and benefits. If a budget is being planned for implementation in the following FY, personnel costs for the next FY, not the current year, should be put into the budget. Although a 2% or 3% increase in salaries may not seem like very much, consider the impact on a budget if 3% of $300,000, or $9,000, had to be found to cover payroll. In a small program with limited sources for additional funds, that amount of money could mean eliminating a position to make up the shortfall. Losing a position is often the downfall of a program with specific time-limited objectives to achieve.

Another area for careful planning is travel costs. Reimbursement for automobile travel can be very difficult to determine because of the unknowns about the location of program clients. Also, reimbursement per mile often changes as the price of gasoline fluctuates. One approach is to determine the longest and the shortest distances for travel within the service area. An average number of miles per trip can then be determined. For example, if the longest round trip is 50 miles and the shortest round trip is 5 miles, the average trip is 27.5 miles. If the reimbursement rate is $0.52 per mile, each trip costs $14.30. With this rate, any number of trips can be calculated for the annual budget.

Specifying Activities

Specifying exactly what activities will be conducted for a new program should be completed before the budget is planned, but in the real world, the work may not be done in that order. Chapter 14 provides you the information to develop an implementation plan and the detail needed for a sound program budget. The problem with planning activities after the budget is planned is that the funds to implement all the activities are rarely adequate. A program planner may omit large segments of activities. For example, a new program often needs advertising to get out the word, but no one's time is allocated for this, as well as no money allocated for printing, distribution of material, or placing advertisements.

Another area often neglected is recruitment of staff. If the program requires additional staff, rather than reassignment of current staff, money will be needed for advertisements, time to screen and interview applicants, and time for orientation and training about the new program. In addition, funds may be needed to reimburse applicants for interview expenses (e.g., travel to the agency).

A well-thought-out implementation plan is invaluable in providing the detail needed to develop a realistic program budget. The number of interventions to be delivered, the amount of time for each, the supplies needed for each intervention, documentation of each intervention, and the time needed for preparation and postintervention activities must be specified to calculate personnel needs. Some national standards may be found to provide guidance, but, in general, the program planner must rely on the input of staff and those who have had experience with the intervention. For example, a commonly used time for home visits is 1.5 hours for all activities, that is, preparation, travel, visit, documentation, and follow-up. If a program of home visiting to 50 pregnant women over a year must have adequate public health nursing time for five home visits to each woman, the number of FTEs is calculated using 1.5 hours per visit. A total of 375 hours, or 0.22 FTEs using the formula presented earlier, would be needed for home visits.

A well-thought-out budget also contributes to a more accurate evaluation. Discussion about cost and program evaluation is covered in Section V.

Including All Budget Items

A complete program budget will contain all items needed for the program, including personnel, nonpersonnel, and donated goods and services. The detail for a budget or budgets must meet the requirements of the funding source, but must also provide the detail needed by the program manager to administer the funds according to the intentions of the program planner; these may or may not be different people.

As pointed out earlier, the program objectives and activities provide the details needed to determine the program budgets. Often only an operating budget is needed, but a capital budget is needed if expensive equipment and/or buildings are part of the program implementation.

Constructing the budgets should begin as soon as ideas are generated about what kinds of personnel, supplies, and equipment are needed. During the program-planning phase, the advanced practice public/community health nurse may need to develop a file of material needed for the budget, for example, supply catalogs, price quotations from suppliers or vendors, and estimates for capital projects. When the budgets are being put on paper or computer spreadsheet, you will need more information about prices and costs for personnel. This is the time to get as much documentation in writing as possible for the budget file. Request salary scales for the staff positions indicated in the plan, obtain policies about benefits, and gather the latest information about the budget process for the agency in which the program will be located.

With the latest information about costs, you will be ready to make specific calculations for the program. Using the two broad categories of personnel and nonpersonnel, list all the items for each category from the program objectives and activities.

PERSONNEL COSTS

Box 13.4 contains the usual categories of personnel items for a personnel budget. Some organizations also have tuition reimbursement and time away for personal business. If groups of employees are members of a bargaining unit or union, wage increases

---

BOX 13.4   PERSONNEL ITEMS FOR A PROGRAM BUDGET

Salaries and wages
    Basic salary and wages
    Overtime wages
    Merit or longevity pay
    Bonuses
    On-call pay
	Workers' compensation insurance
	
	State unemployment insurance
	
	Social Security (FICA)
	
	Medicare

Fringe benefits
    Health insurance, dental insurance
    Life insurance
    Uniform allowance
    Tuition reimbursement
    Vacation and sick leave
    Retirement
	Travel reimbursement
	
	Reimbursement for work-related education
	
	Consultants and contract services

FICA, Federal Insurance Contributions Act.

negotiated in contracts need to be included in the personnel budget. The total amount of time allowed away from work should be included in the budget because it adds time from other positions to complete program activities. If the actual time available for work is not calculated, as shown in Box 13.3, the program will have inadequate staff for full functioning (Murray, 2014).

Another reason for having complete personnel expenses accounted for is that a budget must cover all expenses because there is usually no backup source of money in cases of being over budget or if unexpected expenditures occur. For example, if a staff member becomes ill and is off work for an extended period on paid sick leave, money is usually not available in a program budget to hire a replacement for the extended time of the regular employee's absence. Another example is covering expenses of employees hired with grant money. If the employees are to be terminated at the end of the grant period, for example, in 3 years, all fringe benefits must be paid by the grant budget. This includes unused vacation and sick time at the end of the grant period.

The personnel portion of a budget may contain salary and wages for parts of full-time positions, for example, 10% of the manager's time rather than 100%. Many nonprofit organizations operate with this arrangement of allocating salaries to several sources of funding. For example, the local health department may have five grants from the state health department, a grant from the Centers for Disease Control and Prevention, a grant from the governor's office, and a grant from the Department of Agriculture. The advanced practice public/community health nurse may have a role in six of the funded programs, thus having her salary divided up among the budgets according to the amount of time allocated for each program.

The determination of the amount of time needed for each program should be carefully considered in planning the program and reconsidered when the budget is actually set down on paper. Perhaps the most realistic way to determine the amount of time needed for a specific program is to attach the activities to the specific positions. For example, if the advanced practice public/community health nurse is to supervise the staff, but not have overall management responsibilities, the allocation of time may be similar to the example given in Box 13.5. The 17.5 hours per week translates into over 0.4 FTE. For the other

---

BOX 13.5 EXAMPLE OF TIME ALLOCATION FOR ADVANCED PRACTICE PUBLIC/COMMUNITY HEALTH NURSE FOR PROGRAM STAFF SUPERVISION

Individual staff conferences for clinical supervision	1 hour per day
Staff meetings	2 hours per week
In-service education programs	2 hours per week
Administrative meetings	2 hours per week
On-site demonstration and staff supervision	2 hours per month
Continuing education for self	4 hours per month
Community meetings communications	1 hour per day
Total	17.5 hours per week

almost 0.6 FTE, the advanced practice public/community health nurse may be assigned to administer another program or implement a community program.

When determining the exact activities needed for each position, you need to guard against the tendency to allocate unassigned activities to positions already determined to be full-time work. If a large activity, like program evaluation, is not assigned specifically to someone, it will usually not get done, at least not on a timely basis. In addition, activities should be assigned to positions that will be qualified to complete the activities. If calculations show that more than one position is needed for a group of related activities (e.g., home visiting), the total number of positions needs to be indicated in the personnel portion of the budget. As indicated earlier in the chapter, calculations to determine the exact number of positions should be based on known amounts of time needed for activities, time studies in the agency, or reported activities in the literature. There are many factors that go into determining how much time is needed for a group of activities, so a time study within the specific agency is most helpful, but often costly to conduct. Consultation with similar agencies may be helpful to gain useful information for this part of budget planning.

In implementing a new program, you should always include time for staff orientation, training about the program and interventions, as well as on-the-job coaching, correction of errors in program delivery, and retraining. The personnel costs associated with implementing a new program also have implications for the nonpersonnel part of the budget, for example, copy costs for training materials or travel expenses for outside experts to conduct training.

Fringe Benefits. Although not all organizations have the same package of fringe benefits, you need to consider all possible fringe benefits so as to have a complete budget. Some organizations have a formula for determining fringe benefits as a percentage of salary or wages. Different categories of employees often have different benefit packages depending on bargaining for union contracts, date of hire, and other factors. It may be necessary to use different formulas for calculating fringe benefits for different employee groups. If the calculations need not be included in the budget itself, they need to be retained for monitoring budget expenditures to be certain that money is being spent the way it was planned.

Consultant Services. Another personnel cost for budget inclusion is consultant services. For example, a small program may employ a bookkeeping service on a monthly basis rather than hire a bookkeeper. Other consultant services may be audit services, evaluation services, and clinical expert services. If consultants donate their services, a statement from them indicating the usual salary or fees they would have charged should be used to include the amount as part of the donated or in-kind contributions often required in budget requests to funding sources.

Contract Services. Contract services are other personnel costs to be detailed in a program budget. These services include cleaning services, laundry services, and laboratory or radiology services. Depending on the budget guidelines of the agency, service contracts for equipment, for example, copy and facsimile machines, may be included in personnel or nonpersonnel costs.

NONPERSONNEL COSTS

The major categories of nonpersonnel costs are space, equipment, supplies, travel, telephone, computer services, insurance, and postage. If a program has nonpersonnel costs that do not seem to fall within these categories, it is better to name a new category rather than use a miscellaneous category, which is usually unacceptable to funding sources.

Space Costs. Included in the space category are rent or mortgage payments, utilities (electricity, Internet service, telephone, heat, water, and sewer), building repairs and upkeep (if the building is owned or repairs are not covered by rental lease), and property taxes (if the building is owned and these are not included in the mortgage payment). Cleaning or janitorial services may be included in space costs if not placed under the heading of contract services.

Space needs may also be met by using donated space that is available during specific hours of program operations. Insurance may still be needed. Consultation should be sought about insurance protection needed as well as a written agreement that the organization donating the space agrees to keep current insurance premiums for fire and liability, if it agrees to continue the coverage. The program manager also needs assurance that the donating organization will pay taxes on the property and complete repairs on a timely basis, unless the agreement is otherwise.

Equipment and Furniture. Options for acquiring equipment and furniture are to purchase, lease, or rent the items needed. Borrowing equipment is not often used but may be possible for short-term needs. For example, when a community nursing center was opened in an inner city by a nursing school and a community organization, both organizations loaned furniture and equipment to the center. Donations of computers, children's toys, and furniture were also obtained. The center had to include in the budget the service contracts on the printers and copy and facsimile machines. Any special equipment should be enumerated in budgets, such as computer tablets for use by nurses in the field.

Supplies. Several types of supplies may be needed for a program, depending on the activities and focus. All consumable supplies should be placed in this category, for example, office, copy machine and printer ink cartridges and toner, client records, teaching materials, and small office equipment such as staplers, paper cutters, and hole-punches. If the agency does not have a formula to use for calculating the amount of office supplies for each position, you should get estimates from similar programs to determine a realistic figure for the budget.

Travel. Travel expenses include local travel for staff to deliver the program interventions and off-site travel to attend national conferences and training programs. Local travel needs to be based as much as possible on actual distances. Also, if home visits are part of the program, allowance needs to be made for making several trips without finding some clients at home. Even with appointments, it is common for the nurse to find that clients are not home when the nurse arrives for a scheduled home visit. Methods for calculating mileage were discussed earlier.

A funding source may allow funds for one national meeting per year. By conducting online searches or by calling airlines, hotels, and organizations to get current and projected costs for future meetings, the public/community health nurse can obtain actual costs. If projected costs are not available, at least 5% should be added to current costs for a budget to be implemented within a year.

Telephone. Funds for telephone services add a major item to any nonpersonnel budget. Installation and rental of telephones should be included unless the program purchases the phones. Monthly telephone charges need to be projected on the basis of the use of telephone calls identified in the programs. Long-distance charges are often negligible in local programs. Use of cellular phones is important for some programs, so both cost of the phones and monthly changes should be included in the budget. The use of computers may be part of telephone charges, so it needs to be considered in monthly charges. Restricting phone usage to local calls or restricting most telephones for internal use only saves money from unauthorized use of telephones both during and after business hours.

Computer Services. Funds needed for computer services encompass a variety of areas. Monthly fees for connection to the Internet may be needed to conduct email communication and search for information. Assistance with software programs and other forms of technical support may be needed on an "as needed" basis. Training staff to use program-specific software may be needed and could be included here or under the category of consultants. If the computer equipment is new, a service contract for the hardware may be a good investment.

Insurance. The specific types of insurance needs will depend on the setting of the program to a great extent. For example, if the program is located within an organization, liability, malpractice, fire and hazard, and bonding insurance will already be in place for all programs. If the program is free-standing without a parent organization sponsor or a landlord, the budget will need to contain insurance for all the areas plus more. Members of a governing board are not employees, so a policy to protect the board members against legal actions for errors and omissions should be provided by the organization or program. Many insurance policies have deductibles, so current or reserve funds will need to be set aside to meet the deductible amounts (Rakich, Longest, & Darr, 1992).

If staff use automobiles for conducting program components (e.g., home visits), automobile insurance should be adequate to cover both personal and business-related incidences. Staff may also be encouraged or required to carry personal or professional liability insurance in addition to the organization's liability policies. An expert in insurance coverage should be consulted before the budget figures for insurance are finalized.

Postage. The budget figure for postage may or may not be a large amount of money depending on the framework of the program. However, the needs for postage should be thought through carefully because this is an area often neglected. If next-day delivery of grant proposals will be needed during the budget year, adequate funds should be allocated for this activity. If program evaluation calls for a mailed survey, adequate funds need to be set aside for not just one mailing but probably two follow-up mailings to get adequate return of surveys.

Other needs for postage include mailed reminders of client appointments, announcements of program activities, newsletters, educational material to clients, regular correspondence to other agencies, committee activities (minutes and meeting reminders), governing board activities, fund-raising events, mailings to employees, and results of client diagnostic tests. Even though the volume for any of these may not be great, the omission of several hundred dollars from a budget will present problems in implementation before the budget year is finished.

Other Categories. As mentioned earlier, the category of "miscellaneous" should not be used. If items or services are needed, place them within the categories described or develop new categories. For example, often food or other incentives are used in programs to encourage and reward participants. Most of these items should be placed under "supplies" in the budget. If this is not acceptable to the funding source, some of which prohibit the use of funds for food, another source of funding will need to be located.

The category of participant incentives, payments, or rewards could be used if the funding sponsor allows these budget items. Money for gift certificates, cash payments, tokens for public transportation, payment for child care, and other direct benefits to program participants could be placed in this category. Other types of rewards often used include clothing for infants, children's books, cosmetics for adults, and certificates for use of a fitness club. A careful match of the program goals with participant incentives may result in better program outcomes and satisfied participants. Some people, however, view incentives as bribes that do not encourage behavior change beyond the incentive phase of the program.

A separate budget category may be created for governing board activities. Board members may be paid a fee for attending each meeting. Reimbursement for travel to and from meetings is a usual practice. Often, refreshments or meals are provided or reimbursed, if meetings last all day or members travel long distances to attend. Some programs provide space, telephone, and/or secretarial support for board activities, especially meetings. The provision of childcare during board meetings will encourage more community participation. These items may be included in a separate budget category to allow for an actual accounting for board expenses.

■ FUNDING FOR COMMUNITY HEALTH PROGRAMS

A great deal of funding for community health programs comes from federal, state, and local government taxes. Foundations, private businesses, and health-related organizations fund most of the remainder of community health programs. If the funding for community health programs is short term, communities are deprived of stability for programs that contribute in improving both quality and quantity of life. Of course, short-term funding also results in the demise of programs that are not effective and should not be continued. Often, program evaluations are not adequate for funding sources to be able to distinguish between effective and noneffective programs.

Community health programs are often embedded within organizations that are both health and business oriented. For example, many hospitals and healthcare corporations have begun community health programs as part of their continuum-of-care structures. Thus, prevention and health-promotion programs both bring in new patients and retain patients who are receiving secondary and tertiary interventions. For example, healthcare corporations have developed fitness centers that also serve as cardiac rehabilitation centers for patients discharged from the hospitals that are part of the corporation.

Sources of Funding for Community Health Nursing Programs

If community health nursing services are part of an organization, funding for programs may not be problematic. However, nursing is obligated to carry out the services that are part of many funded programs. Finding sources of funding for innovative or newly identified programs is more difficult. More problematic than finding sources often is the problem of finding time to write the grant applications to obtain the funds. University faculty and students, especially master's and doctoral students, may be very helpful. Students can do the literature searches, compile statistics, contact other agencies for information, and assist with putting the grant application together. Faculty should be asked to help write parts or most of the application. Rewards for faculty include being a coinvestigator or coproject coordinator, writing manuscripts about the program, and presenting the program results at conferences. Sources of funding for joint university–community projects should be explored when looking for funding.

FOUNDATIONS AND FEDERAL SOURCES

Sources of funding for innovative projects are foundations and federal government units, for example, the Centers for Disease Control and Prevention and the Agency for Healthcare Research and Quality. Obtaining funding from foundations and federal agencies is very competitive but can be very generous when implementing a large program. Achieving long-term fiscal viability for such programs is another problem and is discussed in terms of a nursing center in Chapter 20. The solution for many public/community health nursing programs is to use a combination of funding sources (Ervin et al., 1998).

Other sources of funding for programs are nursing organizations and specialty nursing foundations. Several offer small amounts of funding for projects, often research projects; for some organizations, only members may apply, for example, the Association of Community Health Nursing Educators. For example, Sigma Theta Tau International offers several competitive grants once a year to members, usually in the spring. Many local Sigma Theta Tau International chapters have very small grant programs also. The American Nurses Foundation has a grant program that is open to members of state nurses' associations. Several regional nursing organizations promote innovative projects and research through funding small pilot projects. The Internet is a good source of current information about funding opportunities from a variety of sources.

PROGRAM ENHANCEMENT

Enhancing an ongoing program is another approach to obtaining funding for a new program. For example, a small amount of funding can provide the resources needed to augment teaching pregnant women in a prenatal clinic. Additional funding for a smoking-cessation intervention within a prenatal clinic may be obtained from the March of Dimes, American Cancer Society, or American Lung Association. These voluntary agencies have small grant programs at the local or regional and the national levels. Often, short-term funding is all that is needed to provide data to create a permanent program within agency funding.

CORPORATE FUNDING SOURCES

Funds from pharmaceutical companies, medical equipment suppliers, publishing companies, and other health-related businesses are not often used by nursing, but are available to professionals. Advanced practice public/community health nurses should explore these and other businesses for sources of funding. One such source is foundations created by hospitals that received Hill Burton funds and have subsequently closed. These foundations are obligated to use the money left from the sale of the building and other assets for health programs but are forbidden from making a profit from investments. In some instances, local foundations are developed when other nonprofit agencies are sold or stop providing direct services, for example, the Visiting Nurse Association of Chicago. Tax laws dictate how endowments and assets of nonprofit organizations may be dispersed.

■ SUMMARY

Developing budgets is one of the final parts of the program plan. A budget is the numerical expression of the program objectives and activities. Sound budget planning that results in adequate funding is essential for a successful program. You will need to become acquainted with fiscal and accounting terms in order to communicate effectively with fiscal managers and other administrative staff. Several types of budgets are used in healthcare agencies and institutions. Approaches to budgeting included in this chapter are traditional, variable, program, PPBS, and zero based. In-depth knowledge is needed of the specific approach used by the funding agency or employing agency. Program budgeting is the approach used for illustration purposes throughout the chapter, but most agencies use traditional budgeting for FY planning. You will want to become comfortable with understanding the basics of the major approaches to budgeting.

In planning a budget, several factors need to be considered. Rising costs or inflation may result in inadequate funds if an inflation factor is not built into budgets. If a period of time will lapse before the budget is implemented, it should contain figures that reflect the current rate of increase in goods and services. Specific activities to be conducted in the program need to be stated in detail so that accurate costing can be done. All items needed in both personnel and nonpersonnel components of the budget should be placed in a spreadsheet format for complete calculations.

The advanced practice public/community health nurse requires creativity to fund innovative programs to promote community health. The major funding sources are federal, state, and local governmental entities. Foundations, voluntary agencies, and professional organizations are good sources for funding but often provide only small grants for limited time periods. A combination of funding sources is often the long-term solution for fiscal viability of valuable programs to keep communities healthy.

■ SUGGESTED CLINICAL OR PRACTICUM ACTIVITIES

1. In some health agencies, individuals are hired expressly to write grant proposals for funding programs. In other agencies, a committee may be formed to develop a grant proposal. Meet with a public/community health nursing administrator at a local health department to discuss the process used for grant proposal development at the local level. Focus on the role of nursing in assisting with the grant proposal development.
2. In a meeting with a nurse administrator at a local or state health department, explore what she or he thinks the role of nursing was and should be in developing budgets for programs.
3. Review budgets for health department programs. What assumptions and/or factors were considered in the budget development?

REFERENCES

Ervin, N. E., Chang, W. Y., & White, J. (1998). A cost analysis of a nursing center's services. *Nursing Economics, 16*(6), 307–312.

Finkler, S. A., Jones, C. B., & Kovner, C. T. (2013). *Financial management for nurse managers and executives* (4th ed.). St. Louis, MO: Elsevier Saunders.

Finkler, S. A., & McHugh, M. L. (2008). *Budgeting concepts for nurse managers* (4th ed.). St. Louis, MO: Saunders Elsevier.

Finkler, S. A., Smith, D. L., Calabrese, T. D., & Purtell, R. M. (2017). *Financial management for public, health, and not-for-profit organizations* (5th ed.). Thousand Oaks, CA: Sage.

Michalopoulos, C., Lee, H., Duggan, A., Lundquist, E., Tso, A., Crowne, S., … Knox, V. (2015). *The mother and infant home visiting program evaluation: Early findings on the Maternal, Infant, and Early Childhood Home Visiting Program. OPRE Report 2015-11.* Washington, DC: Office of Planning, Research and

Evaluation, Administration for Children and Families, U.S. Department of Health and Human Services.

Murray, M. E. (2014). Budgeting, productivity, and costing out nursing. In D. L. Huber (Ed.), *Leadership & nursing care management* (5th ed., pp. 387–398). St. Louis, MO: Elsevier Saunders.

Office of Disease Prevention and Health Promotion. (2016). *Healthy people 2020*. Washington, DC: U.S. Department of Health and Human Services. Retrieved from https://www.healthypeople.gov

Peers, J. (1979). *1001 logical laws, accurate axioms, profound principles, trusty truisms, homey homilies, colorful corollaries, quotable quotes and rambunctious ruminations for all walks of life*. New York, NY: Fawcett Columbine.

Pyhrr, P. A. (1970). Zero-base budgeting. *Harvard Business Review, 48*(6), 111–118.

Rakich, J. S., Longest, B. B., Jr., & Darr, K. (1992). *Managing health services organizations* (3rd ed.). Baltimore, MD: Health Professions Press.

Robbins, S. P., & Coulter, M. (1999). *Management* (3rd ed.). Upper Saddle River, NJ: Prentice Hall.

Zelman, W. N., McCue, M. J., Glick, N. D., & Thomas, M. S. (2014). *Financial management of health care organizations* (4th ed.). San Francisco, CA: Jossey-Bass.

SECTION IV

Program Implementation

CHAPTER 14

Overview of Program Implementation

■ STUDY EXERCISES

1. Why is it important to have a plan for program implementation?
2. How are the phases of program implementation related to change?
3. Compare and contrast two change models.
4. Describe how the advanced practice public/community health nurse might use the role of change agent in program implementation.
5. What effects may the political environment have on implementation of a program?
6. Discuss the use of a strategy for addressing a specific implementation problem resulting from an adverse political environment.

Learning how to conduct a community assessment, how to develop a program plan, and how to describe needed program resources in a budget have been your goals thus far in mastering skills for advanced public/community health nursing practice. The next challenge is to learn how to implement a program. Program implementation involves the activities of putting the program into place, from gaining acceptance for the program to making revisions when the program is not working as planned.

The purpose of this chapter is to provide you with information and examples of how a program may be successfully implemented. Often thorough community assessments and program planning are followed by inadequate time to plan the program implementation. As pointed out in Chapter 12, program implementation may be part of the program plan, but often more detail is needed than can be or should be provided in a program plan.

During implementation planning, many questions will need to be answered about details, for example, who is responsible for each task. Also, planning for implementation provides an opportunity to update plans for the program. This is especially helpful if any major changes have occurred since the program was planned. It is not unusual for program implementation to be carried out 6 months to a year after program planning is completed. During that time interval, significant changes in the target population, community, economic picture, and numerous other factors may have occurred.

■ MODELS OF CHANGE

The need for using the change process is always present in advanced practice, but the implementation of a new program calls for special attention to change. The ultimate goal of any program is to bring about change. Although all members of the target population are not interested in changing before a program is introduced, one purpose of the program is to help create the desire for change in those community members who would benefit from the change.

Of course, all change must come about because of volitional acts on the part of the program participant. No one can make someone change, often even with force or laws. To be better at facilitating change, advanced practice public/community health nurses require a working knowledge of change models and the process of change.

Examples of the use of change models are noted throughout this book, but often the models are not explicit. Often, too, the advanced practice public/community health nurse does not apply a change model but is knowledgeable about the models and is able to call on that knowledge when needed for specific activities. For example, in analyzing a policy change in the community, the nurse can determine what steps were taken, in terms of a change model, to get the policy adopted.

Change occurs at various levels in a community. Individuals change, but systems also change. Four models for viewing change at different levels, that is, individual, group, and community, are Lewin's (1958) three-phase change model, Chin and Benne's (1976) three strategies of planned change, first- and second-order change (Watzlawick, Weakland, & Fisch, 1974), and Minkler's (1980–1981) change approaches. These models offer the nurse a variety of approaches for conceptualizing how to facilitate change.

Lewin's Three-Phase Change Model

One of the most well-known models of change is Kurt Lewin's three-phase model of change: unfreezing, change, and refreezing (Lewin, 1958). The process of change starts when individuals or groups are dissatisfied with the status quo. In unfreezing, the goal is to assist the target group to become ready to seek change. This may be accomplished in one of the three ways: (a) increasing the driving forces that direct behaviors away from the status quo, (b) decreasing the restraining forces that hinder movement from the status quo, or (c) combining the two approaches (Robbins & Coulter, 1999).

During community assessment and program planning, the advanced practice public/community health nurse gathers information about the target group's readiness to accept change and determines what factors may be effective in bringing about the change.

After unfreezing, the change or intervention is introduced. Any change, such as a new program, requires time to be put into place, so programs must allow time for the intervention to become well established before the program is withdrawn or ended. Refreezing involves establishing a new stability or status quo. The advanced practice public/community health nurse may assist with refreezing by securing long-term funding for a program to permit stabilization of the changes. Monitoring the intervention to maintain quality also assists with refreezing.

This change model is used in combination with other strategies as a template for guiding the total process (Archer, Kelly, & Bisch, 1984). It is also a useful approach for change at various levels, including individual, group, and community.

Chin and Benne's Strategies

Chin and Benne (1976) proposed three strategies for change: rational–empirical, normative–reeducative, and power–coercive. All three are relevant for use with individuals, groups, and communities.

Rational–empirical change strategies are based on the assumption that people are willing and able to make decisions on the basis of empirical information presented to them. If this evidence indicates that they will gain some benefit from the change, people will be especially interested in making the change.

In strategies for normative–reeducative change, the belief is that people have values, norms, and attitudes that influence their behavior. Willingness to change is thus contingent upon people's openness to examine and possibly alter their values, norms, and attitudes. Efforts are needed to assist people to examine these bases of their behavior with the view that they will see situations differently.

The power–coercive approach to change usually involves political or economic sanctions or applications of power. Many examples of these strategies exist in current laws for prevention of adverse outcomes, such as mandatory immunization for children entering school, use of seat belts, and wearing helmets on motorcycles. Although laws may mandate behavior, not everyone follows those laws nor agrees with the right for government to mandate such behavior.

Chin and Benne's (1976) strategies for change are especially useful to the advanced practice public/community health nurse in assessing the status of an individual, group, or community regarding change. For example, if a community has already examined its values, norms, and attitudes about a topic, a rational–empirical change strategy will be more appropriate than a normative–reeducative strategy.

First- and Second-Order Change

These ways to approach change deal with the extent to which a system is changed. First-order change is a change that is accomplished in a system without changing the system itself (Archer et al., 1984; Garon, 2014; Watzlawick et al., 1974). Case management is an example of first-order change. The case management premise is that clients and patients need assistance to deal with various agencies to get what they need. Thus, another layer is developed to deal with systems that are not always responsive to patient requests and needs.

In second-order change, the systems themselves are changed. This type of change seeks to reform systems with new approaches, innovative structures, and new ideas. Second-order change demands that problems and situations be looked at with open minds. Creative solutions are required in second-order change. For instance, over the years, many hospitals have sought to reduce the number of uninsured patients who use their emergency rooms for primary care by redirecting them to a primary care source after they have been treated in the emergency room.

Hospitals have also conducted campaigns to change patient behavior—first-order changes. Few have attempted to make second-order change by altering the emergency care system to accommodate patient behavior, for example, by developing a 24-hour walk-in clinic for nonemergent patients. Instead, time and money have been spent trying to change patient behavior to conform with systems rather than changing systems to accommodate patient behavior—a second-order change.

Minkler's Change Approaches

Minkler's change approaches incorporate some aspects of both Lewin's change model and first-order change. Minkler (1980–1981) proposed three approaches to change: noncontingent, or reformist change; contingent, or tentative change; and unfinished, or changing change. Noncontingent change is primarily first-order change that aims at stability as the final state. An example of a good use of noncontingent change is community antismoking campaigns. Stability and refreezing for antismoking behaviors is a desired outcome that is not likely to require a change to other different behaviors.

Contingent, or tentative change, is subject to further change based on feedback from the environment and the consequences of previous changes. This type of change differs from the noncontingent change in that the change is not refrozen as in the Lewin model. An example of contingent change is trying a pilot program before it is introduced to an entire community. This approach allows for changes to be made up until the program is implemented broadly.

Unfinished, or changing change, focuses on change as a continuous process rather than a stable state to be attained. An advantage of this approach is that it may facilitate movement toward second-order change rather than stop at solutions that are first-order change. Current flux in the healthcare system would lend itself to using unfinished change as an approach to organizational changes and even program plans.

■ PHASES OF PROGRAM IMPLEMENTATION

Five phases of program implementation are discussed next: gaining acceptance of the program, specifying tasks and estimating resource needs, developing specific plans for program activities, establishing a mechanism for program management, and putting the plans into action (Dignan & Carr, 1992).

Gaining Acceptance of the Program

New programs involve change, so resistance to change is to be anticipated by at least some of the consumers of the program and some of the providers of the program. Occasionally, community members who are not intended consumers of the program may resist a new program based on their values or beliefs. Resistance to change is likely to be based on uncertainty, concern over personal loss, and the belief that the change is not a good idea (Goodman, 1982).

As has been emphasized throughout this text, the involvement of community residents is an important part of the process of community assessment and program planning. Involvement of community residents often decreases resistance to change because they have been instrumental in designing the program. Although a community may support a program, community residents may not be accepting of the change to be brought about by a program nor may they want to participate in a new program.

Moreover, it is not always possible to involve community residents. For example, in an outbreak of measles, public health workers may need to quickly develop and implement plans to immunize a large part of the child and young adult population in a county. With knowledge of the community, the public health workers can take into consideration the behaviors, patterns of seeking healthcare, and various other characteristics that relate to the acceptance and use of an immunization program.

If program planning has involved the target population and other pertinent individuals and agencies, a revisit to the appropriate groups is in order when the implementation plan is being constructed. Advice about when and how to begin the program should be obtained from the target community. Often, community members know of events that may conflict with the program initiation. Seeking and paying attention to this type of information will help make the program implementation smoother. Guidance about how to contact community groups and residents should be sought from the target population. Often, this contact with the target community may prevent the circulation of inaccurate information.

Especially in an adversarial political environment, individuals who have little access to information readily believe rumors. An example of this occurred during the implementation of a school-based clinic in a low-income Chicago community. An organization based in a Chicago suburb started a campaign to prevent the opening of the clinic by spreading information that students would be given birth control prescriptions without parental consent or knowledge. A member of the outside organization attended a public meeting about the clinic and vehemently protested the opening of the clinic. Local people involved in planning and obtaining funding for the school-based clinic gave an overview of the services, answered questions, and provided factual information about laws pertaining to treating minors in the state of Illinois. The outcome of this episode was that the clinic was eventually opened and successfully served the school population.

Even though some parents and students had been involved in planning the clinic, many parents were not involved and had not paid attention to information provided earlier. Until the potential threat to parental authority was raised, many parents were not aware of the process required for their children to be treated in a school-based clinic. In addition, when programs are in the planning phase, some people may feel that there is no threat because the program may never become a reality.

STRATEGIES FOR GAINING ACCEPTANCE OF A PROGRAM

Even if community involvement has been part of the planning process, gaining acceptance for the introduction of the program is a key step in implementation. Often, gaining acceptance is needed because time has lapsed since the program was planned. Acceptance may be an issue because of changes in the community since the program was planned. For example, the people who helped plan the program are no longer involved in the community.

Four strategies for gaining acceptance for a program are use of the media, involvement of lay leadership, public relations campaigns, and marketing.

Use of the Media. Media, including television, radio, and printed material, have been used successfully for health-promotion interventions, but may also be productive in gaining acceptance for new programs. The more common, and lower cost, media for health programs include posters, articles in local newspapers, pamphlets, fliers, social media, blogs, announcements in newsletters, and public service announcements on television and radio stations.

Media channels should be chosen to reach the target population (e.g., Spanish-language radio stations) or to reach a total community (e.g., a variety of television, radio, and printed media). Messages need to be tailored to the specific intended audience as well as convey the facts about a new program. Message placement and message design are important factors when using mass media such as network television and nationally distributed newspapers (Flora & Cassady, 1990).

Lay Leadership. The involvement of lay leadership to gain acceptance of a new program involves power and authority. Power is the ability to get others to take actions they would not otherwise take. Authority is the expectation that someone should exert control over others or the means to use power through position, person, or institution (Cox, 2014; Simms, Price, & Ervin, 2000).

Acceptance of a program by community leaders may give credibility to a program as well as encouragement to community residents to participate in the program offerings. If the leader does not hold a formal role in the health or social care system, change is more likely to be successful if the leader is charismatic (Dignan & Carr, 1992).

For the advanced practice public/community health nurse, getting key lay leaders involved in the implementation of the program would provide one mechanism for beginning community acceptance. This approach could also backfire in the sense that lay leaders may not be supportive or accepting of a program that they did not help plan and were consulted about only "after the fact."

Public Relations Campaigns. Closely related to the use of media is a public relations campaign. The difference is primarily in the level of planning and the formality of the campaign. Usually, a consultant is engaged to develop a public relations campaign. This involves having a budget adequate to cover the consultant fees along with the cost of developing and distributing the materials for the campaign.

One example of a public relations campaign, not program-oriented but broadly focused, is National Public Health Week, which is the first week in April. This week could be used as a platform for introducing a new prevention program while making the public more aware of the goals of public health and prevention in general. Materials are available from the American Public Health Association, state public health associations, and the National Association of County and City Health Officials (Kreuter, Lezin, Kreuter, & Green, 1998).

Marketing. Most of the three approaches to gaining acceptance of a program may be folded into a marketing plan. Marketing is a process of identifying wants and needs so that they can be satisfied through exchange (Kotler, 1994; Price & Keene, 2000). To reach the target population effectively, a plan is needed before the program is begun. Marketing nursing services also provides visibility for nursing and its contributions to the quality of life of communities.

The marketing process starts with the identification of the market for the service or product. The community assessment forms a good basis for the analysis of the market for a new program. In addition to the data collected during the community assessment, the advanced practice public/community health nurse will need to obtain more data about the specific targeted population for the intervention contained within the program. For example, if the program is aimed at immunizing young children, information is needed about where they are located. Identifying neighborhoods with young children who are likely inadequately immunized may include neighborhoods without health department services, with few or no primary care providers, with limited day-care services, and with low-income families. These circumstances usually result in limited access to immunization services and few cues to mothers to have their children immunized, at least until Head Start or school enrollment requires completion of all required immunizations.

The next step in developing a marketing plan is to identify characteristics of the target population in order to tailor the marketing material. An effective marketing approach is one that satisfies a defined set of wants of a target group (Cooper, 1994). With immunizations for young children, the wants of the target group may be to have healthy children.

Materials aimed at reaching the target population and focusing on their wants and needs are crucial for an effective marketing effort (Fontana, 1991). To identify content for effective marketing material, focus groups composed of the target group may be held. Questions aimed at bringing out very specific ideas from the various group members will be beneficial for helping to shape the marketing material. For example, with a program for increasing the immunization rates for young children, mothers in a focus group may state that a door-to-door campaign may be most effective because mothers are unable to get out much when their children are not in school. Another approach may be to contact mothers through school-age children by notices sent home or immunization clinics held during school functions.

Once a formal marketing plan is developed, putting the plan into action should be carefully planned to coincide with or before the program implementation. A new program often requires a few days of operation before reaching an efficient working level. A marketing campaign aimed at drawing in clients may become more intensive after the new program is working smoothly.

After complete implementation of the marketing plan, evaluation needs to be ongoing to determine whether the marketing strategies are accomplishing the goals. For example, in a project to immunize children, parents and guardians could be asked how they found out about the need to take the children for immunizations. If the marketing strategies are mentioned and the projected numbers of children are being immunized, some credit for program success may be attributed to the marketing campaign.

Changes in the marketing plan may be indicated as the program is in place longer. Careful monitoring of the marketing plan, as part of the program evaluation, may provide adequate data for the program coordinator and staff to make changes in the marketing strategies. For example, often the clients who use services more consistently are more interested and easier to reach. Clients who are more difficult to reach, or who decline services even though they may be needed, require different strategies for them to take needed action.

The advanced practice public/community health nurse may view the target population in terms of Rogers's diffusion of innovations theory. Individuals may be classified into five categories in terms of innovativeness: innovators, early adopters, early majority, late majority, and laggards (Rogers, 1995). To reach the laggards, more intensive, targeted marketing efforts may be needed, such as providing immunizations in the homes or in homeless shelters of families who do not seek care for their children. At times, solutions to reaching the hard-to-reach populations may be found in the research literature.

Specifying Tasks and Estimating Resource Needs

Tasks to implement the program are identified through a detailed review of the program plan. After this step is completed, the resources needed can be specified.

REVIEW OF THE PROGRAM PLAN

The individuals who will implement the program should review the plan to accomplish three main tasks: (a) determination of intermediate and final products of the program, (b) preparation of a detailed list of activities included in the program, and (c) enumeration of the interrelationships among activities (Dignan & Carr, 1992).

Determination of Intermediate and Final Products of the Program. This step involves a careful review of the program's goals and objectives. A clear explanation of the expected products must be evident in how the goals and objectives are stated. For example, an objective written as "to reduce the incidence of preventable diseases in the community by providing access to primary care" gives a picture of the expected products. The final product is a reduction in the numbers of preventable disease cases; the exact diseases to be monitored would need to be determined. The intermediate products are clinical examinations, treatments completed, and cases of diseases diagnosed early. Numbers of people seen and treated are important indicators of the target populations being reached.

Although this is an example of an intervention at the individual level, the goal is to reduce disease rates for the community. A reduction in disease has reverberations for the total community in terms of economics (e.g., worker absenteeism is reduced, thus increasing productivity) and quality of life (e.g., fewer days of illness for children and adults). In addition, the less money spent on medical care, the more money available for food, shelter, and other necessities of life.

Another example of intermediate and final products is in an immunization program for preschool children. The intermediate products are immunizations, and the final products are diseases prevented or disease-free children. Diseases are prevented not only in the immunized children but also in children who are not immunized because the incidences of the diseases decrease as herd immunity is achieved (Oleckno, 2008).

In the earlier example of the program to prevent deaths from falls among the elderly, the intermediate products are fewer falls and fewer injuries. The final products are fewer deaths or, on the positive side, an increase in the quality of life for elderly through avoidance of injury. This also means an improved quality of life for the families of elderly who are not injured and/or who do not die. In addition, for society, the savings realized from not treating injuries from falls may be used in other ways to improve the quality of life, for example, provide better quality and more food for elderly with inadequate incomes.

Preparation of a Detailed List of Activities. The list of activities is best prepared by the staff who will implement the program. Often, the program planners have very clear understandings of what needs to be done but have not actually written these details into the program plan. The program staff should read the plan and write out activities to accomplish each objective. If the explanation found in the program plan is not adequate, the staff should attempt to meet with a program planner or part of the planning group to seek clarification. When this is not possible, it often helps to meet with someone who was involved in any phase of the planning process.

At times, there may be disagreement about how detailed to make the list of activities. There will probably be turnover of staff during the life of the program, so greater detail is preferred to less detail. The document will then be available for orientation of new staff as well as documentation to use for program evaluation and writing other program plans.

Enumeration of Interrelationships Among Activities. Interrelationships among activities are key parts of the implementation plan. All staff members may not be involved in implementing all parts of a program, so a diagram of the interrelationships among and sequencing of activities will provide an overview of how staff will relate and work together toward a common end. Often, the staff performs activities that are seemingly isolated from what goes on before and after their own activities. This isolation may create rigidity and lack of concern about the "big picture" of the mission of the organization. For example, if the mission of a nursing center is to provide direct access to nursing care, a clerk who turns away a client without an appointment is not in tune with what the center hopes to accomplish in the long term.

Tools are available to guide the task of listing the interrelationships among activities. The two summarized here are the Program Evaluation and Review Technique (PERT) and the Gantt chart (Carstens, Richardson, & Smith, 2013; Green & Kreuter, 2005).

TABLE 14.1 PERT Network for Implementing Exercise Program

Event	Description	Estimated Times in Weeks		
		Optimistic	Most Likely	Maximum
A	Confirm agreements with sites	5	7	10
B	Hire staff and consultant	4	8	12
C	Develop protocols	2	4	6
D	Develop marketing plan	1	2	3
E	Conduct trial-run program	1	2	3
F	Implement marketing plan	2	4	6
G	Develop evaluation plan	1	2	3
H	Implement program	2	3	4

PERT, Program Evaluation and Review Technique.

PERT or PERT network analysis was developed for use in large-scale projects, and is also useful for smaller projects that have numerous steps for implementation. The PERT method uses a flow plan that incorporates sequencing activities on a time axis. Time estimates for completion of activities are done in three ways. The optimistic estimate is the time it will take with minimal difficulties. The second estimate is that which is the most likely, considering past experiences with similar projects. A third estimate is made for the pessimistic time frame that is the time to complete activities if maximum difficulties are encountered. In Table 14.1, the activities that relate to each event are listed along with the estimated time frames for an exercise program.

To develop a PERT network, the program manager must identify every activity for each event and the order in which the events must be completed. Next, the activities must be diagrammed from start to finish with relationships to each other identified. The three-time estimates must be computed, followed by construction of a network diagram (Carstens et al., 2013).

As shown in Figure 14.1, circles indicate events, which are end points that represent completion of major activities. The arrows symbolize the activities, which represent time or resources needed to go from one event to another. The critical path is the longest sequence of activities and events in a PERT network.

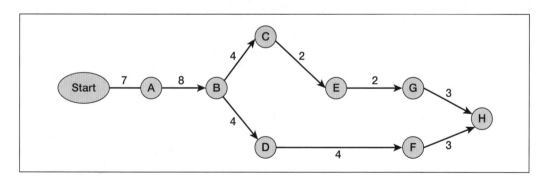

FIGURE 14.1 PERT network diagram.

PERT, Program Evaluation and Review Technique.

Compared with the PERT network, a Gantt chart is a simple tool. A Gantt chart provides a visual timeline for the start and finish dates for each program activity as well as a view of the overlap of activities. An example is shown in Figure 14.2. A useful chart may be developed in terms of months, weeks, days, or hours, depending on the detail needed in explicating the activities. Beginning estimates of personnel requirements may also be determined by using the Gantt chart. By examining the activities for each time period, the type and number of hours may be determined and thus translated into full-time equivalents for each category of staff (Green & Kreuter, 2005).

In addition to constructing planning charts with paper and pencil, several computer programs are available, including Gantt charts (Carstens et al., 2013). Many personal computers have preloaded software to develop timetables and timelines (e.g., Excel).

Determining Resource Requirements. Successful estimation of resource requirements entails complete detailing of program activities and how they are interrelated. A careful and thorough completion of the steps outlined in the implementation process will provide the necessary base for determining resource requirements.

Personnel, supply, and equipment needs may be estimated from the review of activities as detailed in a PERT or Gantt chart. Although a budget was constructed for a program plan, as presented in Chapter 13, the resource requirements will be more detailed at this point in the program implementation process. Also, the details of when specific staff and supplies are needed can be pinpointed more precisely during the implementation planning stage.

During determining resource requirements is also the time to make modifications in the budget and/or program plans if funding does not match the anticipated activities. For example, if program implementation was planned for three sites, but funding allows implementation in only two sites, changes in the plan can be made before the program is implemented, saving time and effort down the line. On the other hand, if more funding is forthcoming than originally budgeted, plans can be expanded to make use of the additional money.

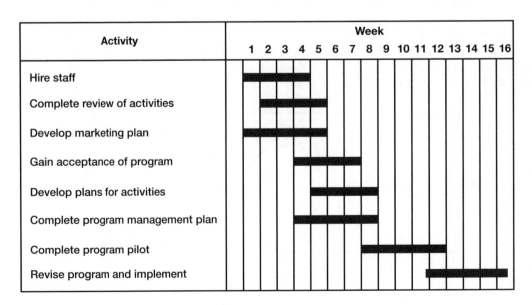

FIGURE 14.2 Gantt chart for implementation activities.

A lapse of time from planning to implementation almost always occurs, so the budget should be carefully reviewed for adjustments in costs of goods and services. Changes in the costs of postage, telephone services, paper goods, and numerous other items may not have been anticipated when the budget was planned. Adjusting the budget to reflect these changes before the program begins will result in fewer surprises as the program revenue or funding is spent.

Developing Specific Plans for Program Activities

A major focus in developing plans for program activities is the marketing plan. In addition to assisting with acceptance of the program, the marketing plan will provide the necessary approach for reaching the target population.

The following questions provide a framework for thinking about the development of the marketing plan:

1. What are the objectives of marketing the program?
2. What is the present status of the program (if it already exists) or the sponsor (if this is likely to affect participation)?
3. What are the best approaches for introducing the program?
4. Who should be responsible for introducing of the program?
5. What indicators of effectiveness of the introduction of the program should be used (Dignan & Carr, 1992; Green & Keuter, 2005)?

The use of these questions will assist in developing a successful marketing plan that involves the target population.

Establishing a Mechanism for Program Management

Establishing a mechanism for program management depends partially on the organization in which the program will be located. If the program will be within a structured organization with well-defined position descriptions and reporting relationships, program management can be established within the existing structure of organization management. If, however, the program is to exist as part of a loosely structured community organization or coalition, a program management system may be needed to foster program implementation and evaluation.

Not all organizational structures require a hierarchical structure for effective functioning, but some structure is needed to accomplish tasks. One of the first decisions for program management is the assignment of responsibility for program coordination. One person may be assigned this task or may function as the point person for the implementation team. The structure of this arrangement will be related to the formality or informality of the sponsoring organization. A program management mechanism or system needs at least these two components: indicators of program status and sources of data.

INDICATORS OF PROGRAM STATUS

Program status may be monitored by time, cost, and performance. All established organizations have systems to monitor each of these indicators in various ways. Existing systems should be used to the extent possible to avoid additional burden on staff for data collection. However, a new program may need to have specific indicators developed for the general indicators of time, cost, and performance (Dever, 1997; Dignan & Carr, 1992).

Although some indicators of time, cost, and performance will be found in the evaluation plan, monitoring is a daily activity that requires standards that demonstrate incremental progress toward objectives and goals. For example, the PERT chart gives the program coordinator three estimates of time for implementation activities. If all activities require the longest time estimate for accomplishment, the cost of implementation will be increased. The budget must be carefully monitored to see that cost is within the allotted amount. Cost overruns may be prevented with careful monitoring and adjustments of activities.

SOURCES OF DATA

To use indicators of program status, data are needed. As mentioned earlier, any existing sources of data should be used to the extent possible to avoid duplication. In addition, any system should incorporate, as often as possible, data-collection mechanisms into daily work so that records do not need to be reviewed for data collection. For example, if one indicator of program status is attendance at group sessions, taking an accurate attendance should be a routine part of the way the sessions are organized. Monitoring attendance on a weekly basis is important for program success, and action must be taken if attendance falls below a specified level. If attendance is low and no action is taken until the evaluation at the end of a year, it may be too late to take corrective action.

Similar diligence is needed with program cost. Overbudget situations may be avoided with careful monitoring, but only if budget statements are regularly produced and distributed to the appropriate individuals. Program coordinators must be certain that personnel who control costs have access to budget information and know what it means.

Indicators of performance may take various forms. Client-satisfaction surveys, self-evaluations, routine performance evaluations, and peer reviews are a few approaches to performance evaluation. Quality and quantity of performance need to be taken into consideration in developing tools for monitoring performance. In addition, performance needs to be monitored carefully in early phases of program implementation to determine whether the program is being implemented as designed.

These indicators of performance may need to be different than those for longer term performance. For example, interrater reliability for the use of certain data-collection tools may be an issue in performance early in program implementation, but not an issue as staff become adept in using the instrument. Table 14.2 has examples of time, cost, and performance indicators that may be used early and ongoing in program implementation.

TABLE 14.2 Indicators of Program Status During Implementation: Time, Cost, and Performance

Indicator Category	Specific Indicator	Sources of Data
Time	Time estimates on PERT chart, time used for interventions	Staff's daily activity reports, observations, client records
Cost	Staff salary to implement set of interventions, supplies used, error rates	Staff's daily activity reports and budget, inventory records, incidence reports
Performance	Client satisfaction, interrater reliability or intervention techniques/methods, client knowledge	Surveys, records of intervention results, interrater reliability studies, knowledge tests before and after intervention

PERT, Program Evaluation and Review Technique.

Putting the Plans Into Action

The last phase of program implementation is putting the plans into action. The two components of this phase are internal implementation and external implementation. If some time has elapsed since the implementation plan was completed, putting the plans into action should begin with a review of the major components of the plans, including the target population, physical space, equipment ordered, forms printed, and funding obtained, as well as a general scan of the community for any changes that need to be considered in the program implementation.

INTERNAL IMPLEMENTATION

Internal implementation has much to do with the previous section about the management system. In addition, other activities need to be conducted for a smooth internal implementation, including, but not limited to organizational change, orientation and training for staff, and a pilot test of the program.

The type of organizational change needed may range from simple to very complex. For example, a new program aimed at providing structured home visits to new mothers and infants will require little, if any, organizational change compared with a program that requires combining two current divisions in a health organization. Regardless of the magnitude of change, resistance is to be expected from staff members, even those who are in support of the change. To some extent, change is difficult for most people and requires energy as well as new information. Models of change are discussed earlier in this chapter.

Orientation and staff training should be planned and conducted in adequate time to allow a pilot test of the major activities that form the core of the new program. The interventions to be used in the new program may need to be adjusted because of the pilot testing, so time for adjustments and retraining staff will be needed. Staff training should include information from the program plan, such as

- Background and rationale for the interventions
- Characteristics of the target population
- Goals and objectives
- Time schedule for implementation
- Protocols of specific interventions
- A trial implementation of the interventions

As much as possible, current staff should be involved in conducting the training to continue the process of acceptance of the new program.

Also, multimedia sources of information should be used if available, for example, a video that demonstrates the use of a new procedure or a self-instructional module for gaining new information. If continuing-education credit is available for such activities, the administration should encourage the acquisition of credit for appropriate professional staff. Training may involve staff becoming certified in the use of some techniques, such as laboratory tests. As much as possible, the training should be completed at the site where services will be delivered to involve as many staff as possible and to have the training process visible to the total staff.

EXTERNAL IMPLEMENTATION

External implementation includes assessment of the target population's readiness for change, involvement of the target population in implementation, and identification of barriers and facilitators of implementation.

Throughout the program planning, the advanced practice public/community health nurse will be involved with the target population for the program. This involvement will continue in implementation by gathering information about readiness for change. Information about two areas needs to be sought and analyzed: (a) events that may have altered the target population's willingness to accept change and (b) changes in the healthcare system that could influence acceptance of the new program (Dignan & Carr, 1992).

Depending on the information obtained, changes may need to be made before the program is implemented. An example is the relocation of the target population. Although this type of change does not often occur quickly, there are instances in which a program was planned for a specific physical location only to discover that the target population no longer lived in the area.

More common is locating a program in an area unacceptable to a segment of the population, for example, locating a community health clinic in an area dominated by a rival gang to a neighboring community. The resulting situation is that people from the neighboring community are afraid to cross the gang boundaries to reach the clinic. Another instance is the placement of a teen clinic in a conspicuous location where the clinic users could be readily observed entering the facility. These are examples of actual situations that resulted in underutilization of facilities. The location of a facility or service is not easily changed, so placement is one crucial factor to check and recheck with the target population.

Changes in the healthcare system are rapid and thus require close monitoring. For example, in past years some states changed Medicaid programs to require that recipients enroll in health maintenance organizations or a managed care entity. A new program would require adjustments before implementation if a major source of revenue was anticipated to be Medicaid reimbursement. Any source of information that helps the nurse keep current about anticipated changes in the healthcare system is important to establish and maintain, but especially during planning and implementing new programs.

◼ ROLE OF THE CHANGE AGENT IN PROGRAM IMPLEMENTATION

The advanced practice public/community health nurse needs to develop and maintain a variety of skills for effective performance as a change agent. A change agent is a leader who stimulates and guides the change process. Change agents are needed to guide the program interventions or innovations past the obstacles involving people. To be effective, change agents need to be identified with the following characteristics: belief that the innovation is critical, persistence to push the innovation ahead regardless of the roadblocks, being a leader in the group that must implement the innovation, and being in possession of good communication skills (Garon, 2014).

In addition to being a change agent, the advanced practice public/community health nurse must identify and work with other change agents. The identification of change agents should be a conscious effort on the part of the advanced practice public/community health nurse. Change agents must be actively involved in the change process. Identification must be followed by assignment to assist with the change process. The leadership for this process must be deliberative if success is to be achieved.

Skills for Role of Change Agent

Many skills come together in the role of change agent, such as group process skills, interpersonal relationships, negotiation skills, and the ability to develop trust. Three sets of skills that are particularly important are communication, visionary leadership, and conflict management (Garon, 2014; Lancaster, 1982).

COMMUNICATION

Throughout nursing preparation and practice, communication skills are stressed as important for effective functioning. For the advanced practice public/community health nurse, communication skills are especially important because of extensive contact with a wide variety of people and organizations. Communication is a process with the basic purpose of effecting change. The public/community health nurse in advanced practice must use communication constantly to convey the essence of practice. Both verbal and written communication are crucial to accomplishing the work of developing healthy communities.

Verbal Communication. The advanced practice public/community health nurse uses verbal communication to lead meetings, make presentations, and facilitate the work of program staff. To be effective, the nurse must develop skills in clear, effective verbal communication.

The difficulty with verbal communication is the inability to edit remarks once they have been stated. Preparation is one key to effective verbal communication. If a formal presentation is to be made, it is logical that the material will be prepared and rehearsed before the date. However, in informal encounters, preparation time may be lacking. Three techniques are often useful to allow time for preparation of verbal responses: seeking clarification, asking others' opinions, and setting up an appointment to discuss the issue (Simms & Ngin, 2000).

Seeking clarification will allow time to think about an answer as well as to ensure that the question or remark was heard correctly. At times, we hear something different than what was said because of our own mind-sets or anxieties. The additional time for clarification will also provide the questioner an opportunity to change or redirect the query.

When others are asked for their opinions, the focus is taken away from the group leader. This technique is desirable to use in situations in which there are no correct answers but multiple opinions. An argument may be avoided or others' ideas may bring out an approach not yet considered. There is rarely one right way to accomplish a goal, so a variety of ideas should be entertained if scientific evidence is not available to provide a logical answer.

At times, the topic under discussion is not appropriate for a group session or is an individual's "axe to grind." The wise leader often avoids a one-to-one discussion in a group setting by requesting that the individual meet with the leader at a different time. A private meeting will allow the leader and the individual to save face in front of the group and air differences in an open environment. The unwise approach is to try to make the individual feel belittled or wrong just to prove a point or to keep power in the group. Although the leader needs power to lead, power gained at the expense of others may squelch group discussion and open the door for disgruntled group members to undermine the work of the group.

Written Communication. Advanced practice public/community health nurses need well-developed written communication skills for responsibilities such as writing reports, preparing grant proposals, and documenting community assessments and program evaluations.

Writing clearly and concisely is hard work. The best exercise for learning to write well is to write often. Asking someone to edit and comment on drafts of your writing helps to improve skills over time. Another recommended technique for improving writing skills is to take a course in writing. Many universities or colleges have courses in writing for publication or technical writing. Continuing-education courses are also available for obtaining the basics of clear written communication.

VISIONARY LEADERSHIP

Leaders attempt to influence the behavior of others, and power is the means used for that influence. Leadership styles vary, but the best leadership style is the one that is needed for a specific time and place. Implementing change requires a leadership style that is flexible or situational (Hersey & Duldt, 1989).

Situational leadership theory is based on research that demonstrates that there is no one best style of leadership, but one of four basic styles may be effective, depending on the situation:

- High task behavior and low relationship behavior
- High task behavior and high relationship behavior
- High relationship behavior and low task behavior
- Low relationship behavior and low task behavior

Directing activities of others is defined as task behavior. Providing socioemotional support by establishing personal relationships with followers is the relationship behavior of leaders. Thus, the amount of task behavior (e.g., high or low) and the amount of relationship behavior (e.g., high or low) depends on the situation.

The theory of situational leadership is based on an interaction among three factors: the amount of direction a leader gives, the amount of socioemotional support a leader provides, and the maturity level of the followers on a specific task. *Maturity* is defined as the capacity to set high, yet attainable, goals; willingness and ability to take responsibility; and the education and experience of the group related to a specific task.

A team composed of health professionals who are mature and work well together may accomplish goals with a leadership style of low task behavior and low relationship behavior. If a team is composed of new employees who are also new to their professions, a leadership style of high task behavior and high relationship behavior may be more effective. The leader who is using situational leadership will need to assess the situation and the skills of followers. A tool for assessing team skills is provided in Chapter 7.

Visionary leadership combines situational leadership with the ability to lead followers to an uncertain but envisioned future. The visionary leader sees things as they should be, not how they are, or how they could be. To be able to communicate that vision to followers is also important because it is easier to accomplish complex tasks with the help of others.

When setbacks or obstacles appear, as they usually will during a project, followers will look to the visionary leader for a morale boost and a plan for dealing with adversity. Discouraged followers can lead to a less-than-positive outcome. The visionary leader sets a "can do" climate for followers and keeps the long-term vision alive.

CONFLICT MANAGEMENT

Advanced practice public/community health nurses are faced with the potential for conflict in any situation in which other disciplines and the community are involved. Conflict is inevitable and is viewed as healthy if not a hindrance to functioning. *Conflict* is defined for purposes of this text as "perceived incompatible differences resulting in some form of interference or opposition" (Robbins & Coulter, 1999, pp. 454–455). Conflict is based on scarcity of power or resources, differences in social position, and different value structures.

Dealing with conflict in constructive ways requires both knowledge and experience. Strategies for conflict resolution include avoidance, defusing, containment, confrontation, lose–lose, win–lose, and win–win (Cohen, 1980). Of these, the latter is the most desirable and may be reached by negotiation or collaboration. Different theorists view negotiation differently. One view is that negotiation is a cyclic interactional process that uses such strategies as persuasion, trade-offs, demands, appeals, compromises, and mutual agreements. Another view is of negotiation as a process of information, timing, power, and pressure to secure a commitment to change behavior (Cox, 2014; Simms et al., 2000).

Collaborative theory views conflict as a creative force that leads to an improved situation to which both sides are committed. This approach advocates that people should bring their differences forward to identify underlying causes and find an alternative that is mutually acceptable to all (Likert & Likert, 1976).

ETHICAL ISSUES IN USING CHANGE MODELS

Whichever change model is used, one must examine the ethical issues involved with the use of knowledge to assist in changing behaviors (Dudley-Brown & Rushton, 2016). Even though people may not be changed without their cooperation, some approaches to change are more apparent to participants than others. Also, informed consent is an important part of any program in which people are involved. These issues, that is, participants' knowledge of the change approach and informed consent, are examined in this section.

Change in program participants may bring about changes in relationships. Often, these changes are not compatible with the ongoing relationship and the comfort derived from the predictability. For example, many smokers are married to smokers. When one person decides to stop smoking, the relationship between the married couple changes also. At times, the smoker may try to sabotage the smoking-cessation attempts of the partner or becomes angry because of the threatened change in the relationship. Another example of change in a relationship may be seen in weight-reduction programs in which it is often a woman who is attempting to lose weight and changes food preparation for the total family.

Behavior changes are not innocent attempts to better someone else's life; they are serious modifications that have far-reaching ramifications for total families, not all of which are positive. Changes at the group and community levels are also not without broader ramifications for a total community. For example, the legislation that banned the use of leaded gasoline in automobiles resulted in leaded gas not being available in almost all parts of the country. Anyone who owned an automobile that used leaded gas would have been forced to buy a new car if leaded gas were no longer available. Often, people with old automobiles did not have the means to purchase new ones.

An ethical approach to a behavior-change intervention is to inform participants about the potential ramifications for families, relationships, and other such areas for consideration before they commit to the program and the intended changes. Most individual behavior changes require support and reinforcement to make and maintain. Program participants need to be given information about how to ask for support from significant others during and after program participation. Many people, for example, have returned to smoking because of a lack of support or sabotage.

■ RELATIONSHIP OF INTERVENTIONS AND PROGRAM IMPLEMENTATION

In program implementation, attention is directed to how the interventions fit within the program, how to effectively implement the interventions, and how to maintain the fidelity of the interventions throughout the life of the program. As discussed in Chapter 12, interventions are the parts of programs that will bring about the intended changes. Programs may be planned with very brief descriptions of the ideas to be implemented but supply inadequate detail to allow for consistency in the actual implementation. For example, the content of a smoking-cessation program described as "help people stop smoking" would not be very helpful to the people who are designated to implement the intervention within the program. This section addresses issues of fitting interventions within programs.

The Fit of Interventions Within Programs

More than one intervention may be needed for a program to achieve its objectives. Examples of this are programs to improve cardiovascular health. These programs may include interventions for lowering cholesterol through diet, weight reduction through diet, smoking cessation, and exercise interventions for nonactive participants. Some participants need to use all the program components, whereas others concentrate on one component.

Regardless of the number of interventions, the program and the interventions must be compatible. Although achieving compatibility will have been part of the planning process, incompatible components are sometimes discovered only when the trial of the program is conducted. For example, if a program participant is to attend three group sessions on pregnancy between the first and second prenatal visits, the second prenatal visit should not be scheduled before the sessions are completed.

In addition, the intervention should be supported by the ongoing activities of the agency. An intervention that is out of place because of the time needed for implementation, the characteristics of the client population, or other factors will often not be successful. For example, a series of group sessions are sometimes not well attended by people who have children and other responsibilities or by those who are in the contemplative phase of change. Educational sessions that are held every day with clients in attendance at a clinic or other activity may be more successful, especially in helping clients move from the precontemplative to the contemplative phase of change (Conn, 1994; Prochaska, Redding, & Evers, 2008).

Another aspect of fit of the intervention with the program is funding. Adequate funding should be obtained to implement the intervention as planned. Cutting comers to conserve funds may result in wasted resources if the outcomes are not achieved. Sustainability of a successful program through continued funding is much more likely if effectiveness is demonstrated.

Implementing the Interventions

A trial run of the interventions is desirable before full-scale implementation. After implementation, activities should be carefully monitored and a formative evaluation conducted. When a smooth level of operations is achieved and the evaluation criteria demonstrate early achievement of outcomes, monitoring may be put on a less intensive schedule.

During implementation, staff need feedback about their performance. Often only negative feedback is given; staff very much need to know that what they are doing is correct and is having some effect. Patterns of performance of individual staff members should be addressed in private conferences. If patterns of performance indicate that several staff members are having problems with the interventions, this may indicate a need for more staff development or a review of the parts of the interventions that are troublesome.

Maintaining Fidelity or Integrity of Interventions

Maintaining the fidelity or integrity of interventions involves seeing that they are consistently carried out as designed (Carroll et al., 2007). During the implementation of an intervention, several issues may arise to interfere with the intervention being implemented in the way it was designed (Kirchhoff & Dille, 1994). For example, new staff members who have not had orientation to the intervention may not use the appropriate techniques or protocols. At times, the intervention may be modified because of lack of time or lack of staff. All these issues and many more may result in the intervention not being implemented as designed.

Mechanisms to maintain the integrity of interventions should be put into place when the interventions are implemented. These mechanisms may be part of the evaluation, part of the management system, or both. Ideally, the mechanisms should involve a combination of techniques so that several aspects of interventions can be monitored simultaneously. For example, daily staff reports could include both numbers of participants and content covered in teaching sessions. This area is covered in more depth in Chapter 15.

Observations of the interventions being carried out are valuable, especially if there are structure and process standards to be met. Clinical practice guidelines are used in some nursing care settings to promote the use of consistent applications of evidence-based nursing care to patients (Stanik-Hutt, 2016). Daily staff activity records should be monitored regularly to determine whether any variations in the interventions are occurring. For example, in one very busy community health clinic, all clients who came to the clinic each day were not being seen before the clinic closed, and many were told to return the next day. Thus, because of pressures to see as many clients as possible, the staff may have cut corners in teaching clients.

Other issues of consistency involve the differences among staff in how an intervention is implemented. Inconsistencies in practice are great among nurses (Madigan, 1998) and perhaps even greater among other staff. If community members are involved, there may be more issues in terms of consistency of implementation that need to be addressed early in the program implementation. One approach to increasing consistency is to hold regular staff meetings to discuss issues with implementation and how to handle the issues. Regular review of protocols and procedures will reinforce the content.

Staff meetings will serve various other purposes, one of which is to build pride in the job being done by the group. Sharing evaluation results, giving positive feedback about group accomplishments, and passing on compliments from clients are important components for group cohesion. Reinforcement helps staff to continue to do a good job in implementing the interventions consistently.

■ POLITICAL ENVIRONMENT AND PROGRAM IMPLEMENTATION

Environment refers to institutions and forces outside an organization that may affect outcomes (Robbins & Coulter, 2016). The political environment is one part of the total environment in which programs exist. The political environment should be monitored for

- Concerns and worries of key decision makers, gatekeepers, and stakeholders
- Changes in other organizations that relate to the program being implemented
- Public policies that may affect program results (e.g., changes in reimbursement) (Robbins & Coulter, 2016; Witkin & Altschuld, 1995)

Strategies for Addressing Political-Environment Issues

Close monitoring of political-environment issues may help to anticipate and prevent any negative affect on a program. However, not all issues in the political environment are predictable nor are they always rational. Thus, strategies will often need to be planned and implemented after issues have arisen. The following strategies may be used to prevent adverse effects on a program, but may also be useful after an adverse situation is detected.

COMMUNICATING WITH STAKEHOLDERS

If the program is at the community level, one strategy to use to prevent adverse effects on a program is regular meetings with community residents. Meetings will be valuable in maintaining support for and confidence in the program. Community members need feedback about program progress and accomplishments. Close contact with the key decision makers, gatekeepers, and stakeholders will reinforce that there are no hidden agendas and everyone is welcome into the fold.

Other techniques to maintain effective communication include a newsletter, an email listserv, and regular articles in local newspapers. Client testimonials about how the program has helped them are an effective method for the public to be able to see how the program is making concrete contributions to the quality of community life.

USING A MARKETING PLAN

An initial, thorough marketing plan will assist with gaining favor for a new program, but may not address all the negative circumstances surrounding a program or an agency nor do all segments of a community respond the same way to messages (Kreuter et al., 1998; Price & Keene, 2000). Political support can and does change even with community approval and backing. An example of this was the demise of a very successful nurse midwifery program in California. Physician opposition gained support from the legislature to close the midwifery practice, thus allowing physicians to move into the area.

In instances of loss of support for a program, several approaches may be taken. The first obvious one is to do nothing if the program can continue to function. If the loss of support means loss of clients, a new or augmented marketing plan may be able to revive the client base. A new marketing plan would need to focus on the areas that have contributed to loss of the client base, for example, a turnover in staff or a change in hours of service.

Another example in which marketing efforts may be effective is in naming a program or service. When a community nursing center was opened in a building that had been a nursing home, many community members thought it was another residence for older people because the name included the words *nursing center*. Several approaches could have been used to change the environment for the program. The name of the center could have been changed to reflect a common community understanding, for example, *family health center* or *healthcare clinic*. Another solution would have been to move the center to a location associated with other healthcare services. The name change is by far the easier solution.

BUILDING COALITIONS

Other strategies for dealing with a negative political environment include working with other organizations to gain support for the program, securing support from other citizen groups, and building coalitions. A *coalition* is a group of people and/or organizations working together to achieve goals that they are unlikely to achieve separately (Dluhy, 1990; Flynn & Rains, 1993; Helvie, 1998). Ideally, a coalition is established during the community assessment or planning process but may still be an effective approach to an adverse political environment.

Coalitions may be formal or informal, temporary or permanent, and they may be composed of individuals or groups of organizations. The composition and duration vary with the goals, the resources, and the commitment of the members. Advantages of coalitions include the ability to reach more people and an expanded resource base (Helvie, 1998).

■ SUMMARY

This chapter presented an overview of program implementation, including its five phases: gaining acceptance of the program, specifying tasks and estimating resource needs, developing specific plans for program activities, establishing a mechanism for program management, and putting the plans into action (Dignan & Carr, 1992).

Program implementation requires knowledge about the change process and change theory. Four useful models of change for this phase in the process include Lewin's (1958) three-phase model, Chin and Benne's (1976) three strategies of planned change, first- and second-order change (Watzlawick et al., 1974), and Minkler's (1980–1981) change approaches.

Successful program implementation requires an effective change agent. Change agents need to possess effective verbal and written communication skills, visionary leadership, and conflict-management skills.

During implementation, attention should be directed to how the interventions fit within the program, how the interventions are most effectively implemented, and how to maintain the fidelity of the interventions throughout the life of the program. The political environment must be carefully monitored during implementation. Strategies and approaches for creating a supportive political environment include meeting regularly with stakeholders, developing coalitions, marketing, and providing information to the public.

■ SUGGESTED CLINICAL OR PRACTICUM ACTIVITIES

1. Meet with two or three community stakeholders to explore their views on how new health or social programs were introduced to their communities and how acceptance of the program was achieved or not achieved.
2. Observe the implementation of a new program and compare it with the proposed written program plan. What employee training was completed before implementation? What adjustments were made? What corrections were made during the implementation?

REFERENCES

Archer, S. E., Kelly, C. D., & Bisch, S. A. (1984). *Implementing change in communities: A collaborative process.* St. Louis, MO: Mosby.

Carroll, C., Patterson, M., Wood, S., Booth, A., Rick, J., & Balain, S. (2007). A conceptual framework for implementation fidelity. *Implementation Science, 2,* 40. doi:10.1186/1748-5908-2-40

Carstens, D. S., Richardson, G. L., & Smith, R. B. (2013). *Project management tools and techniques: A practical guide.* Boca Raton, FL: CRC Press.

Chin, R., & Benne, K. D. (1976). General strategies for effecting changes in human systems. In W. Bennis, K. D. Benne, R. Chin., & K. Corey (Eds.), *The planning of change* (3rd ed., pp. 22–45). New York, NY: Holt, Rinehart & Winston.

Cohen, H. (1980). *You can negotiate anything.* Secaucus, NJ: Lyle Stuart.

Conn, V. S. (1994). A staged-based approach to helping people change health behaviors. *Clinical Nurse Specialist, 8*(4), 187–193.

Cooper, P. (Ed.). (1994). *Health care marketing: A foundation for managed quality* (3rd ed.). Gaithersburg, MD: Aspen.

Cox, K. B. (2014). Power and conflict. In D. L. Huber (Ed.), *Leadership & nursing care management* (5th ed., pp. 159–185). St. Louis, MO: Elsevier Saunders.

Dever, G. E. A. (1997). *Improving outcomes in public health practice.* Gaithersburg, MD: Aspen.

Dignan, M. B., & Carr, P. A. (1992). *Program planning for health education and promotion* (2nd ed.). Philadelphia, PA: Lea & Febiger.

Dluhy, M. J. (1990). *Building coalitions in the human services*. Newbury Park, CA: Sage.

Dudley-Brown, S., & Rushton, C. H. (2016). Legal and ethical issues in translation. In K. M. White, S. Dudley-Brown., & M. F. Terhaar (Eds.), *Translation of evidence into nursing and health care* (2nd ed., pp. 313–322). New York, NY: Springer Publishing.

Flora, J. A., & Cassady, D. (1990). Roles of media in community-based health promotion. In N. Bracht (Ed.), *Health promotion at the community level* (pp. 143–157). Newbury Park, CA: Sage.

Flynn, B. C., & Rains, J. W. (1993). Establishing community coalitions for prevention: Healthy cities Indiana. In R. N. Knollmueller (Ed.), *Prevention across the life span* (pp. 21–30). Washington, DC: American Nurses Publishing.

Fontana, S. A. (1991). Applying marketing concepts to promote health in vulnerable groups. *Public Health Nursing, 8*(2), 140–143.

Garon, M. (2014). Change and innovation. In D. L. Huber (Ed.), *Leadership & nursing care management* (5th ed., pp. 37–54). St. Louis, MO: Elsevier Saunders.

Goodman, P. S. (1982). *Changes in organizations: New perspectives in theory, research, and practice.* San Francisco, CA: Jossey-Bass.

Green, L. W., & Kreuter, M. W. (2005). *Health promotion planning: An educational and ecological approach* (4th ed.). San Francisco, CA: Jossey-Bass.

Helvie, C. O. (1998). *Advanced practice nursing in the community.* Thousand Oaks, CA: Sage.

Hersey, P., & Duldt, B. W. (1989). *Situational leadership in nursing.* Norwalk, CT: Appleton & Lange.

Kirchhoff, K. T., & Dille, C. A. (1994). Issues in intervention research: Maintaining integrity. *Applied Nursing Research, 7*(1), 32–46.

Kotler, P. (1994). *Marketing management analysis, planning, implementation, and control* (8th ed.). Englewood Cliffs, NJ: Prentice Hall.

Kreuter, M. W., Lezin, N. A., Kreuter, M. W., & Green, L. W. (1998). *Community health promotion ideas that work.* Sudbury, MA: Jones & Bartlett.

Lancaster, J. (1982). Change theory: An essential aspect of nursing practice. In J. Lancaster & W. Lancaster (Eds.), *Concepts for advanced nursing practice: The nurse as a change agent* (pp. 5–23). St. Louis, MO: Mosby.

Lewin, K. (1958). Group decision and social change. In E. Maccoby, T. Newcomb., & E. Hartley (Eds.), *Readings in social psychology* (3rd ed., pp. 197–211). New York, NY: Holt, Rinehart & Winston.

Likert, R., & Likert, J. (1976). *Ways of managing conflict.* New York, NY: McGraw-Hill.

Madigan, E. A. (1998). Evidence-based practice in home healthcare: A springboard for discussion. *Home Healthcare Nurse, 16*(6), 411–415.

Minkler, M. (1980–1981). Unfreezing Lewin: The case for alternative change strategies in health education. *International Quarterly of Community Health Education, 1,* 174–177.

Oleckno, W. A. (2008). *Epidemiology: Concepts and methods.* Long Grove, IL: Waveland Press.

Price, S. A., & Keene, D. (2000). Marketing nursing and nursing services. In L. M. Simms, S. A. Price., & N. E. Ervin (Eds.), *The professional practice of nursing administration* (3rd ed., pp. 546–564). Albany, NY: Delmar.

Prochaska, J. O., Redding, C. A., & Evers, K. E. (2008). The transtheoretical model and stages of change. In K. Glanz, B. K. Rimer., & K. Viswanath (Eds.), *Health behavior and health education* (4th ed., pp. 97–121). San Francisco, CA: Jossey-Bass.

Robbins, S. P., & Coulter, M. (1999). *Management* (3rd ed.). Upper Saddle River, NJ: Prentice Hall.

Robbins, S. P., & Coulter, M. (2016). *Management* (13th ed.). Essex, UK: Pearson Education.

Rogers, E. M. (1995). *Diffusion of innovations* (4th ed.). New York, NY: Free Press.

Simms, L. M., & Ngin, P. M. (2000). Effective communication. In L. M. Simms, S. A. Price., & N. E. Ervin (Eds.), *The professional practice of nursing administration* (3rd ed., pp. 227–246). Albany, NY: Delmar.

Simms, L. M., Price, S. A., & Ervin, N. E. (2000). *The professional practice of nursing administration* (3rd ed.). Albany, NY: Delmar.

Stanik-Hutt, J. (2016). Translation of evidence to improve clinical outcomes. In K. M. White, S. Dudley-Brown., & M. F. Terhaar (Eds.), *Translation of evidence into nursing and health care* (2nd ed., pp. 73–93). New York, NY: Springer Publishing.

Watzlawick, P., Weakland, J. H., & Fisch, R. (1974). *Change: Principles of problem formation and problem resolution.* New York, NY: W. W. Norton.

Witkin, B. R., & Altschuld, J. W. (1995). *Planning and conducting needs assessments: A practical guide.* Thousand Oaks, CA: Sage.

CHAPTER 15

Monitoring Program Implementation

■ STUDY EXERCISES

1. What are the basic principles of the community development model? Describe how the model facilitated program implementation in the case described.
2. In what ways do cultural determinants of care affect monitoring of program implementation?
3. What is the role of the advanced practice public/community health nurse in program implementation and monitoring?
4. What data are used to monitor program implementation?
5. What are the advantages and disadvantages of each type of data?
6. Describe components of successful program implementation.
7. What is the role of assessment in program implementation and monitoring?
8. How can the advanced practice public/community health nurse enhance community involvement in and ownership of programs?
9. How does the concept of social justice apply in monitoring program implementation?
10. What factors affect revisions of the program plan?
11. What strategies influence population-focused nursing care?

This chapter explores the role of the advanced practice public/community health nurse in (a) successfully implementing a program, (b) working with community groups to enhance community involvement and ownership, and (c) revising a program plan. Information about monitoring program implementation is provided through examples from a program developed by a faculty member in collaboration with faculty colleagues.

Throughout the chapter, references are made to the development and evolution of a school-based, nurse-managed clinic in a rural medically underserved and health professional shortage area in Indiana (Indiana State Department of Health [ISDH], 1998). From

---

This chapter was originally written by Dr. Joyce Krothe, professor emeritus, Indiana University, for the first edition of this textbook. It has been retained in this edition with minor changes to content and references because it provides a very important example of the many challenges that advanced public/community health nurses encounter when developing and implementing a new program with the community. References were updated where possible. However, much of the original content remains extremely relevant to program implementation today.

inception, the program was supported with funding from the ISDH through a grant to Indiana University School of Nursing, in addition to local sources of funding. Program development and implementation are described in this chapter.

A community–academic partnership led to the development of the nurse-managed clinic. A community development model, as described by Glick, Hale, Kulbok, and Shettig (1996), was used to establish the nurse-managed clinic, with decision making shared between the community and the advanced practice public/community health nurse, who served as the program director. The mission of the clinic was (a) to provide health-promotion and disease-prevention services to county residents who lacked access to healthcare because of financial barriers and (b) to serve as a setting for clinical education for nursing students.

■ COMPONENTS OF SUCCESSFUL PROGRAM IMPLEMENTATION

Comprehensive assessment is the foundation of any community-based program, an essential component of community development theory, and the key to successful program implementation. Equally important is attention to both initial and ongoing assessment of the community, focusing on community strengths and assets as well as on needs. The reconceptualization of health promotion to include a focus on resources within the community was drawn from the 1986 Ottawa Charter (World Health Organization [WHO], 1986). This case provides an example of a program established by advanced practice public/community health nurses to address the public health core functions of assessment, policy development, and assurance (Institute of Medicine [IOM], 1988; Levin et al., 2008).

Kelly (1996) noted that community care is not simply an altruistic form of care, but a culturally significant endeavor. An understanding of and sensitivity to cultural determinants of care were paramount in implementing the program described in this chapter. Community members played a significant role in all phases of program planning and implementation. Advanced practice public/community health nurses served in the roles of program director, clinic manager, and care provider in the clinic. References to nurse(s) throughout the chapter assume the advanced practice public/community health nursing role defined by the Public Health Nursing Section of the American Public Health Association in 1996 and reaffirmed in 2013. Although the examples included in this chapter are specific to the case described, they have implications for other community-based programs. The implications that relate to the three major subject areas are summarized in the boxes at the end of each major section.

The Community Assessment Process

A thorough initial community assessment using existing data sources, as well as key informant interviews with community members, is foundational to initiation of any community-based program and ultimately is a key factor in program success. This process has been described as population-focused assessment, which includes assessment of the epidemiologic, environmental, biopsychosocial, cultural, spiritual, and technical factors affecting and strengthening the population (Baldwin, Conger, Abegglen, & Hill, 1998).

It is essential to involve community members in the assessment process prior to program implementation and on an ongoing basis. This was especially important in the case described because none of the public/community health nurses resided in the community where the clinic was established and were, therefore, perceived as outsiders. Programs based on an assessment conducted with the full participation of the community are more successful over time than are those based solely on professionally conducted assessments (Association of Community Health Nursing Educators, 1999).

The nursing knowledge necessary for successful program implementation most closely fits the definition of situated knowledge described by SmithBattle, Drake, and Diekemper (1997). In this context, "family narratives and community histories convey meaning and preserve context whereby community health nurses gain an insider perspective and begin to understand how social embeddedness shapes and organizes . . . beliefs, actions, choice, and possibilities" (SmithBattle et al., 1997, p. 81). Situated knowledge is the result of advanced educational preparation and experience in a particular community.

Two Indiana University School of Nursing faculty members conducted an initial community assessment of the county where the nurse-managed clinic was established in 1996. The process included attention to environmental and cultural factors and assessment of community support systems, as well as residents' perceptions of health-related problems in their community. The initial assessment process continued for 6 months and included an in-depth analysis of existing health status data, a survey of community school children's health concerns, and approximately 40 open-ended interviews. The assessment process was initiated by the school nurse for the county school corporation; the nurse had expressed concern about the lack of access to adequate healthcare for uninsured or underinsured school children. This individual served as the initial key informant and the liaison to all other members of the community. Most important, she was a lifelong resident of the community and thus recognized as an insider.

Understanding the concept of insider–outsider status is important to understanding successful program implementation in many communities. The focus community was often described as Appalachian, characterized by considerable pride among residents manifested as an attitude that they can take care of their own problems. The residents were described as independent in nature and resistant to services they do not help plan, but willing to work in partnership with people to support programs that benefit their community (Krothe, Flynn, Ray, & Goodwin, 2000). The residents also were described to have positive attitudes toward nurses as providers of healthcare and toward Indiana University, the recipient of grant funds. These were important factors in establishing a partnership with the community and facilitating the residents' transition to leadership roles.

Chalmers and Bramadat (1996) discussed the Alinsky approach of developing local leaders and helping communities come together around an issue. "Alinsky's success relates in part to the insider relationship leaders have with their communities. . . . Health professionals are generally outsiders to the communities they work with" (p. 722). The nurses in this case remained cognizant of this factor by incorporating local leaders in decision making at every stage in the process.

A suspicion of people considered to be outsiders was frequently expressed during the initial assessment process. Also, because of the close geographic proximity of this community to the university, the community had often been the subject of university-sponsored projects and programs. Several community members indicated that they had often participated in projects without the benefit of understanding how their participation had benefitted the community. Glick et al. (1996) described the "town and gown dichotomy" of towns with universities, which often "sets up an insider/outsider mentality" (p. 48). The authors also referred to the distrust that can result when communities perceive they have been promised a service that the university did not deliver.

Although there was a stated desire to work toward success of the clinic, the advanced practice public/community health nurses sometimes felt they were being tested to see whether they would follow through on their promise to be sensitive to cultural factors when implementing clinic services. This phenomenon is thought to have contributed to the length of time required to establish the clinic and to accomplish the desired population-focused outcomes. Health professionals need to acknowledge their status as outsiders and work in partnership with community insiders to achieve success in program implementation.

Description of the Community and Assessment Data

The community where the nurse-managed clinic was established was well known for the beauty of its rural and recreational areas and thriving tourism industry. Almost 38% of the county was dedicated as public land. However, healthcare resources in the community were limited. There were no tertiary-care facilities in the county and residents traveled to four contiguous counties for hospital or specialty care. There were two primary care physician practices available to county residents; however, neither of them used a sliding-fee scale for payment. Some health services were offered at the local health department.

Many of the residents employed in the county worked for small businesses that did not provide health insurance to employees. Residents without health insurance often waited until they were very sick to seek healthcare and, thereby, used more costly services rather than seeking early or preventive healthcare. "Access to care has become one of the major health issues . . . and rural residents are particularly vulnerable because their communities often lack available and/or accessible services" (Anderko, Uscian, & Robertson, 1999, p. 168). Barriers to healthcare for rural residents have been noted as lack of public transportation, inadequate number of healthcare providers, and providers "who may not be familiar with rural community values and culture" (Alexy & Elnitsky, 1998, p. 3).

SOURCES AND METHODS OF DATA COLLECTION

Interviews with approximately 40 members of the community over 6 months and examination of epidemiologic data about community health status indicators supported the need for more accessible and affordable healthcare for community residents. The decision for a school-based, nurse-managed clinic evolved from the community assessment process. Schools were viewed as community access points and as settings that had wide community support and acceptance. They were thought to foster feelings of neighborhood connectedness, and they were well dispersed geographically throughout the community.

Although other settings, such as churches, were considered, it was the community that chose schools as the best setting for the nurse-managed clinics. This is an important factor in successful program implementation. The community should have a voice in choosing the location where services are provided, because this ultimately will affect program utilization and effectiveness.

The public/community health nurse must always be able to support with research evidence actions taken to address the expressed desires of the community. The historical roots of the movement to secure health services for schoolchildren date to Lillian Wald's initiatives in the early 1900s (Barger, 1996; Bell, 1996). More recent literature supports the fact that school-based health services have been shown to improve access to primary care and to be a cost-effective means of delivering primary care to underserved areas (Keeton, Soleimanpour, & Brindis, 2012).

Several questions were raised in the process of negotiating arrangements to use local schools as clinic sites, for example, the issue of whether the clinics would dispense birth control arose frequently. The liaison with the school nurse for the community proved to be invaluable in resolving such issues. The program director would often defer to her to answer politically charged questions in public forums, such as a school board meeting, understanding that her public support of the program would be valued by community members who recognized her insider status.

COMMUNITY ASSESSMENT FINDINGS

During the assessment process, key informants spoke of the difficulty community residents had traveling to the only town in the area where healthcare services were available. For some, the distance was 40 miles, and, furthermore, the hours that services were available were limited. Many residents left the county for purposes of employment and were unable to access services during regular business hours. Another discovery during the assessment process was the perception that the only town in the county where all available health services were located belonged to the tourists. This perception had not been understood by the program director prior to conducting the community assessment. In fact, it probably would have been the preferred site for locating the clinic had the community not been asked to help decide on the location. Thus, the community had a voice in selecting two schools in remote parts of the county for initial clinic services.

The Essential Role of Timing

Meaningful change takes time, and patience over time is an essential ingredient in successful program implementation. Glick et al. (1996) described patience as a "necessary attribute in developing services that are culturally appropriate and community focused" (p. 49). However, timeliness as defined by the community may not coincide with the provider's definition of time or with the funding agency deadline for reporting program outcomes. A period of years may be necessary for successful program implementation and evaluation.

Allowing sufficient time to establish trust and build rapport with a community is highly individualized but essential if the nurse is to build a collaborative partnership with the community. In one study to identify factors influencing successful program implementation, community health nurses indicated that at least 2 years were necessary to establish a base for community development (Bramadat, Chalmers, & Andrusyszyn, 1996). During this time, the nurse must accept the challenge to design interventions to keep the process moving and avoid stagnation.

Perseverance over time and a willingness to take risks are also essential for successful program implementation. SmithBattle et al. (1997) studied the responsive use of self in public/community health nursing practice. This is a "highly developed skill . . . crucial to developing a partnership between the CHN and the client" (p. 76). A period of years was required to plan and successfully implement the program because of the cultural factors in the community described in this chapter.

FUNDING TIME FRAMES AND PROGRAM OUTCOMES

It may be difficult within a program funding time frame to demonstrate that desired outcomes have been achieved. Successful program implementation requires that funding be available for a long enough period of time to adequately assess outcomes. In the case of the program described in this chapter, 1 year of funding would not have been sufficient to make a measurable difference in health status indicators in the community. Too short a funding period for program implementation may lead to a premature negative evaluation of program outcomes and could jeopardize future funding.

Timing is also an important element in securing funding. In the case described, the ISDH had issued a request for proposals to support the development of nurse-managed clinics in underserved areas of the state to meet the *Healthy People 2000* (U.S. Public Health Service, 1990) health status objectives. The faculty completed the community assessment process at about the same time that the state initiative for nurse-managed clinics and a request for proposals were announced.

Adequate time is essential to operationalize the concept of full community participation. Communities are often recipients of time-limited programs from which they realize few benefits, and they may be reluctant to participate in yet another short-lived intervention. This may have explained the fact that initially some community members expressed reluctance to invest time and energy in establishing the nurse-managed clinic. Although it took considerable time to implement, the community development model employed in this case facilitated gaining community support. Other models may have been implemented in a shorter time frame, but it is doubtful that they would have been able to be sustained over time, given the historical and cultural factors involved.

Factors Affecting Program Implementation and Evaluation

Deciding what programs to initiate requires balancing current health status data with the community's perceptions of what constitutes a problem. For example, in this case, the available health status indicators pointed to hypertension as a significant problem of community residents. However, it became evident that many community residents did not perceive it to be a significant problem. They did not perceive their community to have a greater incidence of hypertension than others.

An instrument was developed to assess clients' knowledge of factors that contribute to hypertension as well as factors that may reduce it. The instrument had been pilot-tested in a similar clinic population and shown to have good reliability. Data from a survey of community residents using this instrument showed that residents often failed to make a link between health behaviors and health status outcomes. Thus, to enhance program outcomes in this area, the nurses worked with clients to increase their understanding of the link between health behavior and health status.

INDICATORS OF PROGRAM SUCCESS

Program success should be viewed from multiple perspectives, including effective use of resources in program implementation. Community members may not understand why all available resources cannot be allocated to direct client services. For example, in this case, questions arose regarding a considerable outlay of resources to purchase software for data collection required by the funding agency. Requirements of funding agencies need to be communicated to community residents in order for them to understand decisions related to resource allocation.

The Role of Communication/Interpersonal Skills

High-level communication skills are essential to building community partnerships. Public/community health nurses need to have effective interpersonal skills at both individual and group levels in negotiating with many different entities, if they are directly involved in healthcare delivery. For example, the suggestion of school sites as the location for the nurse-managed clinics led to negotiations with the superintendent of schools, the school principals, and finally with the board of education for the school corporation. The public/community health nurse must also have the ability to communicate with other stakeholders, including community residents, other healthcare and social service providers, and legislators. "Communication is increasingly important in an era that requires documentation of practice outcomes, efficient use of resources and justification to funders" (Keller, Strohschein, Lia-Hoagberg, & Schaffer, 1998, p. 208).

BOX 15.1 COMPONENTS OF SUCCESSFUL PROGRAM IMPLEMENTATION

Comprehensive community assessment

Full community participation

Effective communication skills

Time and patience

Sensitivity to cultural factors

In one study to identify the knowledge and skills required for expert public/community health nursing, participants identified communication skills, group dynamics, and group facilitation skills as essential (Bramadat et al., 1996). "Mutual collaboration between the nurse and the client depends first and foremost on the client being heard" (SmithBattle et al., 1997, p. 78). The community as a whole is the client for advanced practice public/community health nurses, and the nurse must, therefore, ensure that all sectors of the community are heard.

The skill of listening is an essential component of effective interpersonal skills. "Listening conveys respect, trust, and a fundamental regard for people within a community. . . . The notion of having voice and giving voice to, are central to community empowerment . . . authentic listening is often remarkably absent . . . it is more complex than incorporating listening skills on a one-to-one basis . . . it requires the practitioner to be fully present as a co-learner and co-participant, engaged in participatory dialogue with the community" (Sheilds & Lindsey, 1998, p. 28). In this case, the skill of listening was evidenced in, among many other situations, negotiating clinic sites.

Components of successful program implementation are summarized in Box 15.1.

■ ENHANCING COMMUNITY INVOLVEMENT AND OWNERSHIP

The practice of public health is a team effort consisting of a partnership between the public and committed health professionals (Misener et al., 1997). The focus is on relationships rather than place per se. "A health promotion approach to collaborative partnerships . . . involves doing with rather than doing to . . . clients are not mere objects of professional interventions but full partners in the process" (Cameron & Wren, 1999, p. 96). Community in this context is viewed as a vehicle for change.

Using the Concept of Community as Relationships

Although geographic factors are important contextual variables in program implementation, the concept of community as relationships is paramount. John McKnight, a well-known community organizer, distinguished neighborhood as a geographic place from community as it relates to people and their relationships (Sheilds & Lindsey, 1998). Baldwin et al. (1998) traced the shift from defining community as a geographic entity to the focus on the human relationship aspects of community and population-focused nursing.

Working with community groups to enhance their involvement may require an adjustment of language to satisfy the participants' local culture. Budgen and Cameron (1999) referred to this concept as being "multilingual within English" (p. 282). An example of this relates to how the clinic was named. The community health nurses suggested the name Health Promotion Clinic, but the Community Advisory Board (CAB) for the project believed the concept of promotion might not be well understood in relation to health and, in fact, might be perceived negatively by community members. Therefore, they suggested the name Health Support Clinic, which was adopted. This proved to be an important factor in the community's assuming ownership of the clinic.

Diekemper, SmithBattle, and Drake (1999) described the "intentional" perspective of advanced practice nurses working in population-focused care. This perspective includes what researchers identify as multilingual and multiperspective skills. "Nurses who are intentionally practicing from a much broader perspective on behalf of targeted vulnerable populations" exhibit these skills when working with communities (p. 11). This perspective requires the skills of an advanced practice public/community health nurse who can function at the level of program development and evaluation, as in the case described.

Involving the Community in Program Planning

The term *program planning* "is used to encompass the whole sequence of processes that when performed together produce the program and the desired results" (Wilkey & Gardner, 1999, p. 268). Thus, program planning is process oriented and includes assessment, planning, implementation, and evaluation. In addition, this project included the action/dissemination step described by Flynn and Krothe (2000), which enhanced community involvement and contributed to community ownership. This step entailed communicating research findings to various audiences, such as state and local boards, using the findings from practice to inform health policy makers, and taking actions for social change.

Sheilds and Lindsey (1998) noted that the characterization of communities as interpersonal relationships tends to leave unacknowledged the power relationships that are present in communities. These power relationships must be incorporated in program planning. It has been suggested that to decrease the disparities in power that exist in communities, health professionals should focus on the expertise they can offer in partnership with a community, rather than going into the community as the expert (SmithBattle et al., 1997).

Nursing students who had clinical experiences with the clinic often expressed surprise at the power and politics that operated in this small community. One CAB member, a nurse working for a home care agency in the community, resigned from the board stating that prior to serving on the board she had been unaware of local politics affecting decision making about residents' healthcare. For example, a discussion related to the scope of services the clinic could offer was viewed as usurping the role of the local health department by some board members representing that entity. The nurse who resigned viewed this as detrimental to the good of the community and expressed distress that politics would affect decisions for the common good of community residents. However, when politics are understood in the context of attempting to influence the allocation of scarce resources, it becomes clearer. It is the role of the nurse to reframe the function of politics in program implementation in this context.

Expecting change and remaining flexible are important characteristics when working with diverse community groups, and these skills require experienced community health nurses. Kelly (1996) stated "the delivery of care in diffuse community settings requires a more robust knowledge and skill base to withstand the degree of indeterminacy which is likely to challenge practice" (p. 42).

Involving Nursing Students for Educational Experiences

Advanced public/community health nurses provide population-focused services (Levin et al., 2008). Students at both graduate and undergraduate levels need opportunities to develop the necessary skills for care delivered to aggregates, such as geographic or school communities. Population-focused care is a foundation for the public/community health nurse's distinctive contribution to healthcare (Levin et al., 2008).

Students often have learning experiences in established community health programs and do not understand the complexities involved in planning new programs and building community partnerships. In a discussion of population-focused nursing, Baldwin et al. (1998) pointed out that it is unreasonable to expect master's and doctoral-prepared nurses to become leaders in population-focused nursing without grounding and practice at the baccalaureate level.

"Educators need to ensure that the academic preparation of public health nurses at the graduate level is not too insular and narrow in content" (Misener et al., 1997, p. 48). Students need to develop skills in interdisciplinary and multiagency collaboration and integration of health promotion and research (Jacobson, MacRobert, Leon, & McKennon, 1998). The project described in this chapter incorporated undergraduate students in all phases of program implementation and proved to be an ideal situation for modeling the advanced practice public/community health nursing role.

Students often served as a liaison between the community and advanced practice nurses. Community members were eager to participate in planning the students' clinical learning experiences. They suggested clinical learning sites, served as clinical preceptors, and facilitated learning experiences with other health-related community agencies. This was an important factor in building a partnership with the community.

Mitty and Mezey (1998) discussed collaboration between practice sites and academic nursing programs to prepare advanced practice nurses for community-based practice. The authors noted that when nurse practitioners were first introduced into primary care, their affiliation with academic nursing programs facilitated their acceptance and helped them achieve mutually beneficial goals. The community–academic partnership described in this example has facilitated community acceptance of advanced practice nurses.

Implementing a Community Development Model

Chalmers and Bramadat (1996) described several models of community development:

1. The economic model focuses on increasing community control through economic development. It has not traditionally been associated with nursing, but is relevant when one considers the multiple determinants of health and current marketplace forces. The economic model incorporates involvement in the policy process.
2. The education model focuses on community development through formal and informal educational processes. It operates on the premise that once the community is better developed through education, the community as a whole will benefit. Healthcare providers have historically decided what clients needed to know and delivered it with little input from them.
3. The empowerment model is people centered and emphasizes human and social development.

THE EMPOWERMENT MODEL

Empowerment is a mechanism through which communities gain mastery over their affairs and focus on underlying problems. It is the model most closely aligned with nursing and with the community development model implemented in this case. "Empowerment is linked to both primary healthcare and health promotion. Primary healthcare emphasizes individual and community involvement in health initiatives, collaborative efforts, and egalitarian values" (Chalmers & Bramadat, 1996, p. 723). It is a bottom-up model that builds community competence through intersectoral cooperation, fully mobilizing local initiatives and maximizing resources.

SOCIAL CONTEXT IN HEALTH-PROMOTION ACTIVITIES

Health promotion is not just the responsibility of the health sector; it requires incorporating other social resources within the community. Social context is always considered when implementing a community development model; it ensures that local people are the decision makers. Social context links individual health experiences with housing, education, and transportation, thus recognizing that health promotion is a shared responsibility among various community sectors. Health promotion moves beyond specific individual health risks to include social and personal resources within the context of the community. In a community development model, the community as an aggregate has an identity greater than the sum of individuals. Long-term solutions that promote the greater health of the whole community are considered (Cameron & Wren, 1999).

Chalmers and Bramadat (1996) defined *community development* as the "process of involving a community in the identification and reinforcement of those aspects of everyday life, culture and political activity which are conducive to health" (p. 719). They described issues that arise when public/community health nurses practice within a community development model, for example, the structure of organizations in which nurses work. Despite problems that occur, the authors contend that a community development model is an important mechanism to promote health at the community level.

Wilkey and Gardner (1999) stated that "one of the biggest challenges and most frequent omissions in health programming has been the full participation of the community," noting that many practitioners are not familiar with a partnership model and, therefore, reluctant to relinquish control (p. 268). Full community participation is absolutely essential to implement a community development model.

When programs are established on the basis of a community development model, nurses work to create conditions that enable communities to improve their health. Such activities require full community participation. Care begins and ends with the community rather than with health professionals and requires that professionals relinquish control. The public/community health nurse becomes a partner with the community rather than merely a provider of services to the community.

Examples of Community Development

Consistent with the framework of the community development model, the advanced practice public/community health nurses placed great value on the participation of the community in establishing the nurse-managed clinic. Collaboration among various sectors was absolutely essential given the close community ties and the rural nature of the community. Successful population-based programs require interdisciplinary knowledge and collaboration among agencies at the community level. Successful programs require the public/community health nurse to hire and supervise project staff; manage agency resources; develop coalitions with community organizations, healthcare providers, and business and consumer groups; and design programs that affect health at the aggregate level.

ROLE OF A CAB

A CAB was formed and was instrumental in program developments. The board comprised individuals with lifelong ties to the community who were familiar with the cultural context of healthcare in their community. Members of the CAB for the clinic represented a broad spectrum of the community health and social welfare sectors, including the local school corporation, health and social service providers, and consumers. It is important to mention that consumer participation on the CAB was difficult to achieve and remained a challenge throughout the process.

ROLE OF COMMUNITY HEALTH WORKERS

Traditional healthcare models that foster dependency on professionals fail to acknowledge and build upon the strengths that exist in communities. This program used community health workers to build upon the existing strengths in the community. These individuals were lifelong residents of the community and similar to the families served by the clinic. They helped to bridge sociocultural differences between providers and clients and assisted the providers in gaining entry to the community (Roman, Lindsay, Moore, & Shoemaker, 1999).

Social Justice

Roemer (1999) believed that the main objective of public health should be social justice. This program was developed using a community development model and a definition of health that incorporated social justice. This concept is specific to the specialty of public/community health nursing practice, dating to the very beginnings of public health with the activities of Lillian Wald, when living and working conditions were first recognized as essential to community health and well-being (Barger, 1996). Implicit in the notion of social justice is a responsibility to ensure access to healthcare through program and policy development and implementation. The origins of public/community health nursing dictate that "to be relevant it should be embedded in the continuously evolving social environment" (Association of Community Health Nursing Educators, 1999).

In a discussion of Watson's theory of caring, Sheilds and Lindsey (1998) stated that "if community social justice is a value and an ethic, community nursing must address the underlying sociopolitical elements of practice" (p. 27). Roemer (1999) suggested that it is the human care perspective that is crucial in health systems management and attention to issues of social justice that promotes quality health. Principles of social justice were employed in community determination of needs and implementation of the nurse-managed clinic described in this chapter.

Factors that enhance community involvement and ownership are summarized in Box 15.2.

> **BOX 15.2 ENHANCING COMMUNITY INVOLVEMENT AND OWNERSHIP**
>
> Form community partnerships
>
> Incorporate student learning experiences
>
> Implement a community development model
>
> Base actions on social justice
>
> Address power relationships

■ REVISIONS OF THE PROGRAM PLAN

Kelly (1996) suggested two forces at work in the context of healthcare delivery. The first force is one of moving away from the medical model of healthcare toward a more participatory and broader conception of health, consistent with that proposed at Alma Ata for primary healthcare (WHO, 1978) focusing on outcomes. In contrast, a second force is one of economic concern and limiting spending on healthcare, a task orientation for care. Both forces were experienced in implementing the program described in this chapter and resulted in program revisions. These forces continue to be viewed as highly relevant in the current healthcare environment. They are embodied in the Triple Aim of "better care for individuals, better health for populations, and lower per capita costs" (Institute for Healthcare Improvement [IHI], 2017).

Revisions Related to a Managed Care Environment

The advent of managed care affected public/community health nursing practice in the case described in this chapter. Initially, the program director advocated for a family nurse practitioner to provide clinic services, but the community indicated that it was not ready for this level of provider. However, hospitals in contiguous counties purchased the practices of the two physicians in the community and immediately placed a nurse practitioner in both of them. The community was not consulted for input regarding this decision but began to use nurse practitioner services.

Community members expressed positive comments about the in-depth health education and holistic focus of care provided by the nurse practitioners. As they began to use nurse practitioner services, community members expressed a desire to hire a nurse practitioner for the school-based clinic. The acceptance of an advanced practice public/community health nurse occurred because of contextual variables specific to the managed care environment.

The School of Nursing served as the recipient of grant funds for the nurse-managed clinic, so the university administration became increasingly concerned with issues of liability related to the clinic. The program director was asked to consult with an attorney contracted by the school to review existing documentation for the clinic. This resulted in revisions of several of the data-collection tools. Although entirely understandable from the institution's perspective, this created the need for some additional dialogue and negotiations with the community. For example, the local school board had approved a consent form for treating high school students during the school day. Although the form was modeled on other consent forms used by the school corporation, it did not meet the requirements of the university for protection from liability. Thus, provision of services to school students during regular school hours was suspended until a compromise could be achieved and a consent form acceptable to both groups was approved.

Another example of program revision related to the general consent form for client services. The program director attempted to remain sensitive to the community's request to "keep it simple," while also satisfying the attorney's need for adequate information to protect the School of Nursing and clinic employees from liability claims.

Revisions Related to Clinic Funding and Structure

When clinic services were initiated, the CAB established a nominal per family annual fee for services. They felt strongly that families should not be asked to pay out-of-pocket costs for each visit because grant funding was available. However, a sliding-fee scale was eventually necessary for two reasons. First, the grant funding could not totally support the level of services that had evolved. Second, the initial grant funding had been provided to establish the clinic, with the understanding that the ultimate goal was financial self-sufficiency. Demonstrating a local commitment of funding was important to leverage additional resources for expansion of clinic services. This level of community buy-in was important beyond the actual dollars that were collected.

CAB members began to take the initiative in submitting applications for local funding. This was an important step in the community taking ownership of the program. Requiring evidence of community partnerships as a condition of funding is common. Board members submitted applications for funding to several local organizations, such as the county commissioners and local charities.

Another program revision involved the process the CAB undertook to move to a governing board model. This allowed direct oversight in hiring an executive director, budgetary decisions, and policy development. It was a step in turning over control to the community, and a positive indication of community ownership.

Revisions Related to Client Services

Simpson and King (1999) discussed the factors that must be considered in relation to a community's definition of health. The nurse-managed clinic linked community assessment findings with *Healthy People 2000* and targeted identified priorities of the funding agency. However, services had to be modified to address what community members identified as problems, while also addressing the priorities established by the funding agency. Client priorities may differ from those of the professionals. Program modification in relation to the services provided demonstrates sensitivity to community needs.

ILLNESS-RELATED SERVICES

Decisions related to services must be grounded in the community, with community views receiving priority. Although illness-related services were not the primary focus of the program, they were incorporated on the basis of an identified need voiced by the community. It was unrealistic to think that community residents who lacked access to care would be interested only in health promotion and disease prevention–related services to the exclusion of services to address their immediate health concerns. "It is important to note that a population-based practice does not eliminate the individual levels but integrates all three levels (individual-focused, community-focused, and systems-focused) into public health nursing practice" (Keller et al., 1998, p. 208). Therefore, chronic healthcare needs of the clients were addressed, while using every opportunity to discuss health promotion and disease prevention concepts within the larger context of improving the health of the community.

Service to individuals is recognized as one way of improving population outcomes, with individuals viewed within the context of their families and their environment. However, in this case, the primary focus remained the community at large, for example, increasing immunization levels of preschool children through education, promoting healthy lifestyles, and providing community outreach programs to settings such as a local sock factory and a senior center.

Health indicators were used to identify problems. For example, individuals were treated for hypertension and encouraged to incorporate lifestyle changes, but the focus remained on risk factors in the community. The program director and the nursing students collaborated with the school nurse to conduct mandatory hypertension screening of fourth graders and developed worksheets to be completed with an adult at home. Throughout, the staff was cognizant of the fact that changing behavior is a complex process and extends beyond mere provision of information.

ACTION RESEARCH AS BASIS FOR SERVICE CHANGES

An action research approach (Flynn, Ray, & Rider, 1994) was employed in the school clinics. Action research requires dialogue between the providers (in this case, the nurse researchers) and the participants (in this case, the clients and community members). Identifying culturally based health outcomes is a core competency of the public/community health nursing role (Levin et al., 2008). Community residents helped to define a culturally acceptable method of data collection and also helped to define the research questions. The community health workers assisted in data collection, thus fostering the belief that the information collected was relevant to the success of the nurse-managed clinic.

Several data collection tools were used to monitor program outcomes. One of the tools, a client satisfaction survey, had been developed for a previous study of nurse-managed clinics (Ray, 1997). Although the client populations of the clinics were similar, the clients in the school-based clinics in this case were reluctant to complete the questionnaire. They indicated a preference for open dialogue as a mechanism for input, offering comments such as, "If you really want to know what I think about it, why don't you just ask me?" Their input led to a change in data collection methods. An advanced practice nurse who was not affiliated with the program conducted focus group interviews to collect evaluative data in a narrative format. This proved to be a more effective format for data collection.

Sometimes it is necessary to change the format in which research data are collected to obtain reliable and valid data. Budgen and Cameron (1999) described a diabetes program with aboriginal populations in Canada and noted that efforts to modify questionnaires to the community cultural perspective were not successful in that participants disliked completing questionnaires. Thus, data were collected in face-to-face interviews. A phenomenological method allows nurses to understand the lived experience of others within their cultural context (Budgen & Cameron, 1999).

"Program funders sometimes want greater up-front specification of program goals, timeliness, and quantifiable results than is possible" with a community development model (Wilkey & Gardner, 1999, p. 280). The funding agency in this example was very supportive of the program and extended funding past the original 3-year period. They noted progress made at the community's rate of change and considered the cultural context.

COMMUNITY SUPPORT FOR CHANGE

Funding guidelines must meet the approval of community members. During the third year of state funding, there was an opportunity to apply for a new state initiative to establish a full-service community health center. Although the community stood an excellent chance of receiving funding from this source, the CAB did not approve submitting the application because of their concern that a community health center would be perceived as competing with the local providers. The program director could not proceed with the application without the full support of the community. This was especially important considering the small size of the community, approximately 1,500 residents, and the need to maintain positive relationships with the two existing providers. The board and the project director continued to identify appropriate funding initiatives and to develop other proposals collaboratively.

ACHIEVING CITIZEN PARTICIPATION

Armbruster, Gale, Brady, and Thompson (1999) noted that citizen participation is a requirement of the *Healthy People 2000* (U.S. Public Health Service, 1990) objectives: "broad participation promotes ownership, thereby expanding resources and increasing commitment to long-term health promotion activities" (p. 17). Although consumer input is absolutely essential to successful program implementation, participation by consumers on the CAB was very difficult to achieve and remained an ongoing challenge. Simply designating a percentage of positions for consumer representation on the CAB was not adequate to achieve the desired level of representation. The few consumers on the board were often not comfortable speaking up in large meetings. Strategies to involve them in other ways were employed, such as seeking their input on an individual basis and requesting their participation in ad hoc task forces.

Persistence over time is required to achieve the desired level of consumer representation. Most troubling was reaching those who were most hard to reach, the consumers for whom the services were targeted, in this case the uninsured and underinsured residents of the community. One strategy employed was to identify an individual who had the potential to act as a catalyst to engage others. For example, one client was persuaded to have her picture in the local newspaper. She was the director of a local senior citizens' center and well known in the community. She stated, "I wasn't crazy about everyone knowing I had no insurance . . . but I thought it might help others." She became a member of the CAB and subsequently submitted applications to two community organizations to secure funding for clinic services.

USE OF THE MEDIA

Media advocacy is one political tool that can be directed at those most in need of services and is consistent with the goal of public/community health nursing practice to promote healthy public policy. The local weekly newspaper became an effective way to communicate with the community. All families in the community received an advertisement supplement regardless of whether they subscribed to the newspaper; therefore, this section was used for clinic advertisements. Local interest stories were written by the community health workers and included photographs of community residents. The nurses had to relinquish control of the content and editing of the stories in order to maintain cultural relevance.

MESHING COMMUNITY DESIRES AND PROFESSIONALS GOALS

The funding agency required reporting data in a format that was not always accepted by the community. This situation required modifications in how data were collected and aggregated for purposes of reporting. The data were modified for presentation to the CAB, such as in graph and chart format. Nurses need to be adept at interpreting research findings and program statistics in ways appropriate for multiple audiences, understanding each group's unique need for information.

The majority of care provided by advanced practice public/community health nurses was not reimbursable under insurance; therefore, other payment sources such as grants and direct contracts with employers, city and state governments, and others needed to replace the unavailable insurance revenue (Wilkey & Gardner, 1999). In this case, requests for funding were submitted to the county commissioners, as well as to local boards and foundations, and also requests for donations were made through advertisements in the local newspaper.

The first attempt to secure funding from the county commissioners was not successful, which illustrated the need to increase community awareness of the importance of the clinic on a consistent basis. This had been communicated initially but needed to be ongoing. The CAB discussed strategies to increase community awareness of the program's mission. Many of the county commissioners were not familiar with the purpose of the clinic and its role in affecting community health. Some were not aware of the advanced practice role of public/community health nurses and thought of them in more traditional roles such as home visiting. The board decided to develop a brochure that included photographs of clinic staff and clients to be shared with all potential funding sources.

Although externally identified issues must not preclude attention to community-identified issues, addressing them may enhance opportunities for funding. For example, in the case described, the community did not identify hypertension as a problem, but health status data at the county level indicated it was a significant problem. Addressing hypertension facilitated obtaining initial funding to establish the clinic and, thereby, allowed the nurses to address other community-identified health issues as well.

NURSES BRINGING ABOUT CHANGE

Policy development was identified as one of the public health core functions in the IOM report (1988). "Health promotion broadens the conceptualization of health beyond the health care system and emphasizes the prerequisites needed for health. It requires action in the policy arena" (Chalmers & Bramadat, 1996, p. 722). Contributing to development of legislative policies that support healthy communities requires advocacy on behalf of uninsured and underinsured communities. In this case, the nurses worked to secure an agreement with two hospitals in contiguous counties for diagnostic testing. At the same time, they worked to develop the capacity of this community to become their own advocates by encouraging ways to involve consumers in clinic activities.

Community health promotion requires practitioners to engage in collective action for social change. Development of healthy public policy is a participatory process. Viewing health in a social context requires commitment to social change that will improve health and heighten political awareness and involvement in public policy. Providing leadership in policy making has been identified as an essential competency to provide nursing leadership in public health (Misener et al., 1997).

Key points to consider in program revisions are summarized in Box 15.3.

BOX 15.3 REVISIONS OF THE PROGRAM PLAN

Expect and tolerate flexibility

Incorporate marketplace reform

Balance professional and community priorities

Identify multiple funding options with community support

Communicate program outcomes for multiple audiences

■ SUMMARY

The ultimate goal of program implementation can best be summarized in the following quotation: "Go to the people. Live among them. Start with what they have. Build on what they have. But of the best of leaders. When their task is accomplished. Their work is done. The people all remark. We have done it ourselves" (Budgen & Cameron, 1999, p. 267).

This chapter has used examples from the development of a school-based, nurse-managed clinic to illustrate steps for successful program implementation, the role of working with the community, and revisions in the program plan. A community development model provided the framework for establishing a partnership with the community. Essential to this process was the role of the advanced practice public/community health nurses, the development of a community–academic partnership, and careful attention to the cultural factors involved in healthcare in the community. The core functions of public health, assessment, policy development, and assurance (IOM, 1988) were incorporated into the public/community health nursing interventions described in this chapter.

■ SUGGESTED CLINICAL OR PRACTICUM ACTIVITIES

1. Locate a nurse-managed clinic in a nearby community and meet the director to explore the history of the clinic development.
2. How did the community–academic partnership affect program implementation and monitoring in the nurse-managed clinic?
3. What factors are important in keeping the clinic operating?
4. Obtain permission to talk with clients who receive service at the clinic. Seek their opinions about the service and the care provided by nurses.

REFERENCES

Alexy, B. B., & Elnitsky, C. (1998). Rural mobile health unit: Outcomes. *Public Health Nursing, 15*(1), 3–11.

American Public Health Association. (1996). *The definition and role of public health nursing: A statement of American Public Health Association Public Health Nursing Section.* Washington, DC: Author.

American Public Health Association. (2013). *The definition and practice of public health nursing: A statement of American Public Health Association Public Health Nursing Section.* Washington, DC: Author.

Anderko, L., Uscian, M., & Robertson, J. F. (1999). Improving client outcomes through differentiated practice: A rural nursing center model. *Public Health Nursing, 16*(3), 168–175.

Armbruster, C., Gale, B., Brady, J., & Thompson, N. (1999). Perceived ownership in a community coalition. *Public Health Nursing, 16*(1), 17–22.

Association of Community Health Nursing Educators. (1999). *Essentials of baccalaureate nursing education for entry level community/public health nursing.* Pensacola, FL: Author.

Baldwin, J. H., Conger, C., Abegglen, J. C., & Hill, E. M. (1998). Population-focused and community-based nursing—Moving toward clarification of concepts. *Public Health Nursing, 15*(1), 12–18.

Barger, S. E. (1996). The nursing center: A model of community health nursing practice. In M. Stanhope & J. Lancaster (Eds.), *Community health nursing: Promoting the health of aggregates, families, and individuals* (4th ed., pp. 343–356). St. Louis, MO: Mosby.

Bell, R. (1996). Promoting collaboration in community health nursing. *Nursing & Health Care: Perspectives on Community, 17*(4), 186–188.

Bramadat, I. J., Chalmers, K., & Andrusyszyn, M. A. (1996). Knowledge, skills and experience for community health nursing practice: The perceptions of community nurses, administrators and educators. *Journal of Advanced Nursing, 24*(6), 1224–1233.

Budgen, C., & Cameron, G. (1999). Program planning, implementation and evaluation. In J. E. Hitchcock, P. E. Schubert., & S. A. Thomas (Eds.), *Community health nursing: Caring in action* (pp. 267–300). Albany, NY: Delmar.

Cameron, G., & Wren, A. M. (1999). Reconstructing organizational culture: A process using multiple perspectives. *Public Health Nursing, 16*(2), 96–101.

Chalmers, K. I., & Bramadat, I. J. (1996). Community development: Theoretical and practical issues for community health nursing in Canada. *Journal of Advanced Nursing, 24*(4), 719–726.

Diekemper, M., SmithBattle, L., & Drake, M. A. (1999). Sharpening the focus on populations: An intentional community health nursing approach. *Public Health Nursing, 16*(1), 11–16.

Flynn, B. C., Ray, D. W., & Rider, M. S. (1994). Empowering communities: Action research through healthy cities. *Health Education Quarterly, 21*(3), 395–405.

Flynn, B. C., & Krothe, J. S. (2000). Research applications in community health nursing. In M. Stanhope & J. Lancaster (Eds.), *Community & public health nursing: Promoting the health of aggregates, families, and individuals* (5th ed., pp. 253–265). St. Louis, MO: Mosby.

Glick, D. F., Hale, P. J., Kulbok, P. A., & Shettig, J. (1996). Community development theory: Planning a community nursing center. *Journal of Nursing Administration, 26*(7-8), 44–50.

Indiana State Department of Health. (1998). *MUA/HPSA designation area.* Information Services Commission, Office of Policy & Research. Indianapolis, IN: Author.

Institute for Healthcare Improvement. (2017). *IHI triple aim initiative.* Retrieved from http://www.ihi.org/Engage/Initiatives/TripleAim/Pages/default.aspx

Institute of Medicine. (1988). *The future of public health.* Washington, DC: National Academies Press.

Jacobson, S. F., MacRobert, M., Leon, C., & McKennon, E. (1998). A faculty case management practice: Integrating teaching, service, and research. *Nursing and Health Care Perspectives, 19*(5), 220–223.

Keeton, V., Soleimanpour, S., & Brindis, C. D. (2012). School-based health centers in an era of health care reform: Building on history. *Current Problems in Pediatric and Adolescent Health Care, 42*(6), 132–156. doi:10.1016/j.cppeds.2012.03.002

Keller, L. O., Strohschein, S., Lia-Hoagberg, B., & Schaffer, M. (1998). Population-based public health nursing interventions: A model from practice. *Public Health Nursing, 15*(3), 207–215.

Kelly, A. (1996). The concept of the specialist community nurse. *Journal of Advanced Nursing, 24*(1), 42–52.

Krothe, J. S., Flynn, B., Ray, D., & Goodwin, S. (2000). Community development through faculty practice in a rural nurse-managed clinic. *Public Health Nursing, 17*, 264–272.

Levin, P., Cary, A., Kulbok, P., Leffers, J., Molle, M., & Polivka, B. (2008). Graduate education in public health nursing: At the crossroads. *Public Health Nursing, 25*(2), 176–193.

Misener, T. R., Alexander, J. W., Blaha, A. J., Clarke, P. N., Cover, C. M., Felton, G. M., . . . Sharp, H. F. (1997). National Delphi study to determine competencies for nursing leadership in public health. *Image, 29*(1), 47–51.

Mitty, E., & Mezey, M. (1998). Integrating advanced practice nurses in home care: Recommendations for a teaching home care program. *Nursing and Health Care Perspectives, 19*(6), 264–270.

Ray, D. W. (1997). *Identifying outcome measures in the practice setting: Evaluation research in nurse managed clinics.* Paper presented at the Association of Community Health Nursing Educators Spring Institute, Research Workshop, Vancouver, BC, Canada.

Roemer, M. (1999). Genuine professional doctor of public health the world needs. *Image, 31*(1), 43–44.

Roman, L. A., Lindsay, J. K., Moore, J. S., & Shoemaker, A. L. (1999). Community health workers: Examining the helper therapy principle. *Public Health Nursing, 16*(2), 87–95.

Sheilds, L. E., & Lindsey, A. E. (1998). Community health promotion in nursing practice. *Advances in Nursing Science, 20*(4), 23–36.

Simpson, M. R., & King, M. G. (1999). God brought all these churches together: Issues in developing religion-health partnerships in an Appalachian community. *Public Health Nursing, 16*(1), 41–49.

SmithBattle, L., Drake, M. A., & Diekemper, M. (1997). The responsive use of self in community health nursing practice. *Advances in Nursing Science, 20*(2), 75–89.

U.S. Public Health Service. (1990). *Healthy people 2000.* Washington, DC: U.S. Government Printing Office.

Wilkey, S. F., & Gardner, S. S. (1999). The varied roles of community health nursing. In J. E. Hitchcock, P. E. Schubert., & S. A. Thomas (Eds.), *Community health nursing: Caring in action* (pp. 301–334) Albany, NY: Delmar.

World Health Organization. (1978). *Primary health care.* Report of the International Conference on Primary Health Care Alma-ATA, USSR, 6–12 September 1978. Geneva, Switzerland: Author. Retrieved from apps.who.int/iris/bitstream/10665/39228/1/9241800011.pdf

World Health Organization. (1986). *Ottawa charter for health promotion.* Ottawa, Ontario, Canada: Health and Welfare Canada.

SECTION V

Program Evaluation

CHAPTER 16

Overview of Program Evaluation

■ STUDY EXERCISES

1. What is program evaluation?
2. Why is program evaluation important in advanced public/community health nursing practice?
3. What is the relationship of program evaluation to research?
4. What are the purposes of conducting a program evaluation?
5. Describe the application of the various types of program evaluation models used in public/community health nursing practice.
6. What is the relationship of program evaluation to community assessment and program planning, and to the models presented?

The purpose of this chapter is to introduce program evaluation by discussing the history, definitions, purpose, and importance of evaluation for advanced public/community health nursing practice. This chapter includes models useful for conducting program evaluations and examines the relationship of evaluation to community assessment, program planning, and research.

■ HISTORY

Program evaluation is often thought to be a recent phenomenon, as many people date its beginning to the 1960s when the federal government spent large sums of money to evaluate a wide range of human service programs. However, according to Madaus and Stufflebeam (2000), program evaluation began just prior to the 1900s and has developed through at least six different periods. The periods are the Age of Reform (1800–1900), the Age of Efficiency and Testing (1900–1930), the Tylerian Age (1930–1945), the Age of Innocence (1946–1957), the Age of Development (1958–1972), the Age of Professionalization (1973–1983), and the Age of Expansion and Integration (1983–2000).

The Age of Reform

The Age of Reform was set in the period of the Industrial Revolution in both Great Britain and the United States. It was a time of increased social change and interest in social reform. In both countries, it was a period in time when there was great interest in the reform of both social and educational institutions. The reform of public health, hospitals, orphanages, poor laws, and educational institutions was a priority in Great Britain. Reforms relevant to health during this period included Chadwick's Report on the Sanitary Condition of the Laboring Population of Great Britain conducted in 1842, and the 1882 Royal Commission on Small Pox and Fever Hospitals Study, which concluded that infectious disease hospitals should be open and free for all citizens (Pinker, 1971).

In the United States, Horace Mann was a leader in educational evaluation when, in 1845, he evaluated the Boston schools based on performance testing. Joseph Rice conducted an evaluation of spelling performance in large city school systems between 1887 and 1898; his study was identified as the first educational program evaluation in the United States. The foundation of accreditation evaluation was laid in the late 1800s with the establishment of the North Central Association of Colleges and Secondary Schools (Madaus & Stufflebeam, 2000).

The Age of Efficiency and Testing

The Age of Efficiency and Testing was the period in which attention was focused on investigating localized questions regarding social reform and educational management. Many surveys were used during this period to evaluate school and teacher efficiency. The Department of Educational Investigation and Measurement in the Boston schools developed "objective" tests in arithmetic, spelling, handwriting, and English composition. These tests eventually became norm referenced and were used by teachers to evaluate whether their classes were above or below standard (Madaus & Stufflebeam, 2000). Standardized achievement tests were developed after World War I, and school districts used these tests to measure program effectiveness. Throughout the history of evaluation, tests were closely linked to program evaluation (Stufflebeam & Shinkfield, 1985).

During the same period, the American Public Health Association's Committee on Administrative Practice and Evaluation called for public health officers to begin to engage in improved program planning and evaluation in order to change the methods by which public health programs were begun (Pickett & Hanlon, 1990). Thus, the need for program evaluation that had begun in education was now recognized as a need for programs in healthcare.

The Tylerian Age

The Tylerian Age was named for Ralph W. Tyler, who is often referred to as the father of educational evaluation. Tyler conceptualized evaluation as a comparison of intended outcomes with actual outcomes (Madaus & Stufflebeam, 2000). His approach called for the measurement of behaviorally defined learning outcomes rather than organizational and teaching inputs. Tyler's program evaluations were concerned with outcomes rather than individual test scores, so they were not concerned with the reliability of the differences in scores among students. Tyler's work was so well received throughout American education that his ideas dominated educational evaluation for more than two decades (Stufflebeam & Shinkfield, 1985).

The Age of Innocence

The Age of Innocence occurred just after World War II, when American society was ready to enjoy life. Most Americans had experienced both the Depression and World War II and were ready to expand their capabilities and increase their resources. This was the backdrop for great educational expansion, with building new schools, new programs (the advent of the community college), and new services. However, with all this expansion, society had very little interest in holding educators accountable, identifying and addressing the needs of the underprivileged, or recognizing the problems in the educational system (Madaus & Stufflebeam, 2000). Evaluation continued to be a concern of the local school district, and state and federal agencies had yet to get involved in program evaluation.

Regionalized planning and evaluation for health services were just beginning to be called for in the 1940s when the American Hospital Association established its Committee on Post War Planning in 1944. The federal government's first attempt to legislate health-care planning was through the Hill–Burton Act in 1946 (Pickett & Hanlon, 1990).

The Age of Development

The Age of Development came in abruptly with the Russian launch of Sputnik I in 1957. The U.S. government responded to the launch with the National Defense Act of 1958. This Act provided for new and revitalized programs in mathematics, science, and foreign languages. It increased services for counseling and guidance and increased testing programs within school districts (Madaus & Stufflebeam, 2000). Federal funds also were expanded to evaluate these programs. School districts and teachers found themselves no longer able to decide whether to evaluate their programs as they were mandated to conduct evaluations. However, for all the work that was now required, they found that their work was not accomplishing the task of evaluation. Cronbach, in a landmark article in 1963, counseled educational evaluators to reconceptualize evaluation as "a process of gathering and reporting information that could help guide curriculum development" (as cited in Stufflebeam & Shinkfield, 1985, p. 20). Many new models of program evaluation resulted from this period. "These conceptualizations recognized the need to evaluate goals, look at inputs, examine implementation and delivery of services, as well as measure intended and unintended outcomes of the program" (Stufflebeam & Shinkfield, 1985, p. 22).

In healthcare, the same expansion of programs was seen. State governments were given the authority to plan mental health programs to meet population needs through the Community Mental Health Centers Act of 1963 (PL.88–464). The Office of Health Planning was established in 1966 as part of the Department of Health, Education, and Welfare (now the Department of Health and Human Services).

The Age of Professionalization

The Age of Professionalization ushered in the emergence of evaluation as a profession in and of itself. It was found to be related to, but distinct from, research and testing. Questions regarding the education and qualifications of evaluators were abundant. Those who were doing evaluation realized that the methods used in evaluation to achieve results were seen as peripheral to serious research. However, they served the informational needs of clients and dealt with the realities of the situation (Madaus & Stufflebeam, 2000).

The Age of Expansion and Integration

The Age of Expansion and Integration corresponded to the Reagan years and was marked initially by decreased funding of evaluation. However, the field of evaluation expanded and became more integrated with economic growth. One sign of this expansion was the proliferation of program evaluation societies and journals, both nationally and internationally. Evaluation networks from education and evaluation research societies from the social sciences merged, facilitating integration and exchange of evaluation ideas and methods across disciplines. Although the area of program evaluation experienced dynamic expansion, the evidence base for evaluation impact and outcomes in education and human services was limited. The ultimate value of program evaluation is in its "actual and potential contributions to improving learning, teaching and administration, health care and health, and in general the quality of life of in our society and others" (Madaus & Stufflebeam, 2000, p. 18).

■ DEFINITIONS OF PROGRAM EVALUATION

Program evaluation has had many definitions as it has been developed over the last 150 years and is often defined in relation to the setting in which it is used. However, throughout the years and across settings, these definitions have remained consistent as can be seen by the following:

Education focus: "Evaluation is the collection and use of information to make decisions about the educational program" (Cronbach, 1963, p. 672).

Program focus: Program evaluation is a process of making reasonable judgments about program effort, effectiveness, efficiency, and adequacy. It is based on systematic data collection and analysis. It is designed for use in program management, external accountability, and future planning. It is focused especially on accessibility, acceptability, awareness, availability, comprehensiveness, continuity, integration, and cost of services (Attkisson, Hargreaves, Horowitz, & Sorenson, 1978, p. 242).

"Program evaluation is the systematic collection of information about the activities, characteristics, and outcomes of programs for use by specific people to reduce uncertainties, improve effectiveness, and make decisions with regard to what those programs are doing and effecting" (Patton, 1986, p. 14).

Program evaluation is a diligent investigation of a program's characteristics and merits. Its purpose is to provide information on the effectiveness of projects so as to optimize the outcomes, efficiency, and quality of healthcare. Evaluations can analyze a program's structure, activities, and organization and examine its political and social environments. They can also appraise the achievement of a project's goals and objectives and the extent of its impact and costs (Fink, 1999, p. 3).

Objective focus: Evaluation is the process of determining the degree to which an objective of a program or procedure has been completed or met. It usually includes a review of the objectives, and establishing the criteria used to measure the degree of success. Evaluation includes the process of comparing an object of interest with an acceptable standard, as well as concern for effectiveness, efficiency, and quality of activities, and performance (Timmreck, 1995, p. 180).

Outcome focus: Schalock provided a definition of outcome-based evaluation as a type of evaluation that uses person- and organization-referenced outcomes to determine current and desired person- and program-referenced outcomes and their use (*program evaluation*), the extent to which a program meets its goals and objectives (*effectiveness evaluation*), whether a program made a difference compared to either no program or an alternative program (*impact evaluation*), or the equity, efficiency, or effectiveness of policy outcomes (*policy evaluation*) (Schalock, 2001, p. 6).

Commonalities of Definitions

These definitions have the following commonalities:

1. They involve the systematic collection of information about the activities, characteristics, and outcomes of programs.
2. They use of the information to make decisions regarding program improvement and effectiveness.

■ THE RELATIONSHIP OF PROGRAM EVALUATION TO RESEARCH

Although similar to research, program evaluation is not the same as basic research. Basic research is conclusion oriented and conducted to discover new knowledge and to test hypotheses and theories. Program evaluation is decision oriented and is conducted to inform program planners and decision makers about the effectiveness and efficiency of programs while contributing to increased accountability and continuous improvement (Schalock, 2001). Table 16.1 depicts a comparison between research and program evaluation (Issel, 2009; Weiss, 1972).

Evaluation and Advanced Practice

For the advanced practice public/community health nurse, program evaluation must be acknowledged as a professional responsibility. As healthcare dollars continue to be limited and healthcare consumers become increasingly more educated, healthcare providers must prove both the effectiveness and efficiency of programs to garner scarce healthcare dollars. Program evaluation allows the advanced practice nurse in public/community health to document where, how, and under what conditions specific interventions or programs make a difference. This assertion is supported by a logical and rational argument that is supported, in turn, by systematic procedures and methodologies for collecting objective evidence to reach evaluation conclusions.

TABLE 16.1 Summary of How Evaluation and Research Are Alike and Different

Feature	Evaluation	Research
Purpose	Assess program effectiveness, inform decision makers, contribute to continuous quality improvement	Generate new knowledge, test hypotheses and theories
Measures	Qualitative and quantitative measures or instruments that may be program specific	Qualitative and quantitative instruments, usually with established validity and reliability
Outcomes	Specific to program objectives; may be compared with other programs or national objectives	Generalizable if design meets criteria
Primary audience	Stakeholders, for example, community members, agency administrators, funding agencies, and others who make decisions about programs	Scientific and academic communities

Sources: Issel, L. M. (2009). *Health program planning and evaluation: A practical, systematic approach for community health* (2nd ed.). Boston, MA: Jones & Bartlett; Weiss, C. H. (1972). *Evaluation research: Methods for assessing program effectiveness.* Englewood Cliffs, NJ: Prentice Hall.

Evaluation research is also the responsibility of the advanced practice public/community health nurse (APHN). It requires the nurse to use the knowledge and competencies from the disciplines of epidemiology, administration, research methods, and political science to address the critical question: "Does this program, treatment, or intervention make a difference?" Evaluation research refers to the process of collecting and analyzing data that increase the ability of the researcher to prove rather than to assert findings.

Evaluation research frequently requires the consent of participants; thus, the APHN in public/community health nursing has the ethical responsibility to inform participants of the risks and benefits of their participation. Evaluation research is a specific form of research with the primary goal of testing the application of knowledge rather than the discovery of new knowledge. Both evaluation and evaluation research are integral parts of the advanced practice role in public/community health nursing.

▪ PURPOSES OF PROGRAM EVALUATION

Program evaluations are conducted for the main purposes of identifying problems and limitations as the program progresses and for assessing program accomplishments. Although the staff involved in program implementation does not always welcome program evaluation, it is as important as program planning and implementation.

Reasons for Conducting a Program Evaluation

Although the major purposes of conducting program evaluations are clear, the reasons for conducting program evaluations are numerous and not always clearly stated. At times, individuals or groups who are opposed to a program's existence may call for a program evaluation. Other reasons for program evaluations may have political undertones but may be publicly stated as a means of showing accountability. The APHN should be aware that program evaluation may serve one purpose but be conducted for many reasons.

The following are possible reasons for conducting a program evaluation:

1. To demonstrate that the program is meeting the identified goals and objectives
2. To determine whether the program's outcomes are in line with the goals and objectives
3. To determine whether the identified need(s) for which the program was designed is being met (or has not changed)
4. To justify current or projected expenditures (e.g., personnel, equipment, workflow, supplies)
5. To determine the costs of the program in terms of money, people, and/or time spent
6. To see whether the identified timeline is on target
7. To determine whether priorities are set correctly and meet the needs of the project and organization
8. To obtain evidence that demonstrates the effectiveness of the program
9. To gain support to expand the program
10. To compare different types of programs regarding methods, effects, and/or cost

Although the preceding list gives many reasons for conducting a program evaluation, the primary purpose of evaluation is to assess the outcomes that can be determined to be a result of the program.

■ MODELS TO GUIDE PROGRAM EVALUATION

APHNs use a variety of program evaluation models. Time and space do not allow for a comprehensive listing. Four models chosen as exemplars in this introductory chapter are Donabedian's (1966) paradigm, Stufflebeam's (2000) Improvement-Oriented Evaluation (context, input, process, product—CIPP), Green's (1999) PRECEDE–PROCEED model, and *Public Health Nursing: Scope and Standards of Practice* (American Nurses Association [ANA], 2013). Each model is presented with a brief discussion of its advantages and limitations of each. Other evaluation models are discussed in Chapters 17 and 18.

Donabedian's Paradigm

The Donabedian paradigm was originally adapted from educational evaluation and developed for analyzing the quality of medical care (Donabedian, 1966). Donabedian used the components of structure, process, and outcome as they related to ensuring the quality of medical care. Although it was originally developed as a quality-assurance model, the Donabedian paradigm was easily adapted to program evaluation as programs can be evaluated in terms of structure, process, and outcome. The model's relevance and direct applicability to the evaluation of the quality of nursing care have also been acknowledged (Bloch, 1975; Dachelet, 1984; Donabedian, 1969).

STRUCTURE COMPONENT

The structure component of the paradigm identifies the administrative and organizational structure of a program. The evaluation of structure includes examination of the following program elements: the organizational chart, the credentials of the staff members, the size of the staff to effectively run the program, the adequacy of the physical facility and equipment, the fiscal resources, and the ability of the program to relate to programs within the organization and the community. The underlying assumption of the evaluation of the structure is that if a program is well organized, competently staffed, well equipped in an appropriate facility, and fiscally stable, and has a focused program, the structure is in place for good outcomes to occur. The advantage of the structure component of the Donabedian paradigm is that it is concrete and the information is often readily available. Its major limitation is that the cause–effect relationship is poorly established between structure and outcome.

PROCESS COMPONENT

The process component of Donabedian's paradigm relies on counts of program activities and on what the program does. The original definition of *process* was based on what health-care professionals do when providing quality care. The evaluation of the process component includes data such as number of visits made, number of group sessions conducted, number of activities completed, and number of clients seen. These data are often obtained from clinical records, appointment logs, billing records, and activity reports (Dachelet, 1984). The process evaluation component assumes that if an adequate amount of effort is expended, then adequate results will be achieved. It, therefore, requires that a consensus be determined regarding what is considered poor, fair, adequate, good, or excellent before the evaluation process begins. The advantage of process evaluation is that the data are often both countable and easily accessible. The limitation of process evaluation is that there often is a tenuous relationship between what is good process and what is good outcome. However, research findings are providing data to determine what effective process is and what it is not.

OUTCOME COMPONENT

The outcome component of the paradigm relies on evaluation based on outcomes. Program evaluation based on outcomes measures results of the project or program. For advanced public/community health nursing practice, this component is often used to measure the health status of individuals, families, groups, or populations who participated in the program. Program goals for healthcare are usually written in terms of how the recipients of the program will improve their health. The advantage of this component of the paradigm is that outcome studies provide data on the extent to which the program achieved its identified goals. The limitations for using this method are that these studies often require evaluation research methodology, which requires rigorous research designs, financial resources and time, and valid and reliable methods of evaluation of health status that are often not available for all areas of study.

Stufflebeam's CIPP Model

Stufflebeam conceptualized the CIPP Model (context, input, process, product) as an educational evaluation model to assist school districts to evaluate programs that were funded by the Elementary and Secondary Education Act of 1965. Although the purpose of this Act was to provide funds to school districts across the United States to improve the education of disadvantaged students and to upgrade the system of elementary and secondary education, it also required educators to evaluate their funded projects (Stufflebeam & Shinkfield, 1985). The CIPP Model provides a system view, whether it is in education, human services, or healthcare. The model is based on the view that the most important purpose of evaluation is not to prove but to improve. In this model, evaluation is seen as a tool by which to help programs work better for the people they are intended to serve (Stufflebeam & Shinkfield, 1985). The CIPP Model is composed of four types of evaluation: context, input, process, and product.

CONTEXT EVALUATION

The purpose of context evaluation is to identify the strengths and weaknesses of some object, such as an organization, program, target population, or person, to provide direction for improvement (Stufflebeam & Shinkfield, 1985). The objectives of context evaluation are as follows:

1. Define the institutional context; identify the target population and assess their needs.
2. Identify opportunities to address the identified need; diagnose the problems that underlie the need.
3. Determine whether the proposed program objectives are sufficient to meet the assessed need (Stufflebeam & Shinkfield, 1985).

The methods used for context evaluation include survey development and analysis, needs assessment, document review, hearings, and the use of the Delphi technique (Stufflebeam & Shinkfield, 1985). The assessment of the population to be evaluated can range from individual clients of the healthcare organization to the healthcare facility itself (e.g., a rural clinic, the home care division of a health department) to an aggregate served by the healthcare organization (e.g., pregnant adolescents, senior citizens).

The evaluator needs to investigate prior interventions and their outcomes, review previously developed programs, and determine the anticipated duration of the program, what resources are available, and the cost–benefit ratios. Information gathering on these topics should go on throughout the context evaluation, and at the end of context evaluation, a diagnosis should be generated. The information collected during the context evaluation should then serve as a guide to the development of an activity, which might be a health education offering, a research project, or a new program to be offered by the organization (Kennedy-Malone, 1996). The outcome of context evaluation should be that priorities for the program or project are established.

INPUT EVALUATION

The purpose of input evaluation is to help prescribe a program to bring about needed change (Stufflebeam & Shinkfield, 1985). The objectives of input evaluation are to identify and assess the system's capabilities, alternative program strategies, procedural designs for implementation, budgetary needs, and time schedules.

Methods used during an input evaluation include an extensive review of the literature regarding programs developed in other settings that have successfully met needs similar to the ones identified during the context evaluation; visitation to similar program sites; identification of staff and material resources in the agency or from the larger community; and procedural designs for relevance, feasibility, and economy (Stufflebeam & Shinkfield, 1985). Pilot programs and/or research trials may need to be conducted to test the design, relevance, and cost-effectiveness of the program.

During this type of evaluation, the APHN may consult with outside experts or even make site visits to other successful programs. She or he will often ask nurses employed in the agency what their experiences have been when a new program or project has been started. Budget departments and program planners must also be involved to ensure program accountability. From these individuals, the nurse will develop a team that will prepare the program plans for presentation. Well-developed plans for a cost-effective and relevant program should be the result of input evaluation (Kennedy-Malone, 1996).

PROCESS EVALUATION

The purpose of process evaluation is to provide an ongoing check of the implementation of the plan. The objectives of process evaluation are to identify or predict in the process of implementation any defects or problems with the design or implementation, to provide information for any preprogrammed decisions, and to keep a record of ongoing activities and events (Kennedy-Malone, 1996; Stufflebeam & Shinkfield, 1985). In other words, process evaluation is the method for checking on the implementation of the program or project. Stufflebeam stated that the lynchpin of a sound process evaluation is the process evaluator (Stufflebeam & Shinkfield, 1985).

To implement these objectives, the project evaluator needs to accomplish the following activities:

1. Develop advisory committees composed of community residents who are interested and involved with the community that the program or project intends to serve (e.g., members of Planned Parenthood, a local teen center, high school health teachers, and community center personnel for a teen pregnancy prevention program).
2. Ask the advisory committee for feedback throughout the planning phase of the project. Advisory committee members can also serve as possible referral sources for the program.
3. Document ongoing activities (such as contracts, client responses to the program, time spent by staff, cost of supplies) as these activities are an important part of

process evaluation. These records may assist program personnel to support the continuation of the program or project; they will also assist in building a case to add personnel.

If a program is successful, accurate records from the stage of process evaluation will assist and encourage others to develop similar programs (Stufflebeam & Shinkfield, 1985). The outcome of this stage of process evaluation is that the program is implemented and refined (Kahn et al., 2014; Kennedy-Malone, 1996).

PRODUCT EVALUATION

The final stage of the CIPP Model is product evaluation. Its purpose is to measure, interpret, and judge the attainments of the program. The objectives of product evaluation are to relate outcome information to the program or project objectives and to context, input, and process information (Stufflebeam & Shinkfield, 1985). Stufflebeam (2000) stated that it is a re-evaluation or recycling of information. Methods used for product evaluation include the comparison of program or project outcome to some type of national standard or established criteria; the reporting of product evaluation findings to consumers of the program or project, advisory board members, and supervisory and key personnel of the agency supporting the new program or project; and identification and reporting of program or project cost-effectiveness. The outcome of this stage of evaluation is the report of the program or project on which the decision to continue the program or project will be based.

A full implementation of the CIPP Model addresses the following questions:

- What needs were addressed, how pervasive and important were they, and to what extent were the project's objectives reflective of assessed needs (addressed by context information)?
- What procedural, staffing, and budgeting plan was adopted to address the needs; what alternatives were considered; why was it chosen over them; and to what extent was it a reasonable, potentially successful, and cost-effective proposal for meeting the assessed needs (addressed by input information)?
- To what extent was the project plan implemented, and how and for what reasons did it have to be modified (addressed by input information)?
- What results—positive and negative, as well as intended and unintended—were observed, how did the various stakeholders judge the worth and merit of the outcomes, and to what extent were the needs of the target population met (product information) (Stufflebeam & Shinkfield, 1985)?

In conclusion, the CIPP Model uses a continuous process of context evaluation with input, process, and product evaluation on an "as-needed" basis. The evaluator continuously examines the program milieu while intermittently focusing on all factors brought to the situation by participants, all ongoing activities, and all consequences of the program as the need arises (Sarnecky, 1990). The four types of evaluation used by the CIPP Model (context, input, process, and product) can be used to assess programs in the planning stage as well as programs that have already been developed and implemented.

The PRECEDE–PROCEED Framework

The PRECEDE–PROCEED framework was developed in the 1970s as a systematic planning process to enhance the quality of health education interventions. The acronym PRECEDE, the original part of the framework, stands for predisposing, reinforcing, and enabling constructs in educational diagnosis and evaluation. The PRECEDE part of the model was based on the idea that an educational diagnosis should precede an intervention plan, comparable to how a nursing diagnosis precedes a nursing treatment plan and intervention. The term *diagnosis* was used in the original model to describe each phase of the PRECEDE planning process. Although the authors continue to state that diagnosis is still an appropriate term to describe the process in each phase, the term is associated with clinical procedures and is problem oriented. Thus, the term *diagnosis* used in the original model has been changed to *assessment* in the 1999 revised model as it is a positive approach that focuses "on aspirations and strengths, not just on needs, weaknesses, deficits, problems, and barriers" (Green & Kreuter, 1999, p. 34).

The PROCEED (policy, regulatory, and organizational constructs in educational and environmental development) part of the model was added in 1991. It was added because it became evident that the emergence of and need for health-promotion interventions went beyond what was considered the traditional approaches to changing unhealthy behaviors (Green & Kreuter, 1991, 1999). In 2005, the model was revised to include ecological and participatory approaches and incorporate new knowledge from genetics (Green & Kreuter, 2005).

The revised PRECEDE–PROCEED model is an eight-phase process that can be used as either a conceptual framework for practice or a planning model. Brief descriptions of each of the first five phases of the framework are given as an overview as each of these phases supports the evaluation phases. The evaluation part of the model is the final three phases: process, impact, and outcome.

SOCIAL ASSESSMENT

The purpose of the social assessment, phase 1, is to determine perceptions of people regarding their own needs and quality of life. Multiple data sources are used to collect information, including interviews with key informants, focus groups with community members, windshield observations, and surveys. A program relevant to the identified population can be designed by understanding the community's concerns.

EPIDEMIOLOGICAL, BEHAVIORAL, AND ENVIRONMENTAL ASSESSMENT

Phase 2 assists program planners to identify which health problems are the most important for the targeted population or aggregate within the community. The epidemiological assessment uses the analysis of secondary data, as well as existing data sources, such as vital statistics, state and national health surveys, medical records, and registries, to provide indicators of morbidity and mortality within the population. Genetics is part of the revised model. These indicators assist the planners to specify aggregates within the population who are at high risk (Green & Kreuter, 2005).

During phase 2, the planner sets priorities and develops program goals. Decisions for setting these priorities should be guided by the desires of community members, health problems with the greatest impact, and those for which solutions are available. The outcome of phase 2 should be a goal statement of the program's benefits and measurable objectives that answer questions such as: "Who will do how much of what by when? How much of what—for instance, conditions, circumstances, policies—will be changed by when?" (Gielen, McDonald, Gary, & Bone, 2008, p. 410).

The purpose of the behavioral and environmental assessment in phase 2 is to identify the behavioral and environmental risk factors that relate to the health problems selected during the epidemiological assessment phase. The behavioral risk factors are those lifestyle behaviors that place individuals at risk and contribute to both the occurrence and the severity of the health problem. The environmental risk factors are the physical and social factors that are external to individuals and most frequently outside their control (Green & Kreuter, 2005).

Once all the behavioral and environmental risk factors are identified, each factor should be rated on relevance and association to the health problem. The factors should also be rated on their ability to be changed. Targets for intervention are then chosen based on the ratings of each factor. Phase 2 is completed by the development of measurable objectives written to specify either the desired behavioral effect or environmental change.

EDUCATIONAL AND ECOLOGICAL ASSESSMENT

During phase 3, the educational and ecological assessment phase, the predisposing, reinforcing, and enabling factors are identified (Green & Kreuter, 2005). These factors both initiate and sustain the change process and predict the likelihood that the behavioral and environmental changes will occur. Predisposing factors are those that provide the rationale and/or the motivation for a behavior and may include the person's feelings of self-efficacy, knowledge level, attitudes about the subject, personal preference, and abilities. Reinforcing factors are those that have previously given the person either reward or positive incentives to continue the behavior and may include support of a significant other, influence of peers, or external rewards (e.g., a raise or promotion). Enabling factors precede the change and support and/or allow the motivation to be realized and can affect behavior either directly or indirectly. Programs to build new skills needed for behavior change, services to support the change, and resources to support the behavioral and environmental outcomes are enabling factors (Gielen et al., 2008).

As in phase 2, the predisposing, reinforcing, and enabling factors should be rated in terms of importance and capacity for change, after which priority targets for interventions are identified. At the end of phase 3, measurable objectives must be written to identify (a) how many clients/patients will know, believe, or be able to demonstrate the identified change by a certain point in time; and (b) what type of resources (money, in-kind services, collaboration of community agencies) will be available to whom (agency, person, or group) by what point in time. This process is built on a thorough knowledge base of the current literature, an understanding of an appropriate theoretical base, and information from the target population (Green & Kreuter, 2005). A good example of the use of this phase of the model is seen in the work of Smith, Danis, and Helmick (1998) presented in Box 16.1.

BOX 16.1   EXAMPLES OF PREDISPOSING, REINFORCING, AND ENABLING FACTORS

Gielen et al. (2001), in their randomized trial of enhanced anticipatory guidance for infant injury prevention, identified predisposing, reinforcing, and enabling factors from parent interviews. The authors identified a *predisposing factor* of extremely favorable attitudes of parents toward childproofing. *Reinforcing factors* were identified as routine injury-prevention counseling by pediatricians and social support networks that felt childproofing was important. The *enabling factors* identified by them were access to safety supplies and skills or assistance to use the supplies effectively.

ADMINISTRATIVE AND POLICY ASSESSMENT AND INTERVENTION ALIGNMENT

Phase 4 of the PRECEDE–PROCEED model is identified as the phase of administrative and policy assessment and intervention alignment. The purpose of this phase is to delineate the intervention strategies and make final plans for their implementation. During this phase, the policies, resources, and circumstances that are needed for implementation and sustainability are identified. The intervention strategies are based on phase 3 development, and the necessary resources (such as time, people, or money) are identified as to their accessibility and availability. Barriers to implementation must be assessed and addressed during this phase. Organizational policies and/or regulations that might affect implementation must also be identified and planned for during this phase; in addition, resource limitations, staff abilities, and time constraints are also assessed (Green & Kreuter, 2005).

IMPLEMENTATION

Phase 5 of the model is implementation. Little detail is discussed about implementation. Green and Kreuter stated that the phase of implementation merges with the stages of evaluation as monitoring the implementation process is the first step in process evaluation. They went on to state that the necessary ingredients of implementation are a good plan, an adequate budget, good organizational and policy support, good training and supervision of staff, good monitoring in the process evaluation stage, experience, sensitivity to people's needs, flexibility, an eye fixed on long-term goals, and a sense of humor (Green & Kreuter, 2005).

PROCESS EVALUATION

Phase 6 is the phase of process evaluation. This is the first stage in the evaluation process as it is often the first type of information available. During this phase of evaluation, all program inputs, activities, and reactions of the stakeholders are examined. Process evaluation is also used to examine to what extent the intervention was implemented according to protocol or guidelines. Program goals and objectives are examined to make sure they are plausible and specific to the project. Resources are examined to see whether they are adequate. Stakeholders (e.g., board members and recipients of the program) are asked to evaluate the program plans.

The critical products of process evaluation are a descriptive picture of the quality of the elements of the program that is being implemented and a measurement of what is going on as the program proceeds (Green & Kreuter, 2005). Process evaluation measures what the program does and assumes that if a certain amount of effort is expended, then certain results will be achieved. To do this, however, a consensus is required on what amount of effort represents a good performance. Examples of the type of process evaluation data reported are number of group sessions conducted, number of people counseled, and number of home visits made. This type of evaluation is often referred to as *formative evaluation*.

IMPACT EVALUATION

Phase 7 of the PRECEDE–PROCEED model is impact evaluation. Impact evaluation is the second level of evaluation in the model and addresses the immediate effect the program has on behaviors targeted for change. Impact evaluation also measures the effect the program has on the predisposing, reinforcing, and enabling factors. The clarity, specificity, and plausibility of the behavioral and educational objectives developed in phase 2 (epidemiological, behavioral, and environmental assessment) and phase 3 (educational and ecological assessment) provide the foundation for evaluating program impact (Green & Kreuter, 2005).

OUTCOME EVALUATION

Outcome evaluation is the focus of phase 8 of the model. Health status and quality-of-life indicators designed in the early phases of the model now become important for measuring program outcomes. These measures are usually identified in terms of pregnancy rates, immunization rates, disease and disability rates, and mortality rates. Social indicators usually include unemployment rates, school dropout rates, homelessness, and elderly persons living independently.

Outcome evaluation is the essential element of evaluation research. The ability to detect changes with either impact or outcome evaluation is dependent on the specificity of the standards, the precision of measurement, the size of the desired effect, and the size of the population on which the measures are taken (Green & Kreuter, 2005). Outcome evaluation provides direct data on the extent to which objectives of the program were achieved.

Standards of Public Health Nursing Practice

The final evaluation model to be discussed in this chapter is not really a model but standards of practice for public health nursing. *Public Health Nursing: Scope and Standards of Practice* (ANA, 2013) is useful to public health and community health nurses at the baccalaureate and master's level to validate the quality of and/or to improve their practice.

The nurse prepared at the master's or doctoral level is considered a specialist in public health or community health nursing and has the educational background and clinical experience to work with populations on the prevention of disease, injury, and disability and the formulation of health and social policy. The specialist in public health and/or community health nursing also has proficiency in planning, implementing, and evaluating health programs and services (ANA, 2013). Standards 1 through 5 are applicable to community or population assessment and program implementation. As you read them, you will find that they are like three models discussed previously, as they require assessment, diagnosis, outcome identification, planning, and implementation.

Standard 1. Assessment: "The public health nurse collects comprehensive data pertaining to the health status of populations" (ANA, 2013, p. 28). For this standard, the APHN is required to conduct an assessment in partnership with population representatives and in collaboration with other healthcare professionals. The assessment is supported by scientific knowledge and epidemiological methods with consideration of the multiple determinants of health, values, needs, beliefs, and meaning of health of the population (ANA, 2013).

Standard 2. Population Diagnosis and Priorities: "The public health nurse analyzes the assessment data to determine diagnoses or issues" (ANA, 2013, p. 30). For this standard, competencies include that the advanced public/community health nurse will use complex data and information to identify health assets, needs, and risks of populations. The APHN, in partnership with members of the population, formulates population-focused diagnoses and sets priorities (ANA, 2013).

Standard 3. Outcome Identification: "The public health nurse identifies expected outcomes for a plan specific to the population or situation" (ANA, 2013, p. 31). Competencies for the advanced-level nurse focus on the use of scientific evidence. Outcomes are stated in measurable terms and achievable through evidence-based practices. Also, outcomes reflect the incorporation of factors such as cost-effectiveness, continuity of services, and satisfaction of stakeholders (ANA, 2013).

Standard 4. Planning: "The public health nurse develops a plan that prescribes strategies and alternatives to attain expected outcomes" (ANA, 2013, p. 32). For this standard, the advanced-level nurse is expected to apply strategies within the plan that contain evidence, expert nursing knowledge, and public health content. The nurse is also expected to lead the multisector team, participate in integration of resources for the planning process, and contribute to continuous improvement of planning process systems (ANA, 2013).

Standard 5. Implementation: "The public health nurse implements the identified plan" (ANA, 2013, p. 34). Competencies for this standard require that the advanced public/community health nurse interpret surveillance data, incorporate new knowledge and strategies, design solutions to barriers, modify the plan when needed, advocate for needed resources, champion new collaborative relationships, and ensure dissemination of the plan (ANA, 2013).

Standard 6. Evaluation: "The public health nurse evaluates progress toward attainment of outcomes" (ANA, 2013, p. 42). Competencies for this standard direct the advanced-level nurse to design an evaluation with others, including stakeholders and representatives of the population that is the focus of the program. The nurse is also expected to use the results of an evaluation to address needed changes in policy, procedure, programs, or services.

These standards not only identify the competencies for assessment, program planning, implementation, and evaluation, but also set the standard for evaluation of the practice of public/community health nursing.

■ THE RELATIONSHIP OF PROGRAM EVALUATION TO COMMUNITY ASSESSMENT AND PROGRAM PLANNING

As one examines the models of program evaluation, except the Donabedian paradigm, similarities of community assessment, diagnosis, planning, implementation, and evaluation become clear. The Donabedian (1969) paradigm relates only to program evaluation. The standards use the wording of assessment, diagnosis, planning, implementation, and evaluation, so the other two will be cited as they relate to each of the activities.

Community Assessment

Community assessment requires the assessment of the health status of the population via data, resident input, and professional judgment. The standards require the public/community health nurse to do this in partnership with community representatives and other healthcare professionals (ANA, 2013). In the CIPP Model, the operating context must assess needs and opportunities and diagnose problems underlying the needs and opportunities as part of context evaluation. The PRECEDE–PROCEED model, phases 1 and 2 (social; epidemiological, behavioral, and environmental), are the means to assess the population status and needs (Green & Kreuter, 2005).

Diagnosis

Diagnosis requires the analysis of the collected data and attaches meaning to it in partnership with the people. The standards for public/community health nurses require nurses to target populations using a variety of information sources and to identify and prioritize problems that are amenable to public health nursing interventions and agreeable to the population (ANA, 2013). The CIPP Model uses context evaluation methods to diagnose problems underlying the needs and opportunities. The PRECEDE–PROCEED model diagnoses the problem or problems found during phase 3 (educational and ecological assessment) and groups them on the basis of educational and ecological strategies that are likely to be employed in health-promotion programs.

Planning

Planning requires the development or use of evidence-based interventions that will improve the health status of the identified population. Public health nursing standards require the nurse to be involved with policy development, assisting in the development of plans to address health concerns, recommending programs or interventions to meet identified needs, working with policy makers to address the needs of communities, serving as an advocate, providing training and programs to meet identified health needs, and the provision of leadership (ANA, 2013). The CIPP Model moves to input evaluation to meet the requirements of planning. Input evaluation requires the identification and assessment of system capabilities, all available data and strategies, as well as designs for implementing the strategies (Stufflebeam, 2000). The PRECEDE–PROCEED model identifies phase 5 (administrative and policy assessment) as the planning phase. Now the planner is ready in phase 4, having all the organized assessment information and the organizational and administrative capabilities and resources, for the development and implementation of the program (Green & Kreuter, 2005).

Implementation

Implementation provides access and availability of interventions through programs, policies, and services (Green & Kreuter, 2005). Public health nursing standards require the public health nurse to collaborate with other health and human service agencies to provide personnel and services to all people consistent with their needs, monitor and improve both availability and quality of services and providers, and assist communities to implement and evaluate the intervention plans (ANA, 2013).

The CIPP Model does not describe implementation, but designates process evaluation for implementing and refining the program design and procedures. During process evaluation, the evaluator monitors any procedural barriers, collects information for program decisions, and describes the actual process of implementation (Stufflebeam, 2000). Phase 5 (implementation) in the PRECEDE–PROCEED model manages the implementation of the program or project. The PRECEDE part of the model requires that the implementation of the program adapt to changing local circumstances, personalities, opportunities, and feedback from the three phases of evaluation (Green & Kreuter, 2005).

Evaluation

Evaluation monitors the health status of the community on a systematic, ongoing basis. Public health nursing standards require that the nurse continuously and systematically collect data according to both epidemiological and scientific methods to determine the effectiveness of the interventions in relation to the outcomes. The advanced public/community health nurse is also required to collect information to improve existing programs and services (ANA, 2013).

The CIPP Model uses product evaluation to complete this task of the evaluation process. Product evaluation requires the evaluator to relate outcome information to program objectives and to context and process evaluation information. The PROCEED phases 6 through 8 (process, impact, and outcome evaluation) assess the extent to which the program was implemented according to guidelines; changes in predisposing, reinforcing, and enabling factors; and effect of the program on health (Green & Kreuter, 2005). In addition, PROCEED evaluation ensures that the program will be accountable to policy makers, administrators, consumers, or clients who need to know whether the program met their standard of acceptability, accessibility, and accountability.

The Donabedian paradigm uses the evaluation modes of structure, process, and outcome, similarly to the PROCEED model, and the CIPP Model's process, product, and product evaluation components. Donabedian's structure component identifies the administrative and organizational structure of a program, so the process component evaluates data, such as number of visits made, number of group sessions conducted, number of activities completed, and number of clients seen, whereas the outcome component relies on evaluation-based measurement of the outcomes of the program.

■ SUMMARY

In this chapter, the historical background of program evaluation was covered from its educational beginning to its use in healthcare and other social service arenas. Program evaluation was variously defined by different authors from different disciplines. The similarities and differences between evaluation and research were depicted in the text and in Table 16.1. The purposes for conducting program evaluation were delineated, and four models of program evaluation were described. Comparisons between the various models and the process of community assessment, diagnosis, planning, implementation, and evaluation served as the concluding portion of this chapter.

■ SUGGESTED CLINICAL OR PRACTICUM ACTIVITIES

1. Using the aspects of program evaluation presented in this chapter, analyze program evaluation plans at a local health department, state health department, a nonprofit community organization, and/or a local governmental program.
2. In reviewing program evaluation reports, examine limitations of the evaluations and the reports. Discuss with a program evaluator how evaluation plans could be improved.
3. Discuss with an advanced public/community health nurse how evaluation results are used to change and/or improve programs.

REFERENCES

American Nurses Association. (2013). *Public health nursing: Scope and standards of practice* (2nd ed.). Silver Spring, MD: Nursesbooks.org.

Attkisson, C., Hargreaves, W. A., Horowitz, M. J., & Sorenson, E. (Eds.). (1978). *Evaluation of human service programs.* New York, NY: Academic Press.

Bloch, D. (1975). Evaluation of nursing care in terms of process and outcome: Issues in research and quality assurance. *Nursing Research, 24,* 256–263.

Cronbach, L. J. (1963). Course improvement through evaluation. *Teachers College Record, 64,* 672–683.

Dachelet, C. Z. (1984). Program evaluation in community health nursing. In J. A. Sullivan (Ed.), *Directions in community health nursing* (pp. 241–269). Boston, MA: Blackwell.

Donabedian, A. (1966). Evaluating the quality of medical care. *Millbank Memorial Fund Quarterly, 44*, 166–206.

Donabedian, A. (1969). Some issues in evaluating the quality of nursing care. *American Journal of Public Health, 59*, 1833–1836.

Fink, A. (1999). *Evaluation fundamentals: Guiding health programs, research, and policy.* Newbury Park, CA: Sage.

Gielen, A. C., McDonald, E. M., Gary, T. L., & Bone, L. R. (2008). Using the PRECEDE–PROCEED model to apply health behavior theories. In K. Glanz, B. K. Rimer., & K. Viswanath (Eds.), *Health behavior and health education: Theory, research, and practice* (4th ed., pp. 407–433). San Francisco, CA: Jossey-Bass.

Gielen, A. C., Wilson, M. E., McDonald, E. M., Serwint, J. R., Andrews, J. S., Hwang, W. T., & Wang, M. C. (2001). Randomized trial of enhanced anticipatory guidance for injury prevention. *Archives of Pediatrics & Adolescent Medicine, 155*(1), 42–49.

Green, L. W., & Kreuter, M. W. (1991). *Health promotion planning: An educational and environmental approach* (2nd ed.). Mountain View, CA: Mayfield.

Green, L. W., & Kreuter, M. W. (1999). *Health promotion planning: An educational and ecological approach* (3rd ed.). Mountain View, CA: Mayfield.

Green, L. W., & Kreuter, M. W. (2005). *Health promotion planning: An educational and environmental approach* (4th ed.). San Francisco, CA: Jossey-Bass.

Issel, L. M. (2009). *Health program planning and evaluation: A practical, systematic approach for community health* (2nd ed.). Boston, MA: Jones & Bartlett.

Kahn, K. L., Mendel, P., Weinberg, D. A., Leuschner, K. J., Gall, E. M., & Siegel, S. (2014). Approach for conducting the longitudinal program evaluation of the US Department of Health and Human Services national action plan to prevent healthcare-associated infections: Roadmap to elimination. *Medical Care, 52*(2 Suppl. 1), S9–S16. doi:10.1097/MLR.0000000000000030

Kennedy-Malone, L. M. (1996). Evaluation strategies for CNSs: Application of an evaluation model. *Clinical Nurse Specialist, 4*(10), 195–198.

Madaus, G. F., & Stufflebeam, D. L. (2000). Program evaluation: A historical overview. In D. L. Stufflebeam, G. F. Madaus., & T. Kellaghan (Eds.), *Evaluation models: Viewpoints on educational and human services evaluation* (2nd ed., pp. 3–18). Boston, MA: Kluwer Academic Publishers.

Patton, M. Q. (1986). *Utilization-focused evaluation* (2nd ed.). Beverly Hills, CA: Sage.

Pickett, G. E., & Hanlon, J. J. (1990). *Public health administration and practice* (9th ed.). St. Louis, MO: Mosby-Year Book.

Pinker, R. A. (1971). *Social theory and social policy.* London, England: Heinemann Educational Books.

Sarnecky, M. T. (1990). Program evaluation part 1: Four generations of theory. *Nurse Educator, 15*(5), 25–28.

Schalock, R. L. (2001). *Outcome-based evaluation* (2nd ed.). New York, NY: Kluwer Academic/Plenum Publishers.

Smith, P. H., Danis, M., & Helmick, L. (1998). Changing the health care response to battered women: A health education approach. *Family and Community Health, 20*(4), 1–18.

Stufflebeam, D. L. (2000). The CIPP for evaluation. In D. L. Stufflebeam, G. F. Madaus., & T. Kellaghan (Eds.), *Evaluation models: Viewpoints on educational and human services evaluation* (2nd ed., pp. 279–318). Boston, MA: Kluwer Academic Publishers.

Stufflebeam, D., & Shinkfield, A. (1985). *Systematic evaluation.* Boston, MA: Kluwer Nijhoff.

Timmreck, T. C. (1995). *Planning, program development and evaluation.* Boston, MA: Jones & Bartlett.

Weiss, C. H. (1972). *Evaluation research: Methods for assessing program effectiveness.* Englewood Cliffs, NJ: Prentice Hall.

CHAPTER 17

Developing a Program Evaluation Plan

■ STUDY EXERCISES

1. What factors should be considered in delineating evaluation questions?
2. How does one set standards for program evaluation?
3. How are standards operationalized?
4. Discuss issues related to internal and external validity of evaluation designs.
5. Why is it important to collect baseline data for a program evaluation study?
6. What roles do interdisciplinary team members and community residents play in program evaluation studies?

Ideally, a program evaluation plan is developed along with the program and implementation plans. This is not always possible, so the evaluation plan may be written after the other plans, but well before the program is due to begin. The formal program evaluation plan brings together all the ideas and data- collection methods that will be used to detect the program effectiveness as well as projected outcomes of the program. The evaluation plan also identifies the resources needed to carry out the evaluation. In this chapter, you will learn about the components of a program evaluation plan and how such a plan is developed.

■ FOCUSING THE EVALUATION

Program evaluations serve many purposes, for example, appraising the process of delivering services, determining the effectiveness of services, or examining the changes in the population served. There are numerous possibilities for the direction of an evaluation, so it is important to narrow down the focus of the evaluation before taking any other steps. The focus of evaluation should take into account the following:

- The types of information that demonstrate the effects of the program
- The role that evaluation results may have in program operations
- Protection from bias
- The criteria used in the evaluation (Dignan & Carr, 1992; Veney & Kaluzny, 1998)

Shaping the evaluation questions and setting standards provide part of the necessary focus for a program evaluation.

Shaping Evaluation Questions

The evaluation questions determine the direction of the evaluation study by concentrating efforts on the areas most important for the program. Answers to evaluation questions thus provide data about a program's features and merits. Sources of evaluation questions are the program goals and objectives (Fink, 1993). A careful alignment of the evaluation questions with the goals and objectives gives the evaluator more confidence that the evaluation is actually addressing what the program is intended to accomplish.

Evaluation questions also set limits for the evaluation study. All aspects of a program could not possibly be studied, given time constraints and resources, so some limits are required. For example, it is often interesting to know what effect a program had on the participants after the program has ended. It is not usually practical to conduct long-term evaluations because of the amount of resources needed to carry out such studies. Most funding sources would prefer to use resources for new programs or for reaching more people with services. Therefore, most program evaluations must settle for questions that help to determine program effects during or immediately before or after a program has terminated.

Evaluation questions may address several different areas of a program, including participants and program effectiveness; program activities, organization, and effectiveness; program costs; and program environment (Fink, 1993).

EVALUATION QUESTIONS ABOUT PARTICIPANTS AND PROGRAM EFFECTIVENESS

Often the goal of public/community health nursing programs is to reach an underserved population, so a demographic description of the program participants is a key factor in the program evaluation. Answers to questions about age, place of residence, gender, and income level indicate whether the program is reaching the intended audience. Sample questions about participants are as follows:

- What are the demographic characteristics of the program participants?
- Where do the participants reside?

A second key question concerns the effectiveness of the program with various segments of the population. Was the program equally effective with all ages of participants? Were males and females equally able to achieve the projected outcomes? If children were involved, was the program effective across the age range and with both genders? These are some questions that may be answered in an evaluation study.

EVALUATION QUESTIONS ABOUT PROGRAM ACTIVITIES, ORGANIZATION, AND EFFECTIVENESS

Evaluation questions may also address the program's specific activities and organization. These areas require exploration to determine, to the extent possible, what relationship they have to program effectiveness and whether the program may be applicable to other settings.

Although program activities are spelled out in the program plan, it is often the case that the program was not implemented exactly the way it was planned. In addition, changes in personnel, funding, clientele, and the physical plant; external environment events, such as a similar program opening nearby; and other factors may necessitate program changes after implementation. Examples of evaluation questions about program activities and organization are as follows:

- What were the chief activities of the program?
- What changes were made in activities during the implementation of the program?
- How well was the program managed?

EVALUATION QUESTIONS ABOUT PROGRAM COSTS

An evaluation of program costs may be a review of the program's resources, a cost–benefit analysis, or a cost-effectiveness study. Evaluation of program costs may examine the resources used in delivering the program, such as the personnel, equipment, supplies, and facilities to produce the outcomes, such as immunizations or better pregnancy outcomes. A *cost–benefit analysis* examines the relationship between costs and monetary outcomes, such as the amount of dollars saved related to potential healthcare costs. When the examination is of the relationship between costs and substantive outcomes, such as better pregnancy outcomes, the evaluation is termed a *cost-effectiveness study* (Shi & Singh, 2015).

Inclusion of questions about costs in program evaluation is controversial for several reasons. There are numerous difficulties in defining costs and measuring benefits. Analytical methods to answer questions related to cost are not generally agreed upon by experts. If the cost analysis is conducted at the same time as the overall evaluation, the complexity of the evaluation study greatly increases (Fink, 1993).

Another difficulty in cost studies is the long time span often needed to determine any results from the program. For example, if a cardiovascular risk-reduction program is funded for 3 years, an improvement in cardiovascular outcomes, especially death rates, may not be seen because of the limited length of time. Long-term studies are needed to determine long-term outcomes. Thus, a program goal to decrease deaths from cardiovascular disease would probably not be possible to achieve in a 3-year program. On the other hand, shorter term objectives can be measured by the evaluation questions. Sample evaluation questions about program costs are as follows:

- What was the total program budget?
- Was the budget adequate to meet all expenses?
- What was the revenue generated by the program activities?

EVALUATION QUESTIONS ABOUT PROGRAM ENVIRONMENT

The *program environment* includes the agency or institution in which the program takes place as well as the social and political environments external to the agency. The type of agency, its location, and the funding sources are important aspects of the program evaluation. Changes in the social and political environments over the course of a program may also affect program outcomes. For example, changes in health policy, alterations in funding levels, new technology, new medications, and other such innovations may have a great effect on the population being served by the program.

The *internal environment* for the program is a key factor in program performance. Organizational structure, turnover in key staff, recruitment of staff, and organizational support of the program are a few of the areas that should be examined for potential evaluation questions. Although there is overlap between areas of internal environment and program activities and organization, the evaluator may be interested in how an event or change may have influenced program performance in more than one way. For example, another new program in the community might result in changes in the program to be evaluated; also, the changes in the program may have an influence on program effectiveness. Some sample questions about program environment are as follows:

- What changes occurred during the program that may have influenced program effectiveness, for example, staffing changes, changes in funding?
- What, if any, external environment events that occurred during the program may have influenced program effectiveness?

After the evaluation questions are written, the staff who designed and/or will implement the program should review them. Often, the same people write the program plan and the evaluation plan. If different staff are involved in these tasks, this review provides some confirmation that the questions are indeed addressing the content of the program. If there is a change in the program plan, the review provides direction for aligning the evaluation with the altered program.

Setting Evaluation Standards

Standards used in program evaluations are "specific criteria by which effectiveness is measured" (Fink, 1993, p. 25). To be useful, standards must be measurable and are similar to objectives in this dimension. Standards differ from objectives in that standards are quantitative and set levels to be achieved in the program operation. Evaluation standards are often developed on the basis of measureable program objectives. The more specific the standards are, the easier they are to measure. For example, an improvement in the exercise level of participants could be specified as a 20% increase in the amount of time spent each week in activities that improve cardiovascular functioning. The level of exercise would be measured for each participant both before and after the program to determine how many achieved the 20% increase. Then, a summary of the level of achievement for the total group could be determined.

Evaluation questions provide the basis for setting standards. After evaluation questions are written, standards may be determined for what is to be achieved. Standards may be set for structure, process, and outcome components as one way to examine the quality of the care provided in the program. *Structure* refers to the human, physical, and financial resources needed in planning a program, such as staff and their qualifications, equipment, the setting, and how the care is organized. *Process* is the activities carried out by the staff to provide care to the program participants. *Outcomes* are the end results of the care provided, such as physical status, quality of life, and social functioning (Donabedian, 1969).

An example of an evaluation question and related structure, process, and outcome standards are presented in Box 17.1.

Several approaches may be used to set standards. This section addresses four approaches: historical or past performance, research findings, comparisons, and norms or epidemiologic data (Fink, 1993; Timmreck, 2003). There is some overlap among these approaches,

---

BOX 17.1   EXAMPLE OF EVALUATION QUESTION AND RELATED STANDARDS

Evaluation question: To what extent did the community nursing center increase the immunization level of children aged 2 years and younger in the community?

Structure standard: Immunizations will be given to all children regardless of payment source or amount.

Process standard: Immunizations will be administered to all children who present to the nursing center and are not currently in their immunization status.

Outcome standard: A total of 80% of the children seen at the nursing center will be fully immunized at the end of the 6-month period.

but they will be treated individually to illustrate their qualities. Also, it may be desirable to use more than one approach to set various standards.

STANDARDS BASED ON HISTORICAL OR PAST PERFORMANCE

Evaluation of a program's performance may be compared with previous performance or the performance of a similar program. Historical standards are useful for programs that have been functioning for a while and have stabilized in terms of resources and activities. One drawback to historical standards is that the evaluator has little scope of knowing whether the original performance, which forms the basis of the standard, was at the right level. Thus, standards developed on the basis of history may be too low or too high. Examples of standards developed on the basis of history or past performance are presented in Box 17.2.

STANDARDS BASED ON RESEARCH FINDINGS

These types of standards are absolute or theoretical standards that may be unattainable. Often, research findings are achieved under ideal conditions that cannot be obtained and maintained in the real clinical or community settings. Standards developed on the basis of research findings may be useful as long-term goals or as a reminder of the "gold standard." However, unattainable standards may result in lower employee morale because their efforts, no matter how intense, may not produce the level specified in the standard.

Examples of standards developed on the basis of research findings are as follows:

- The number of children aged 6 months through 5 years with blood-lead levels exceeding 5 mcg/dL will be zero.
- The mean serum cholesterol level among adults aged 20 through 74 will be no more than 200 mg/dL.

BOX 17.2   EXAMPLES OF STANDARDS BASED ON HISTORY OR PAST PERFORMANCE

Sample evaluation question: Did the program achieve more than it did last year?

Standard: The number of participants during 2016 in the Stretch Your Life program will be 10% more than in 2015.

Sample evaluation question: Was performance the same even with fewer resources?

Standard: The number of children immunized in 2016 will equal the number in 2015.

Sample evaluation question: Did outcomes improve with new methods?

Standard: The number of newly diagnosed cases of tuberculosis will be 20% less than last year.

Sample evaluation question: What was the level of performance compared with previous performance?

Standard: Waiting time in the nursing center will decrease by 10 minutes per client appointment from last quarter.

STANDARDS BASED ON COMPARISONS

Standards developed on the basis of comparisons are often convincing because they compare the performance of groups. These comparisons may be of the same group over time, of similar groups, or among several groups at one time. For example, the performance of one group that received the intervention may be compared with the performance of another group that received the regular care. This approach to standard setting is useful with interventions that have been inadequately tested to determine whether they are effective or with which groups they are effective. Examples of standards developed on the basis of comparisons are as follows:

- Program costs at all sites will stay within 5% of the budget.
- The level of program activity will remain the same as the last fiscal year.
- The amount of increase in knowledge about diabetes will be the same in all adult groups.

Even if an evaluation shows that one group is different from the others, one cannot claim that it was the program that caused the difference. Three questions need to be addressed to have some confidence that the program was effective:

1. Were the groups similar at the beginning of the program?
2. Was the difference between groups large enough to be meaningful?
3. Were the levels of achievement by the groups meaningful in terms of practical implications?

STANDARDS BASED ON NORMS OR EPIDEMIOLOGIC DATA

A norm is a model or pattern considered to be typical for a specific group. Many norms are determined through the collection of epidemiologic data. Norms can be items such as the average weights at specific heights for people in specific age groups or with specific blood pressures.

The use of norms or epidemiologic data for setting standards is useful in many areas. For instance, if the objective of the program is to reduce low-birth-weight rates, data on birth weights would be useful. Comparisons with other parts of a state and country are possible with the use of norms. The *Healthy People 2020* (Office of Disease Prevention and Health Promotion, 2014) document provides a source of information to set standards on the basis of norms.

One key to the successful use of norms is to be certain that they were developed using the same or a similar population to which they will be applied. For example, a norm only for men will not apply to women. Norms for one race will not always apply to other races. Different age ranges also require different norms. What is normal for 20- to 24-year-old people is often not the case for 40- to 45-year-old people. Examples of standards set on the basis of norms are as follows:

- No more than 5% of infants will be born weighing less than 2,500 g.
- No more than 25% of people aged 20 years and older will be overweight.

■ BUILDING EVALUATION DESIGNS

Evaluation design refers to the structure built to objectively appraise a program's effectiveness. Building the design is based on five areas: the evaluation questions and standards, the independent variables, inclusion and exclusion criteria, control group, and measures (Fink, 1993).

Linking Evaluation Questions and Standards to the Design

The evaluation design serves to link the evaluation questions and standards with mechanisms by which they can be implemented. For example, standards that call for changes to occur in the participants over a period of time will require a design in which measurements are taken at least twice. If change is projected for a total community, measurement of a comparable community is needed to demonstrate that the program had some relationship to the change and not other factors such as television programs.

Incorporating Independent Variables

In evaluation design, independent variables are defined as explanatory or predictor variables because they explain or predict the outcomes of the program. Independent variables are viewed as independent of the program and part of the evaluation design (Fink, 1993).

The independent variables provide the items for data collection in the design. For example, a program aimed at improving the quality of life of elderly living in the community by decreasing their isolation has the independent variables of age, gender, and health status of the participants. These independent variables (and perhaps others) are used to examine the outcomes of the program as in the following example:

Evaluation question: Which participants benefit more from the program?
Standard: A statistically significant difference in quality-of-life scores with older males in poor health having higher scores.
Independent variables: Program participation, age, health status, gender.
Outcome (dependent variable): Improved quality of life as demonstrated by an increased score on the quality-of-life instrument.
Evaluator's prediction: Participants with lower quality-of-life scores (those who are older, in poorer health, and males) will have a greater benefit from the program compared with participants beginning the program with higher scores.

If a specific program is aimed at participants who vary in age, income, race, and gender, the evaluation study may need to be divided into more than one group to determine whether the program was equally effective over all program participant groups. If a program is implemented to have an effect on a total community, a sample of participants is needed for the evaluation study because every community member cannot be included. This area will be addressed in more depth later in the section on sampling for evaluation studies.

Adding Inclusion and Exclusion Criteria

A program may not be equally effective for all participants, so the evaluator may need to set criteria that determine who will be included or eligible for the evaluation study. For example, a program designed to increase the number of pregnant women starting care in the first trimester may be offered to all pregnant women, but the evaluation may be focused on primiparous women because of the special purpose of the program. Likewise, age may be a factor in such a program. A program aimed at pregnant teens will have different content from one focused on increasing prenatal care among women who are older and/or have experienced more than one pregnancy.

Eligibility criteria may also be used to exclude program participants who are especially inappropriate for the program evaluation. For example, many programs require a specified level of participation in order for any effect to be possible. A smoking-cessation program can hardly be successful if participants did not attend the sessions. For example, the evaluator might want to exclude persons who had attended only one of three sessions.

Using a Control Group

The experimental group receives the program intervention. A *control group* either receives another program or does not receive the program intervention, but still participates in the evaluation. For example, an evaluation may compare the intervention group with a control group from a community that is not part of any known organized program.

The important part of using a control group is to determine that the two groups were similar before the intervention, for example, in age and gender. Meeting this criterion requires the intervention and control groups be measured both before the program begins and again at the end of the program.

Taking Measures

As mentioned earlier, measures may be taken before and after a program. In addition, measures may be needed during the program. In the example of the program to decrease isolation of community-dwelling elderly, a measure of the quality of life would be needed before the program and at the end of the program. If the program were to continue indefinitely, two or more measures of the quality of life using the same instrument should be taken at specified time intervals, such as every 6 months in the program, for each participant.

The specific time for taking measures is dependent on when effects of the program are anticipated to occur. A period of 6 months may be too long a time for a program designed to decrease isolation, but not long enough to see a difference in the smoking behavior of a community or to see a decrease in the infant mortality rate.

If long-term effects are projected for a program, a data-collection plan needs to be set up and carefully monitored to ensure that accurate data are continuously collected. Usually, evaluation plans for specific programs are not projected to be conducted for longer than 5 years (Fink, 1993).

■ UNDERSTANDING EVALUATION DESIGNS

After determining initial answers to the areas that contribute to an evaluation design, the evaluator is ready to decide on the actual design that best suits the evaluation study. For this discussion, two broad categories of evaluation designs are addressed: experimental and observational.

Experimental Designs

Experimental designs are used to give the evaluator some control on program elements that may influence the outcomes. Experimental designs consist of four types: true experiments, quasi-experiments, before and after designs, and historical controls.

TRUE EXPERIMENTS

True experimental designs are used to infer causation. In true experiments (also called *controlled trials* or *randomized controlled trials [RCTs]*), participants are randomly assigned to a new program or to a control group that may receive the current program or no program. The groups are compared at the same point in time on the variable or outcome of interest, for instance, smoking rates or immunization rates (Grove, Burns, & Gray, 2013).

The true experiment is the only design by which causation can be inferred. However, to generalize the results of the evaluation, evaluations of the program in different locations with a variety of participants over a period of years are needed.

Although the true experiment is an ideal design for a credible evaluation, there are numerous drawbacks of using this design in programs developed for public/community health nursing services:

- Ethical concerns about randomly assigning participants
- Lack of time and money to plan and conduct such extensive evaluations
- Difficulty in recruiting and retaining enough participants for two or more groups
- Lack of resources to conduct evaluations at more than one site (Fink, 1993)

QUASI-EXPERIMENTAL DESIGNS

The purpose of quasi-experimental designs, like experimental designs, is to examine causality. However, the quasi-experimental designs are not as powerful as true experiments for establishing causality. In service settings, quasi-experimental designs are alternatives to the tight control required for experimental situations that often are not possible or ethical.

Quasi-experimental designs are nonrandomized, concurrent controls without random assignment to intervention and control groups (Grove et al., 2013). Numerous biases are introduced with this design. If preexisting groups are used as the control group, bias is often present because the group members are likely to have similar characteristics that may affect the outcomes. If groups are constituted through invitations to participate, those who join groups may be different from those who do not volunteer to be involved.

BEFORE AND AFTER DESIGNS

Before and after designs, or pretest/posttest designs, are quasi-experimental designs within which the participants serve as their own control group (Grove et al., 2013). The group of participants is measured on the appropriate variables before the program begins and then at the end of the program or other specified time.

Bias may also be introduced in these designs. Program participants may be especially enthusiastic to participate in a new program and, thus, be motivated to do well. Employees, too, may be motivated to do well because of the novelty in their work or the consequences of poor outcomes, such as loss of funding if the program is not successful.

To develop a sound evaluation with self-controls, the design requires appropriate measurements that are taken with accurate timing and frequency. For example, if results are expected after 2 months in a program, measurements taken at 1 month may make the program appear ineffective.

HISTORICAL CONTROLS

Evaluation designs with historical controls use data available from sources other than the current program. For example, norms of weight, blood pressure, and laboratory values may be used to compare with program outcomes. Although these norms are useful, the evaluator needs to be mindful that a potential problem is present if there is no comparability between the historical group and the evaluation group (Fink, 1993).

Observational Designs

In program evaluation, observational designs provide descriptive data about the program participants and the program. Compared with the control over program elements that characterizes experimental designs, observational designs attempt to capture a picture of the program elements. The two observational designs presented in this section are survey and cohort (Fink, 1993).

SURVEY DESIGNS

Survey, or cross-sectional, designs are used to obtain information about programs at one point in time. This information is often baseline data obtained before a program begins to provide a picture of the characteristics of the program participants. Later data are collected about program participants to compare with the baseline data. The information from a survey design may be used in guiding program development. For example, a satisfaction survey could be used to discover what, if any, areas of a service need to be changed. A survey study could also be done to determine the knowledge level in a population about a specific subject, for example, the need to start prenatal care in the first trimester.

Designing a survey to collect data for cross-sectional evaluations can be very time-consuming. A frequently used survey or measure for public/community health nursing programs is one for knowledge. A survey to measure knowledge about a topic would need to be pretested for content, reading level, and understandability. Often, pretesting will point out items that are not clearly stated or are not measuring what is intended by the evaluator. These are areas of reliability and validity that are used to determine the accuracy of instruments for use in evaluation. Instrument reliability and validity are discussed in Chapter 18. Also, if a survey is not well designed, the evaluator may end up measuring something different than the intended factors.

COHORT OR CASE-CONTROL DESIGNS

A group of people who have something in common and stay together as a group over time is termed a *cohort*. A case is an individual, group, family, or community (Valanis, 1999). Both cohorts and cases are studied over time in cohort or case-control prospective evaluation designs to determine the extent of a program's long-term effects (Fink, 1993).

Studies involving cohorts and cases are expensive to conduct and have difficulty retaining participants over long periods of time. In addition, bias is introduced because people who chose to participate over the long term may be different from those who were not willing to participate.

■ INTERNAL AND EXTERNAL VALIDITY OF EVALUATION DESIGNS

Evaluation designs are used to structure the examination of program effects. Internal and external validity may be considered with evaluation designs to strengthen confidence in the findings of the evaluation study. *Internal validity* refers to the extent to which the effects or outcomes of the program are a result of the program and not other extraneous factors. *External validity is* the extent to which the findings of the study can be generalized beyond the participants in the study (Fink, 1993; Grove et al., 2013).

When building the evaluation study design, the advanced practice public/community health nurse will want to consider how the design can incorporate details that strengthen internal validity and, if appropriate, allow for external validity. The following discussion provides suggestions about evaluation design that may assist you to develop a stronger evaluation study.

Threats to Internal Validity

Internal validity allows the evaluator to tell whether the program was the reason for the outcomes or whether some other outside factor or event influenced the participants to achieve the outcomes. For programs that take place in the real world with real people, issues of validity are especially difficult to address. Consideration of the threats and possible prevention of the threats through design details will enhance the evaluation effort. The threats to internal validity addressed are maturation, history, instrumentation, testing, and attrition (Campbell & Stanley, 1963).

MATURATION

If a program is intended to produce long-term effects that are anticipated over a number of years, the maturation of the participants should be considered in the evaluation design. Often, programs directed at children must deal with this threat to validity because children mature or change during the course of the program. Adults also change over time. The question of whether the program or maturity caused the change (program outcome) needs to be addressed in the design of the evaluation.

There are several ways to deal with this threat. The first is to include controls in the design. If the intervention group is compared with a similar group without the intervention, the evaluator has more confidence in the outcomes that favor the intervention group.

Another method is to collect data over a short period of time, which decreases the chance that the outcome is due to maturity over time. However, a short period of time will not totally eliminate the effect of maturity that occurs continuously in all people but is more rapid in children.

Prospective designs also tend to favor an unbiased evaluation because they contain data collected before, during, and after the program. If changes occurred after the program began, they may be attributed to the program if other safeguards are in place. A combination of these approaches may be needed to decrease the threat of maturity to internal validity (Campbell & Stanley, 1963).

HISTORY

Another threat to internal validity is history, or what happens during the life of the program. Any number of events may occur between the first and second measurements of participants' outcomes to bring into question whether or not the program caused the results. For instance, a new health policy may bring about exactly what a program intended to accomplish. Changes in healthcare coverage, changes in reimbursement, national health behavior campaigns, similar local programs offered by other organizations, and self-instruction are examples of events that make it difficult to separate the effects of a program from outside influences.

Documenting other events and changes during a program's life is one way to track such possible threats to validity. These alternative explanations for the outcomes of a program should be discussed in evaluation results.

INSTRUMENTATION

It is important to use tools or instruments that are reliable and valid in order to have useful, accurate data. Instrumentation is the process of developing or choosing tools for measuring the items that are the focus of the evaluation study (Waltz, Strickland, & Lenz, 2017).

The first challenge in addressing internal validity and instrumentation is to find tools that are reliable and valid. The unreliable tool will produce unreliable or questionable results. If the tools used to collect data are not calibrated in the same way, for example, scales that weigh inconsistently, results will be questioned. Evaluators may need to develop the tools for a specific project. Often, a one-item tool may be adequate for some aspects of evaluation. For example, asking participants about their level of satisfaction with a program may be all that is needed to measure their satisfaction. Another example is to ask program participants how their health status has changed during the program. This could be phrased as: "Would you say your health has improved, stayed the same, or become worse since you started coming to the program?" One-item tools allow for minimal statistical analyses.

Another challenge to instrumentation is to use the instruments consistently. The evaluation results may be inaccurate if the scorers or observers are not consistent in their tasks of applying the measurements. Scorers who are lenient will produce scores that favor the program, whereas harsh or overly strict scorers will produce scores that put the program in an unfavorable light (Grove et al., 2013). One way to decrease the threat to internal validity from instrumentation is to train the scorers and observers. The advanced practice public/community health nurse then needs to perform periodic tests to determine the level of agreement among scorers, which is to calculate interrater reliability. If the agreement among scorers falls below a preset level, more training is needed (Waltz et al., 2017).

Accuracy in transcribing scores or other data from paper to the computer, or another data-compilation source, also needs to be addressed. A second person can be assigned to spot-check a specified percentage of each day's data entries for accuracy. Techniques for checking accuracy may be needed at several points in the data-processing steps.

TESTING

If tests are used to obtain data about the success of an educational program, the evaluator should be alert for the effects of cumulative test taking on internal validity. Testing is closely related to instrumentation because tests are often the instruments used to obtain data about the success of an educational program. The evaluator must always be cognizant that the initial tests may affect the scores of subsequent tests. In other words, test takers become better at taking tests, which increases their scores. They may also remember the questions from one test to another, which may increase their scores.

Administering the same test within a short period of time increases the effects of test taking on subjects. If possible, a gap of time should pass before the second administration of the same test. Another approach is to place the test items in random order so that the test appears changed.

ATTRITION

Attrition is the loss of participants from a program. Participants who drop out of a program may differ from those who remain. This difference in people may be the reason the program seems to have optimal outcomes rather than the program itself. The threat of attrition to internal validity is often difficult to address because those who drop out are not available for measurement of program effects.

If attrition is anticipated, gathering baseline data from all program participants is all the more important. Collecting data before the program begins will provide some information for comparison of the participants who remain in the program with those who do not remain. For example, age, gender, income, education, and other characteristics of the two groups can be compared to see whether there are any differences in these factors.

Threats to External Validity

External validity is the extent to which the activities of a program may be successfully implemented at other sites with other groups of participants (Grove et al., 2013). Three threats to external validity are reactive effect of testing, interactive effects of selection and the experimental intervention (program), and multiple-treatment interference (Campbell & Stanley, 1963).

REACTIVE EFFECT OF TESTING

The reactive effect of testing, or interactive effect of testing, occurs when a pretest increases or decreases the participant's responsiveness to the intervention. This change in responsiveness makes the results for a pretested group unrepresentative of the effects of the intervention for the untested population from which the experimental participants were selected. This type of threat to external validity may be seen in programs that measure attitudes, for example, and attempt to change them.

One approach to deal with this threat is to use an evaluation design called the *Solomon four group*. This design requires random assignment of participants to four groups. One set of an experimental group and a control group is administered the pretest and one set of groups is not. All groups take the posttest. This design controls for the effect of pretesting.

The Solomon four group design is not used often because it is difficult to obtain the large number of participants for such a study. Conducting such a study is also demanding and expensive because of the need to collect data from various sites and introduce the program simultaneously to two groups (Buckwalter & Maas, 1998).

INTERACTION OF SELECTION AND PROGRAM

People who choose to participate in a program may be different from those who do not participate. The effect of self-selection of program participants may not be evident when a program is being conducted and may not appear to be a problem until a program replication is attempted. Programs that are effective with one group of participants may not be effective with different groups. For example, older adults who are already involved in exercise may volunteer to participate in a program to increase their exercise. If the same program is introduced to sedentary adults, the participation rates may be lower and participants may drop out before the program ends.

To determine whether there are differences between those who participate and those who do not, information about the characteristics of both groups should be collected (Grove et al., 2013). With these data in hand, the program evaluator may be able to make recommendations about changes needed before a program is implemented in other sites with different groups of participants.

MULTIPLE-TREATMENT INTERFERENCE

Programs with multiple interventions can be challenging to evaluate because of the difficulty of keeping the effects of each intervention separate. Programs implemented to address community problems or situations often deal with multiple risk factors in populations that contain a variety of aggregates. To deal with this array of variety, advanced practice public/community health nurses often develop programs that contain several types of interventions. For example, a program to decrease the risks of heart disease may have interventions to increase exercise, decrease dietary fat content, and stop smoking. If the interventions are introduced sequentially to the same group, the effects of previous interventions will still be in effect. The evaluation attempts will be further complicated by the fact that all participants may not partake equally of all aspects of the program (Grove et al., 2013).

The evaluator is thus left with an evaluation study in which the effects of the separate interventions and the effect of the various interventions together are difficult to identify. One approach to this challenge is to evaluate each intervention separately for each group who participated at the specified level (e.g., attended three of four sessions). Even though the compounding effect of participating in more than one program segment will not be erased, the evaluator may be able to determine which type of people benefitted most from which interventions.

If each intervention is evaluated separately, each program segment may be looked at for potential implementation at other sites with other participants. This approach increases the possible external validity of program parts if not the total program.

SAMPLING FOR EVALUATION STUDIES

When it is not possible to conduct an evaluation study that includes all program participants, a sample, or a portion, of the total population is chosen. A population may be people, institutions, or systems. For example, an evaluation study of a population of school-based health clinics may include 25% of the clinics in the state.

The purpose of using a sample is to apply the findings to the total target population of the program without the expense and time required to include all program participants. Using a sample also allows the evaluator to tailor the study to focus on specific items, such as the effectiveness of the program by age groups (Fink, 1993).

This section addresses criteria for inclusion and exclusion from the sample, methods of sampling, size of the sample, and discussion about the sampling unit.

DEVELOPING CRITERIA FOR INCLUSION AND EXCLUSION

Criteria should be used to include or exclude people or items from the evaluation study sample. Inclusion and exclusion criteria were discussed earlier in terms of the program itself. Now, attention turns to the criteria to be used for including and excluding people or items from the sample for the evaluation study. For example, if the program is aimed at decreasing cardiovascular disease risk in school-age children, will the evaluation include children of all ages, children who attended certain aspects of the program, and both boys and girls? These types of decisions need to be made before the study begins in order to have a systematic approach to choose and gather data about the evaluation study sample.

The evaluator usually establishes the criteria for the evaluation, but the involvement of staff and community members may be beneficial to determine any unanticipated variations in program participants. For example, if a program attracted only people in their late teens even though it was designed for all ages of teens, this variation needs to be addressed in the evaluation design.

Guidance for establishing the inclusion and exclusion criteria is provided by the independent variables, which were discussed earlier in this chapter (Fink, 1993). For example, if a cardiovascular disease risk-reduction program is intended for both boys and girls, criteria are needed to determine which boys and girls should be included in or excluded from the sample. Possible criteria may include the ability to read at a specific grade level and attendance at sessions. Children would be excluded if they did not read at grade level and/or did not attend the sessions. Thus, findings from the evaluation study would be applicable to boys and girls who read at grade level and attended the sessions.

Using Probability-Sampling Approaches

There are two general types of sampling methods: probability and nonprobability. Probability sampling, or random sampling, means that every member of the population has a chance higher than zero of being chosen for the sample. This approach to sampling is preferred if a goal of the evaluation is to draw conclusions about the generalizability of the program (Fink, 1993). The discussion of nonprobability sampling follows this section. The term *random sample* is often used for a probability sample. Four designs for random sampling are used: simple random sampling, stratified sampling, cluster sampling, and systematic sampling (Shi, 2008).

SIMPLE RANDOM SAMPLING

Every member of the population has an equal chance of being chosen in simple random sampling, so this type of random sample is considered relatively unbiased. Although many techniques may be used to obtain a random sample, usually a table of random numbers or a computer-generated list of numbers is used to choose individuals from a list of the population.

An example of choosing a random sample is to list all school-based health clinics in the designated study area and number them. Using a table of random numbers and starting at a random place in the table, the first numbers found in the table would be used as the number of the clinics for the sample.

STRATIFIED SAMPLING

When a simple random sample is not adequate to obtain representation from the various parts of a population, stratified sampling can be used. The subgroups are chosen because of the belief that they are related to the dependent variable or outcome of the program (Fink, 1993).

In advanced public/community health nursing practice, the nurse is aware that income, age, health status, education, and other factors are often related to outcomes and need to be considered in program evaluations. Thus, subgroups may be needed to adequately examine program effectiveness. An example is the relationship of education to program outcomes. The evaluator may want to stratify program participants by educational levels in order to have enough people with various levels of education.

Another situation is examining programs in different settings. For example, if school-based health clinics from both rural and urban areas were to be included, the population of clinics could be divided into these two subgroups or strata. Then, a random sample could be selected from the rural subgroup and from the urban subgroup. This would allow the evaluator to examine each subgroup separately and compare them on the basis of specific criteria.

CLUSTER SAMPLING

Cluster sampling is used in large studies that involve many sites. To perform cluster sampling, the population is divided into batches. The population may be counties, cities, institutions, or organizations. The sampling unit is randomly selected and data collected for the site. Each site is treated as a unit in data analysis.

This type of sampling is expensive but has been used in several large-scale studies with evaluation teams at the various sites (Dawson & Trapp, 2001).

SYSTEMATIC SAMPLING

The method of systematic sampling may be used when a list of the total population is available. To determine the number of individuals to draw from the list, the evaluator must know the number on the list and the sample size needed. Then, the population is divided by the desired sample size to obtain k, the size of the gap between selections. Starting with a randomly selected point, every kth individual on the list is drawn for the sample. The starting point may be chosen from a list of random numbers or from the throw of a die. For example, if 100 people attended the program and 20 names were desired for the evaluation, then dividing 100 by 20 would select every fifth name from the list (Grove et al., 2013).

This method provides a random but unequal chance for all members of the population to be included in the sample. In addition, the evaluator should be aware that the list may be ordered in such a way as to exclude certain groups, for example, an ethnic group with names beginning with one letter of the alphabet. The order of the list should be random to avoid biases in terms of alphabetical or other ordered lists.

Using Nonprobability-Sampling Approaches

Nonprobability sampling is commonly used in nursing research studies as well as in evaluation studies when resources and/or factors prohibit the use of probability sampling. Every element in the population does not have an opportunity to be selected in nonprobability sampling. This approach to sampling increases the possibilities that the sample is not representative of the population (Shi, 2008).

Four types of nonprobability sampling are convenience sampling, quota sampling, random assignment to groups, and purposive sampling. The advantages and disadvantages of each method are explored next.

CONVENIENCE SAMPLING

Convenience, or accidental sampling, is used when a quick, relatively inexpensive method of nonprobability sampling is needed. This type of sampling may be used to pilot evaluation tools, train data collectors, conduct exploratory studies, or include hard-to-reach populations, such as homeless people.

Convenience sampling is a method in which participants are chosen because they are available. Therefore, some members of the population have a chance of being chosen and some do not. A convenience sample is not representative of the target population, so the results of the evaluation may not be generalized to the total population.

Selection of a convenience sample may be done in several ways. Typically, it is a group formed as part of a project, such as every person attending a stop-smoking class, every second person who attends a clinic on a certain day, or every person who participated in an exercise program (Grove et al., 2013).

QUOTA SAMPLING

Quota sampling may be used in conjunction with, or instead of, convenience sampling to include types of subjects who may be underrepresented by convenience sampling. Specific numbers of the likely underrepresented groups, such as minorities, women, or the poor, are included in the sample. The quotas may be adjusted to be representative of the numbers found in the target population. This approach is preferable to and could often be used instead of convenience sampling.

Although quota sampling is an improvement over convenience sampling, bias may still be present. In addition, evaluation results are limited to the study site. An advantage of quota sampling is that adequate numbers of a specific subgroup may be added to perform statistical analyses. For example, if convenience sampling could not include an adequate number of men, quota sampling could be used to increase the number of men needed to perform the designated statistical tests (Grove et al., 2013).

RANDOM ASSIGNMENT TO GROUPS

When a convenience sample is obtained for a study, participants are often randomly assigned to intervention and control groups. Although this approach is used to decrease the risk of bias, one review of RCTs and cohort studies found no evidence of harmful or beneficial effects in random versus nonrandom assignment (Vist et al., 2005).

A table of random numbers or the toss of a coin may be used for assignment to groups, but unequal group sizes may result from these techniques. Techniques or adjustments may be used to balance the group sizes, such as stratified random sampling, if this is a desired situation (Grove et al., 2013).

Random assignment to groups may be useful for short-term programs that will be evaluated almost immediately, for example, a new education program to increase knowledge about a specific topic. The two groups could be pretested and posttested within a short period of time to decrease the influence of learning from other sources.

PURPOSIVE SAMPLING

In purposive sampling, the evaluator uses judgment to select subjects or elements for the study. The evaluator may select typical or atypical situations or people. This type of sampling is especially useful for qualitative evaluations or the qualitative aspects of an evaluation. This method provides an opportunity to gain in-depth information about aspects of a program. For example, information from atypical participants may provide guidance for revising the program to attract a broader range of participants.

One disadvantage of purposive sampling is that there is no way to evaluate the judgment of the evaluator in choosing subjects. This approach leaves much room for bias; for instance, the evaluator may choose only those people who benefitted most from the program (Fink, 1993).

■ COLLECTING BASELINE DATA

Standards need to be in place before a program begins so that baseline data can be collected on the basis of the evaluation study design. Baseline data often include characteristics of participants, such as their age, gender, income, education, and place of residence, as well as data about their health status that are intended to be affected by the program (such as knowledge, exercise behavior, or weight). If any changes in the target population are anticipated as a result of program interventions, information should be collected at the first visit or it could be contaminated by program activities.

Obtaining Baseline Data Using Different Approaches

Baseline data may be obtained from participants or from the community assessment or a combination of these. One common approach to obtain baseline data is to ask participants about themselves at their first visit to the program. This approach is most appropriate for programs directed only at those who come to the program.

Often, programs and services developed by advanced practice public/community health nurses are intended to have an effect on a total community or an aggregate within a community. If this is the case, approaches to collection of baseline data must go beyond only those who come to the program. A good source to initially consult is the community assessment. As is often the case, the target population has not started to receive services, so it is not accessible to the evaluator for baseline data. However, baseline data may have been collected as part of the community assessment.

Sometimes, a review of health or social service records will provide adequate data about the target group. For example, a review of health records will show the immunization levels of children and adults being seen in a primary care clinic. The participants who come to an immunization program may not be the same people, but the record review gives general information about the group targeted for the new program, that is, the people who are served by the primary care clinic.

Another approach to baseline data collection is through face-to-face or telephonic surveys. Good candidates for these techniques are groups who meet regularly (such as church organizations, civic clubs, or children's groups) and clients of other agencies or institutions. Survey forms may be left in waiting rooms along with a collection box for the completed forms. Although these techniques will not obtain a 100% response rate, they may be appropriate for a particular program. The precise baseline data to collect will be determined partially by the evaluation design used.

■ INVOLVING INTERDISCIPLINARY TEAM MEMBERS AND COMMUNITY RESIDENTS

Evaluations are often complex and time-consuming. The involvement of several people in the evaluation is not only desirable but also often necessary to complete the work within a reasonable time period. The involvement of members of the interdisciplinary team in the evaluation process is a natural extension of the cooperative efforts to develop a program plan and implement a new program. Leadership by the advanced practice public/community health nurse for teamwork is explored in this section.

Involvement of community residents in an evaluation study may be an unusual situation for most advanced practice public/community health nurses. However, if you want to promote the idea of community ownership of the program, the community should be involved every step of the way. Although the type and depth of involvement of community residents in an evaluation study may vary, three suggested groups of activities are providing advice, designing evaluation tools, and encouraging participation in the evaluation study.

Providing Leadership of the Interdisciplinary Team for Program Evaluation

As mentioned earlier, involvement of the interdisciplinary team begins long before the evaluation is planned and executed. Some decisions about who should be involved and how they should be involved are needed as one of the first steps in leading the evaluation activities of the team. Three areas in particular benefit from this leadership direction: team assignments, monitoring the accuracy of data and information, and avoiding bias.

MAKING TEAM ASSIGNMENTS

The team leader is responsible for assigning duties to each team member. In making assignments, you should try to promote the strengths of team members and balance workloads. As with other aspects of the program-planning process, team members need to be asked what parts of the evaluation study they would like to be involved in. The leader who meets individually with each team member can gain a great deal of information about the individual's strengths, interests, goals, and weaknesses. Mutual agreement on assignments is more possible with this approach.

Training for data collection and other aspects of the evaluation activities will be needed, so the time for initial and ongoing training should be calculated into assignments.

MONITORING ACCURACY OF DATA AND INFORMATION

The advanced practice public/community health nurse provides leadership for overseeing the systems for monitoring the accuracy of data and information. The evaluation loses its usefulness without credible data. Thus, the team leader works with team members to provide smooth implementation of the data-collection systems. Team members can be very instrumental in monitoring data collection in numerous ways. Team members may supervise employees who collect data, such as the clerk who registers people for the program. Team members may collect data themselves as program implementers. They may also enter data into a computer, transfer data from one report to aggregate reports, type reports, or perform any number of other tasks that are required for program reporting.

Accuracy of data may be monitored by various methods. If several people are collecting the same data, interrater reliability checks may be needed throughout the data-collection period. Interrater reliability of data being collected may be determined by having the team leader and a team member collect the same data at the same or closely related times. For example, if interviews are conducted with participants to collect data about program satisfaction, the team leader could accompany the team members and record responses at the same time. The extent of agreement between the two interview records could be calculated.

This approach accomplishes two goals. First, the interrater reliability can be calculated by various means, such as percentage of agreement (Waltz et al., 2017). If the reliability is low (e.g., below 70% agreement), the team leader would have an opportunity to discuss the reasons why it is low, provide retraining, or change the assignments for data collection. Second, observations of data collection provide the team leader with firsthand information about the progress of the program.

AVOIDING BIAS AND IMPROVING CONSISTENCY

The team leader is responsible for overseeing that the data-collection processes are free from bias and provide consistent data. Bias in data collection is often very subtle. The tendency of a data collector to gently lead a respondent to more positive or negative responses is not always obvious to the data collector herself or himself or to others. Some raters are inconsistent in how they rate participants. Other raters may be very lenient or very strict (Waltz et al., 2017).

Leaders who want to protect against bias and inconsistency must train data collectors. Training is not a one-time occurrence but requires constant updates, training new team members, and offering refresher courses for lapses in accuracy or consistency.

A second approach for improving consistency and decreasing bias is monitoring the data on a regular basis. The team leader or a designated team member needs to check data for accuracy, note any unexpected trends, perform interrater reliability checks, monitor legibility of handwritten information, and monitor timeliness of data submission.

Involving Community Residents

A frequently desired outcome for program stability is community ownership. Community ownership may be seen as important for program effectiveness as well as long-term maintenance. Part of the approach to encourage community ownership is through involvement of community residents at every step of program planning, implementation, and evaluation (Minkler & Wallerstein, 2008). Community ownership may be either psychological or fiscal. Even without community ownership, the involvement of community residents in program evaluation is valuable for several reasons.

Programs that are not acceptable and accessible to community members are not very useful. People who attend the programs may not have difficulty accessing the program, but it is necessary to listen to the people who do not attend. Community members may provide the input for those who are not represented as program participants.

Community residents can increase the acceptance of a program by word of mouth and a greater understanding of the program focus. Involvement in the evaluation process also serves as an important educational experience for most people and carries beyond the actual program evaluation.

Community residents may have a variety of roles when participating in program evaluation. These roles are designed to give voice to the community and may depend on the program focus, characteristics of the community, desires of community residents, strengths of the residents, and need during the evaluation (Minkler & Wallerstein, 2008).

A group of community residents may be designated as advisory to the evaluation team. Views of community residents should be considered in areas such as which evaluation approaches may be best received, which aspects of the program may require special attention, and potential problem areas.

Some community residents can be involved at the outset in designing the evaluation tools. This involvement may range from posing evaluation questions to pretesting the actual tools developed by the interdisciplinary team. At times, team members and community residents should meet together to work on specific tasks.

Community residents may also be involved in encouraging others to participate in the evaluation effort by returning surveys or other evaluation items. It is desirable to have a good level of participation in the evaluation study with an unbiased response. The advanced practice public/community health nurse should be mindful that involved community residents do not exert undue influence on others.

■ SUMMARY

A program evaluation plan can be developed by following a series of steps for developing evaluation questions and standards, building an evaluation design, and deciding on a sample. Consideration for collecting baseline data must be given early in the evaluation design so that adequate data are available for all desired aspects of the evaluation. The internal and external validity of the evaluation design must also be considered. The evaluator should be especially concerned with internal validity if the program will not be replicated at other sites.

Involvement of interdisciplinary team members and community residents is important for developing a meaningful and acceptable evaluation study. Contributions of community residents will assist the advanced practice public/community health nurse to target areas of particular interest to the community as well as assist in conveying the importance of cooperation during the evaluation effort.

■ SUGGESTED CLINICAL OR PRACTICUM ACTIVITIES

1. Identify a community-based program evaluation at a clinical site. Interview a nurse or community planner at the site about program evaluation planning. Describe the purpose of the evaluation, the questions or standards used to guide the evaluation, and the evaluation design. To what extent was the evaluation guided by an evaluation plan? How might these elements of program evaluation be improved?
2. Using the same community-based program evaluation identified in activity #1, discuss procedures used in sampling and threats to internal and external validity. How might these threats have been addressed by modifications of the evaluation plan?
3. Using the same community-based program evaluation identified in activity #1, describe the involvement of community residents in the program evaluation process. As an advanced public/community health nurse, how would you enhance the engagement of community residents?

REFERENCES

Buckwalter, K. C., & Maas, M. L. (1998). Classical experimental designs. In P. J. Brink & M. J. Wood (Eds.), *Advanced design in nursing research* (2nd ed., pp. 21–62). Thousand Oaks, CA: Sage.

Campbell, D. T., & Stanley, J. C. (1963). *Experimental and quasi-experimental designs for research*. Boston, MA: Houghton Mifflin.

Dawson, B., & Trapp, G. R. (2001). *Basic and clinical biostatistics*. New York, NY: McGraw-Hill.

Dignan, M. B., & Carr, P. A. (1992). *Program planning for health education and promotion* (2nd ed.). Philadelphia, PA: Lea & Febiger.

Donabedian, A. (1969). *A guide to medical care administration, Vol. 2. Medical care appraisal: Quality and utilization*. New York, NY: American Public Health Association.

Fink, A. (1993). *Evaluation fundamentals: Guiding health programs, research, and policy*. Newbury Park, CA: Sage.

Grove, S. K., Burns, N., & Gray, J. (2013). *The practice of nursing research: Appraisal, synthesis and generation of evidence* (7th ed.). Philadelphia, PA: Saunders.

Minkler, M., & Wallerstein, N. (Eds.). (2008) *Community based participatory research for health: Process to outcomes* (2nd ed.). San Francisco, CA: Jossey-Bass.

Office of Disease Prevention and Health Promotion. (2014). *Healthy people 2020*. Washington, DC: Author. Retrieved from https://www.healthypeople.gov/

Shi, L. (2008). *Health services research methods* (2nd ed.). Clifton Park, NY: Delmar.

Shi, L., & Singh, D. A. (2015). *Delivering health care in America: A systems approach* (6th ed.). Burlington, MA: Jones & Bartlett.

Timmreck, T. C. (2003). *Planning, program development, and evaluation: A handbook for health promotion, aging, and health services* (2nd ed.). Sudbury, MA: Jones & Bartlett.

Valanis, B. (1999). *Epidemiology in health care* (3rd ed.). Stamford, CT: Appleton & Lange.

Veney, J. E., & Kaluzny, A. D. (1998). *Evaluation and decision making for health services* (3rd ed.). Chicago, IL: Health Administration Press.

Vist, G. E., Hagen, K. B., Devereaux, P. J., Bryant, D., Kristoffersen, D. T., & Oxman, A. D. (2005). Systematic review to determine whether participation in a trial influences outcome. *British Medical Journal, 330*(7501), 1175–1179. doi:https://doi.org/10.1136/bmj.330.7501.1175

Waltz, C. F., Strickland, O. L., & Lenz, E. R. (2017). *Measurement in nursing and health research* (5th ed.). New York, NY: Springer Publishing.

CHAPTER 18

Measuring Program Effectiveness

■ STUDY EXERCISES

1. Why is program effectiveness an important part of program evaluation?
2. Describe some measures of program effectiveness.
3. What criteria are used to select measures of program effectiveness?
4. How is the reliability of a measure related to the ability to determine program effectiveness?
5. What is the relationship between reliability and validity of an instrument?
6. What is the relationship of program evaluation to quality-assessment and quality-improvement activities?
7. How may nursing classification systems be used in program evaluation?

As discussed in Chapter 17, program evaluations are completed for many purposes. This chapter concentrates on program effectiveness, or the extent to which a program achieves its objectives, as one approach to program evaluation. Program effectiveness evaluations assist the advanced practice public/community health nurse to make informed decisions about program management.

Throughout the years, evaluations of healthcare have tended to be concerned with structure and process almost to the exclusion of examining outcomes of programs. Current interest is in whether programs make a difference. This chapter presents aspects of program effectiveness to focus on evaluating program outcomes.

■ DEFINITION OF PROGRAM EFFECTIVENESS

The world of evaluation contains a great many "e" words: efficiency, efficacy, effort, and effectiveness. Most of these terms refer to some type of desired result. One way to look at program effectiveness is as success in performing a program (Chen, 2015). Did the program reach the projected or expected outcomes? Outcomes are usually associated with clients, consumers, patients, or other participants in the program. However, the outcomes may be a result of a change in policy, a change in status of a community, or the development of a coalition. The relationship of the program to the desired outcome, that is, whether the program caused the outcomes, is not always apparent from the evaluation, but the design of the evaluation study may help to determine the cause, if possible, of the outcomes.

The discussion of program effectiveness in this chapter concentrates on quality of care and desired outcomes, two parts of the definition of effectiveness.

Quality of Care

Structure and process are two components of care quality useful in evaluating the effectiveness of a program. In the quality of care model proposed by Donabedian (1969), the definition of structure is the human, physical, and financial resources needed to provide healthcare. These resources include the physical facilities, personnel, equipment, supplies, policies, and procedures involved in providing healthcare. The process component of care quality refers to the activities of healthcare personnel in the provision of care to patients. Donabedian (1969) included patient–provider interaction and the technical aspects of care as elements in the process component of the structure–process–outcome model of care quality. Both structure and process are important for program effectiveness, so the evaluator will be interested in measuring both or having results of the quality of care studies about both components.

Quality-assessment and quality-improvement activities contribute to both meeting the criteria for a sound program and the program evaluation. The data about the structure and process provide some ideas about how the program is operating and what has been done to ensure that it is on target for meeting the outcomes.

Program Outcomes

Outcomes are the third component in the quality of care model developed by Donabedian (1966) over five decades ago. His definition of *outcomes* refers to the end results of care to the patient. Although individual patient outcomes may be the desired results of some programs, outcomes are used more broadly in program evaluation to refer to outcomes for the program that are often related to a group or community. As mentioned earlier, outcomes may also involve changes in policy or in the environment.

Outcomes that are attributable to a specific program are very difficult to prove. Thus, the program evaluator is interested in designing a program evaluation study in such a way as to maximize the potential for detecting changes that may be attributed to the program activities. Dealing with the challenges of such a task is the subject of the next sections.

■ MEASURING PROGRAM EFFECTIVENESS

In Chapter 3, the authors presented examples of measures for outcomes of care of the community in three different conceptualizations: community-as-client, community-as-relational-experience, and community-as-resource. In keeping with this framework, suggested measures are next discussed in depth to make them useful to the advanced practice public/community health nurse in program evaluation.

Community-as-Client Measures

Measures derived from epidemiology dominate the examples of measures to use with the community-as-client conceptualization. Morbidity, mortality, infant mortality, and prevalence and incidence rates are important in understanding the disease and injury patterns in a community. The bases of understanding rates, ratios, and proportions come from both biostatistics and epidemiology. This section contains selected measures of program outcomes based on these fields.

MEASURING MATERNAL AND INFANT HEALTH

The infant mortality rate has been used for many years as a barometer of how a country takes care of the most vulnerable segment of society. The infant mortality rate is still a valuable indicator, especially in large urban populations, but has lost some of its power because of the low infant mortality rates observed in many parts of the United States. It is notable, however, that U.S. health indicators, including infant mortality, lag far behind other nations (National Research Council and Institute of Medicine, 2013). Low numbers of deaths (e.g., less than 20) result in unreliable rates that are difficult to interpret (Centers for Disease Control and Prevention [CDC], 2016). Low rates of death, disease, and injury are good news but often do not allow for meaningful statistics to measure program effectiveness.

Infant mortality rates are also not as useful when examining program effectiveness in a small population. A few infant deaths will result in high rates but may be an inaccurate picture of the community over time. Another disadvantage of using infant mortality is that the numbers needed to develop the rates are available only after almost 2 years for each cohort. Program evaluations often need other indicators of effectiveness or change.

Other useful measures are birth weight, weeks of gestation, trimester of initiation of prenatal care, and number of prenatal visits. These measures may be obtained in a shorter time frame than infant deaths and are often more readily available. For example, birth weight may be obtained from the birth certificate, the hospital or clinic record, and, at times, from the mother herself.

Measures of maternal health and behavior may also be used to evaluate the outcomes of programs aimed at improving the health of infants and mothers. For example, the measure of adequate prenatal visits may be used as a measure for a program to improve pregnancy outcomes. If participants do not go for prenatal care, program objectives cannot be achieved. Weight gain of pregnant women can be used as an outcome measure of a program on teaching self-care during pregnancy.

MEASURING COMMUNITY HEALTH

Many programs are aimed at improving the health status of a total community via various components. For example, a program to increase exercise participation may include adults and children. Measures of exercise in the total population are then valuable for gauging program effectiveness. To determine the success of a community-wide exercise program, baseline data would be needed before the program begins. Parallel data could be used for comparison at various points in the program. For example, the number or percentage of people by age categories who exercise would be compared before and after the program.

Smoking cessation for a total community is another example of a prevention program involving all ages of smokers. Calculations of smokers could be done with percentages and rates. Although not as accurate, other measures of smoking may be to monitor sales of cigarettes, electronic cigarettes, and/or tobacco.

Other programs for total communities include seat-belt use, nutrition, immunizations, and safe driving. Records showing statistics before and after the program may be used to measure the use or attainment level for these indicators of community health. Calculating rates for numerous indicators of program success provide a clearer picture of the magnitude of change.

Examples of goals, objectives, standards, and measures of program effectiveness for community-as-client are presented in Box 18.1.

BOX 18.1   COMMUNITY-AS-CLIENT: MEASURES OF PROGRAM EFFECTIVENESS

Goal: To decrease the infant mortality rate

Objective: By 2020 the infant mortality rate for the county will be 5.6 or fewers deaths per 1,000 live births.

Standards

1. No more than 7.8% of the infants born in 2020 will be of low birth weight.
2. Seventy-eight percent of pregnant women will begin prenatal care in the first trimester.

Measures

1. Infant mortality rate: Infant deaths per 1,000 live births for the county
2. Birth weight: Percentage less than 2,500 g
3. Percentage of women who begin prenatal care in the first trimester

Community-as-Relational-Experience

Programs within the context of community-as-relational-experience deal with power relations as well as interpersonal relationships. Advanced practice public/community health nurses who are interested in community-as-relational-experience are involved in policy and community development. Programs developed to address community-as-relational-experience are concerned with shifting power and making second-order changes.

A program to increase involvement of community members in the political process may result in tangible outcomes that should be captured in the program evaluation. The establishment of a coalition, passing an ordinance to decrease lead-based paint in housing, forcing cleanup of hazardous waste sites, and an improved water supply are examples of achievements at the community level that are measurable.

In addition, measures that estimate the magnitude of preventing adverse outcomes, such as disease or injury, as a result of the community involvement may be used to demonstrate cost savings. For example, the prevention of each case of lead poisoning in a child saves the cost of diagnosis and treatment as well as the expense of special education if damage results from late treatment.

MEASURING SOCIAL DETERMINANTS OF HEALTH

For programs developed within the community from the relational experience perspective of advanced public/community health nursing practice, social determinants of health are important indicators of outcomes. Social determinants include economic status of individuals and families, economic health of the community, and employment statistics.

Indicators of economic status may include median income, per capita income, family income, and total community income. For low-income communities, the percentage of the population with incomes below the poverty level is an important indicator for change. Especially important is the percentage of children at the poverty level. Improvements in income levels for low-income communities are indications that health status may also be improving.

Usually, improvements in income mean lower unemployment rates and higher employment rates. Although these indicators may be heartening, one must be wary of higher employment rates if they are in low-paying jobs that are enough above the poverty level to eliminate the family from eligibility for other programs such as food stamps, WIC, and Medicaid. A low-paying job just above the level for entitlement program benefits means that a family often lacks health insurance, paid sick time, and savings for any crisis, such as car repairs or an illness.

In the past two decades, concern had again entered public debate about the number of people who were without insurance coverage. The increase in the number of low-paying jobs without health insurance benefits contributed to the growth in the number of people uninsured. In addition, people who had been taken off the welfare rolls as a result of welfare reform were often without health insurance. With the implementation of the Patient Protection and Affordable Care Act (ACA, 2010), the percentage of persons uninsured decreased from 16.0% in 2010 to 8.8% in 2016 (CDC, 2017). However, concerns were again raised about potential increases in the number of uninsured with the 2016 administrative and congressional threats of repealing and replacing the ACA, also known as *Obamacare*. Indicators, such as percentages of the population with and without health insurance, provide broad parameters about social determinants of health.

The educational level of the population may also be used as a measure of outcomes for community-as-relational-experience. Programs aimed at keeping children in school, such as asthma education, teen parenting, and day care for teenage parents, should consider the inclusion of dropout rates or retention rates as indicators of program success. Other components of educational achievement are graduation rates, school attendance improvement, and number of general education diplomas awarded.

An example of using a measure of community-as-relational-experience is provided in Box 18.2.

Community-as-Resource

The conceptualization of community-as-resource focuses on community strengths and capacity. The community is seen as coming together to share support systems and resources. Measures are multidimensional to reflect both the complexity of the community-as-resource conceptualization and the practice of the public/community health nurse. Both qualitative and quantitative measures are needed for evaluating the outcomes of a program implemented within the community-as-resource approach.

BOX 18.2 COMMUNITY–AS-RELATIONAL-EXPERIENCE: MEASURE OF PROGRAM EFFECTIVENESS

Goal: To improve access to healthcare for uninsured residents of the county

Objective: To connect 10 people per month to primary care providers through the Access to Care program

Standard: At least 10 people per month will make appointments with primary care providers

Measure: Ten appointments per month with new patients referred from the Access to Care program are documented by written reports from providers

The types of measures may include tools to capture the type and number of resources within a community, changes in risk factors, connectedness among community members, and accounts of change. Using McKnight and Kretzmann's (2012) approach to mapping community capacity, increases in number and types of resources available within and to a community could be measured to demonstrate the success of a program. The types of resources could be compared with those identified as needed in the community assessment. An example of this type of measure is an increase in primary care providers. Quantifying these changes could be done in proportions, such as a change from one primary care provider for every 10,000 residents (1:10,000) to one for every 5,000 residents (1:5,000).

Changes in risk factors may be quantified as discussed in the preceding section that contains epidemiological approaches as well as indirect measures. For example, the number of restaurants and grocery stores that sell nonfat milk could be compared before and after a program to improve the nutritional status of a community. Other indicators of a change in risk factors include decreases in the number of arrests for driving under the influence of alcohol or drugs, treatment for opioid abuse, and decreases in the number of cases of child abuse.

Accounts of change may take many different forms in the evaluation of programs within the conceptualization of community-as-resource. Theoretical models may be used to guide the use of measures of change before and after a program, for example, the number of people who moved from precontemplation to the stage of contemplation in the transtheoretical model (Prochaska & DiClemente, 1985). Other accounts of change may be recorded on tools that measure self-reports of attitudes, behaviors, and feelings.

Box 18.3 provides an example of measures to use with community-as-resource.

■ SELECTING EXISTING MEASURES FOR PROGRAM EVALUATION

In selecting from among existing measures for program evaluation, the advanced practice public/community health nurse will need knowledge about the properties of instruments to choose wisely. The primary concern about instruments is reliability, but validity should also be considered. Locating existing measures may pose a challenge because no one source is available. This section presents a review of reliability and validity and provides a summary of sources of measures to use in program evaluation.

BOX 18.3 COMMUNITY-AS-RESOURCE: MEASURES OF PROGRAM EFFECTIVENESS

Goal: To improve access to low-fat, nutritious foods for community members

Objective: To have low-fat foods listed on the menus of all public food establishments

Standards

1. School lunch programs will offer low-fat or nonfat milk choices every day on school lunch menus.
2. All restaurants and cafeterias in public buildings and healthcare facilities will offer low-fat or nonfat menu choices.

Measure: A monthly count of the number of low-fat or nonfat foods offered on a sample of menus for schools and public food service establishments

Understanding Properties of Instruments

A major concern of a program evaluator is to locate instruments that measure the outcome of interest with reliable and valid results. All instruments contain some measurement error; it is impossible to develop a perfect tool. In addition, the administration of instruments by less-than-perfect people in less-than-perfect situations results in more error (Waltz, Strickland, & Lenz, 2017).

Given these limitations, finding the right instrument means locating one that is reliable and valid for the intended purpose, and is also correct for the administration circumstances. For instance, an instrument to measure the knowledge of people with diabetes and their families that requires paper-and-pencil testing and demonstration of skills with insulin administration may be reliable and valid for testing knowledge about diabetes. However, the practical limitations of the clinical setting may make it very unlikely that the test could be administered according to the directions of the test developers. A brief paper-and-pencil test of knowledge and skills may be a better alternative.

RELIABILITY

A measure is said to be reliable if it measures a phenomenon consistently (Waltz et al., 2017). Reliability is a characteristic of the instrument or measure under certain circumstances with certain subjects. An instrument is not considered reliable for all testing situations. When using any instrument, the evaluator will want to run statistical tests to determine the reliability of the instrument in the specific situation.

Three types of reliability are stability, homogeneity, and equivalence. Stability, or test–retest reliability, is the consistency of repeated measures. The use of this type of reliability requires that the characteristic being measured remain the same from one test time to the next. This type of reliability is usually used with paper-and-pencil tests and physical measures.

Homogeneity, also known as *internal consistency,* is the extent to which the items in an instrument measure the same construct. Internal consistency is expressed as the Cronbach's alpha coefficient and may range from 0.0 to 1.0. When the data are dichotomous, the Kuder–Richardson formula (K-R 20) is used instead of the Cronbach's alpha. A test for internal consistency is used with paper-and-pencil tests as well as other cognitive measures.

Equivalence reliability focuses on comparing two versions of the same paper-and-pencil test or two observers measuring the same event. *Interrater reliability* is the term used when two or more observers rate the same event. When two paper-and-pencil instruments are compared, the reliability is referred to as *alternate forms* or *parallel forms.* Interrater reliability is used in clinical settings when more than one rater is using the same instrument. Although there is no standard for acceptable interrater reliability, any value less than 0.80 should raise questions about the reliability of the data (Grove, Burns, & Gray, 2013).

VALIDITY

An instrument is said to be valid to the extent that it reflects the construct being examined. Validity is a matter of degree; it is not absolute. A measure that has been tested for validity in some circumstances may not be valid in others. Thus, the characteristic of validity does not refer to the instrument itself, but to the use of an instrument in specific situations. In addition, validity testing is not a one-time event. Validity is continuously evaluated each time a measure is used.

Although types of validity are discussed in the literature (e.g., content, predictive, and construct), validity is now considered a single broad method referred to as *construct validity* (Grove et al., 2013). Construct validity is the fit between conceptual and operational definitions of variables to determine whether instrument actually measures what it declares to measure.

Various means of testing the validity of an instrument used in specific circumstances may be reported in the literature. Content-related validity may be determined using the index of content validity developed by Waltz and Bausell (1981). Other techniques of testing validity include factor analysis, evidence from contrasting groups, convergence, divergence, discriminant analysis, prediction of future events, and prediction of concurrent events (Grove et al., 2013). Several of these techniques use correlation procedures to determine the relationships between the instrument under study and another known instrument. Correlations may vary between 0.0 and 1.0; a level of .70 or more is indicative of an adequate validity for use of the instrument in another study (Nunnally & Bernstein, 1994).

Criteria for Selecting Instruments

An evaluator wants to find the most appropriate and strongest available tools or instruments to measure the dependent variable (program outcome) to give a program the fairest evaluation. The outcome of the evaluation study will be limited by the ability of the instrument to detect differences in the program participants or in the events that are being measured. Given the objectives for selecting instruments mentioned previously, the following criteria are recommended:

1. Adequate reliability and validity reported
2. Instrument measures what you want it to measure
3. Readability at the level of the population to be studied
4. Similar population used with the instrument earlier
5. Reasonable time required for completing and scoring the instrument
6. Acceptable amount of training needed to administer the instrument
   (Grove et al., 2013)

Often, an instrument is located that is almost, but not totally, suitable for the purpose needed. The evaluator will be tempted to make changes in the wording of a few items, add a few items, or delete a few items. If any changes are made, the evaluator must bear in mind that the reported reliability and validity data are no longer applicable to the changed instrument. Testing to determine the reliability and validity for use of the altered instrument should be done before it is used in an evaluation study.

Sources of Measures for Program Evaluation

Several books have been published with discussions of and actual instruments to use in various studies. A list of books containing instruments is provided in Box 18.4. Often these tools may be used without written permission if profit from their use is not intended. Sometimes, a small fee is charged to obtain copies of the instruments ready for use.

The second major source of information about instruments is research articles. Although the instrument itself may not be found in the article, often, enough information is provided to determine whether instrument will meet the need. Usually, the author can be contacted for more information, including the instrument and directions for use and scoring.

Another source of instruments is the computer Internet site HaPI (Health and Psychological Instruments Online). Other computer sites may be found by exploring

---

BOX 18.4   SOURCES OF INSTRUMENTS FOR EVALUATING PROGRAM OUTCOMES

Beaton, S. R., & Voge, S. A. (1998). *Measurements for long-term care: A guidebook for nurses.* Thousand Oaks, CA: Sage.

Beere, C. A. (1990a). *Gender roles: A handbook of tests and measurements.* Westport, CT: Greenwood.

Beere, C. A. (1990b). *Sex and gender issues: A handbook of tests and measurements.* Westport, CT: Greenwood.

McDowell, I., & Newell, C. (1996). *Measuring health: A guide to rating scales and questionnaires* (2nd ed.). New York, NY: Oxford University Press.

Nunnally, J. C., & Bernstein, I. H. (1994). *Psychometric theory* (3rd ed.). New York, NY: McGraw-Hill.

Reeder, L. G., Ramacher, L., & Gorelnik, S. (1976). *Handbook of scales and indices of health behavior.* Pacific Palisades, CA: Goodyear.

Rinke, L. T. (1987). *Outcome measures in home care. Volume I:* Research (Pub. No. 21–2194). New York, NY: National League for Nursing.

Strickland, O. L., & Dilorio, C. (2003). *Measurement of nursing outcomes* (2nd ed.) *Volume II: Client outcomes and quality of care.* New York, NY: Springer Publishing.

Strickland, O. L., & Dilorio, C. (2003). *Measurement of nursing outcomes* (2nd ed.). *Volume III: Self-care and coping.* New York, NY: Springer Publishing.

Ward, M. J., & Lindeman, C. (1979). *Instruments for measuring nursing practice and other health care variables: Volume* 1 (Publication No. HRA 78–53 [Vol. 1]). Hyattsville, MD: Department of Health, Education, and Welfare (DHEW).

Ward, M. J., & Lindeman, C. (1979). *Instruments for measuring nursing practice and other health care variables: Volume* 2 (Publication No. HRA 78–54 [Vol. 2]). Hyattsville, MD: Department of Health, Education, and Welfare (DHEW).

---

various key words in different search engines. Local university libraries may also have programs constructed for users at that particular site. Exploration of local sources may lead to other sources.

Other instruments may be located in doctoral dissertations, master's theses, unpublished reports, and evaluation studies. *Dissertation abstracts* may be located in at most university libraries and online on the web. Unfortunately, most instruments for measuring phenomena in nursing practice concentrate on changes in the individual. There are instruments directed to individual change that may be used to aggregate change for groups or even communities.

If an appropriate instrument cannot be located, the next step is to develop a new measure to meet the specific need for the evaluation study. Although this is not recommended, there are approaches to make this task easier and the outcome more useful. The following section offers suggestions and pitfalls to avoid.

■ DEVELOPING NEW MEASURES FOR PROGRAM EVALUATION

Developing a new measure is usually very time-consuming and requires a period of testing before it can be used with confidence in a study. The long lead time required for instrument development and testing—sometimes as much as a year—needs to be addressed before the program is implemented. Once the program has begun, as pointed out earlier, baseline data needed for a specific aspect of program evaluation may not have been collected. If the newly developed instrument was not available for baseline data collection, the opportunity for before and after comparisons may be lost.

To avoid these disappointments, the advanced practice public/community health nurse will need to begin instrument development during the phase of writing the evaluation plan. If there are staff members with experience in instrument development, they, as well as consultants, should be involved if funding permits. University faculty experienced with instrument development and testing should also be invited to participate as consultants, experts, or advisors, even if funding is not available to pay them. Often, faculty will donate time if they can be involved in writing and publishing an article about the instrument. Also, faculty may be able to secure funding to assist with the process.

Steps in Developing an Instrument

This section provides an introduction to the steps involved in developing an instrument. The reader will find useful assistance from other sources for details or information not included here (DeVellis, 1991; Steiner & Norman, 2008; Waltz et al., 2017).

IDENTIFYING THE FOCUS OF THE INSTRUMENT

Probably the biggest hurdle for the developer of an instrument is to be very clear about what the instrument will measure. This may sound simplistic but can lead to many hours of frustration if this first step is not completed. For example, if satisfaction with the program is the topic for the instrument, how will satisfaction be defined? Will it be a global satisfaction measure, that is, cover all aspects of the program? Or will each aspect of the program be measured for satisfaction, such as interaction with the staff, adequacy of information, and location of the program?

If an acceptable definition of the concept to be measured is not in the literature, there are formal techniques for identifying the focus of the instrument. One technique is concept analysis, which requires that the attributes or characteristics of a concept be identified (Grove et al., 2013; Meleis, 2012). A concept analysis of patient satisfaction has been published and may be useful (Mahon, 1996). Many other concept analyses can be located in the literature as well as other descriptions of various concepts or constructs for the topic of instrument development.

DEVELOPING ITEMS FOR THE INSTRUMENT

Once the focus of the instrument is decided, the next step is to design the instrument. In this step, developing items for the tool is a good place to start. Items for the tool should be written to reflect as fully as possible the concept to be measured. For example, if knowledge of proper diet is being measured, nutrition, portion size, and regular meal times should be included. As the wording of the items will require testing and rewriting, the concern is to write at least two times the number of items desired in the final tool. Through testing and revision, half of the items may be eliminated (Nunnally & Bernstein, 1994).

REVIEWING INSTRUMENT ITEMS

The next step in instrument development is to have the items reviewed by others for content, understandability, reading level, and cultural relevance. Items should then be revised on the basis of the suggestions. In addition to experts in the content area, members of the group to be studied should review the items.

IDENTIFYING SCALES TO MEASURE THE ITEMS

After writing items to reflect the concept, the advanced practice public/community health nurse needs to identify a way to measure the items. Commonly used for knowledge tests are yes/no scales, multiple-choice questions, and true/false statements. For other types of tools, Likert scales (e.g., to what extent do you agree on a scale of 1–5) are commonly used. The type of scale to be used will depend on several factors, including the amount of detail needed for the program evaluation, the reading comprehension of the program participants, the availability of statistical analysis programs, the statistical analysis skills of staff or consultants, and the time available to complete analyses (DeVellis, 1991; Fink, 1993; Spector, 1992).

TESTING THE DRAFT OF THE INSTRUMENT

The next step is testing the draft tool with a few people like those who will complete the instrument for program evaluation. Getting comments from these participants verbally or in writing will provide information for revising the items. If time allows, a field test of the instrument should be done next with as many people as time and resources allow. The number of people recommended for a field test is 200 (Nunnally & Bernstein, 1994). If it is not possible to obtain such a wide field test, a test with fewer people should be completed.

The data from the field test should be analyzed through item analysis to determine which items perform best on the instrument. The best-performing items should be retained and the others eliminated (Nunnally & Bernstein, 1994). The reliability of the new instrument can also be calculated if the number of responses is large enough.

Validity studies for the new instrument should be carried out after the reliability is determined but may be done simultaneously with the reliability study. However, the evaluator in the service setting often does not have the resources to conduct these additional studies. This is the point at which the assistance of university faculty may be particularly helpful.

An alternative to a simultaneous or separate study is to conduct a validity study at the same time data are collected for the evaluation study. To accomplish this, additional data can be collected from the evaluation study population. For example, if evaluation of satisfaction with the program is measured by a 10-item survey, a second satisfaction tool with known reliability and validity could also be used. The results of the 10-item instrument and the other instrument are then correlated to determine the degree of agreement between the two. A moderate-to-high level of agreement (a correlation coefficient of 0.70–1.0) gives the evaluator confidence about the initial validity of the new instrument. There are numerous other techniques for testing validity (Waltz et al., 2017); consultation may be needed to determine which technique or techniques are appropriate.

Acceptable reliability and validity of a new instrument provides the beginning information about the tool to be used in other studies, but additional testing is needed, as discussed earlier. Every time an instrument is used, reliability and validity estimations, if possible, should be part of the statistical analyses.

■ RELATIONSHIP OF PROGRAM EVALUATION TO QUALITY ASSESSMENT/QUALITY IMPROVEMENT ACTIVITIES

In Chapter 16, quality-assessment and quality-improvement activities were discussed as part of program evaluation or a type of program evaluation. Moreover, quality assessment and improvement may be considered as a separate group of activities that may inform the evaluation study. This section provides suggestions for integrating quality-assessment activities with the evaluation study for efficiency and benefit to the program.

What Is Quality?

What is quality? This question is often asked and volumes have been written to elucidate the answer. One definition is the degree that health services for individuals and populations increase the possibility of preferred health outcomes, and that the health services are consistent with current knowledge (McGlynn, 1997). Another source of information is an analysis of the concept of quality conducted by Mandzuk and Mcmillan (2005).

One part of a definition of quality often neglected is that it involves value judgments. What one person calls *quality* another may refer to as *mediocre*. We need only examine various tastes in music, houses, clothes, and other material possessions to see this in practice. Another aspect of value judgments is that the environment greatly influences what each of us perceives as quality. For example, advertising constantly bombards us with images of what are good products and influences us to buy them. These products may or may not be good, but we often do not know how they compare with others because we do not purchase and try a wide variety of similar products.

The same is often true for healthcare. Most people do not sample the care provided by various providers before they decide who will do the surgery or treat them for hypertension. People change healthcare providers when they are unhappy with the provider and/or the care given, if there is a choice in providers. Often, there are few choices because of either lack of availability, lack of transportation, or other factors that make changing providers either impractical or impossible.

Quality-Assessment Activities

Given that many stakeholders are interested in quality of healthcare, how can a program go about doing that which will result in quality? First, some studies have shown that consumers of healthcare are as interested in the caring component of care quality as they are in the technical component (Ludwig-Beymer et al., 1993).

Thus, the program evaluator may be interested in both the technical quality and the qualitative aspects of quality, such as caring, compassion, and kindness. All these qualities and more can be appraised through the activities of a quality-assessment and quality-improvement (QA/QI) program. The results of the QA/QI program are used to improve the program, but also should be used to provide information about the program evaluation study. One of the difficulties using the results of quality-assessment studies to improve the program is that changing the program may make it very different from the one that was started. Thus, pinpointing which part of the program resulted in the desired outcomes would be almost impossible if adjustments were continuously made during the life of the program. To avoid this situation, QA/QI activities should be geared to keeping the fidelity of the program interventions without modifying the original configurations of the interventions and program design.

For example, a program designed to decrease smoking in an adult population should not be changed to incorporate other smoking-cessation techniques after the program delivery has begun. The introduction of additional interventions will make it difficult to determine whether the original program or the added elements were related to any changes in participants. Replication of programs with continuous changes imposed on the interventions is not possible, nor would it be a good use of resources.

Rather than change the interventions, the QA/QI activities should be geared to keeping the interventions as close as possible to the program plan by monitoring the structure and process criteria and standards established for the program. Standards for QA/QI components should be written to reflect the program intentions for quality; for example, program participants should have all preprogram measures taken at the specified time, and program facilitators should be trained to deliver the intervention as it is explained in the program plan.

These types of standards not only reflect the program as planned but also guarantee that the program is implemented with quality. This focus is on structure and process standards for the QA/QI activities that will contribute to a stronger program and provide valuable data for the program evaluation. The documentation about QA/QI using structure and process standards is used to provide background for the evaluator about maintenance of fidelity and management of the program during the life of the program.

■ USING NURSING CLASSIFICATION SYSTEMS IN PROGRAM EVALUATION

Nursing classification systems assist with the organization and documentation of nursing care. These tools are related to patient classification systems that originally provided approaches for predicting nurse staffing needs for hospital shifts (Abdoo, 2000). Patient classification tools are used extensively in inpatient settings but have not been as popular in public/community health nursing care.

Developments in the past decades have turned to comprehensive systems for classifying patient diagnoses, interventions, and outcomes. Saba (1992) and McCloskey, Bulechek, and others (Johnson, Bulechek, Dochterman, Maas, & Moorhead, 2001; Johnson & Maas, 1997; McCloskey & Bulechek, 1996) developed useful systems for individuals in hospitals, home care, and ambulatory settings. The North American Nursing Diagnosis Association (NANDA) system was established in the early 1970s and has been continuously updated (Herdman & Kamitsuru, 2014).

In 1986, the American Nurses Association initiated action to compile a classification system for nursing practice to submit to the World Health Organization for possible inclusion in the tenth edition of the *International Statistical Classification of Diseases and Related Health Problems* (Carpenito, 1995). As a culmination of the work, the list of diagnoses was created in 1996 as the International Classification of Nursing Practice (ICNP) Alpha version, and was last updated in June 2015 (World Health Organization [WHO], 2017).

Since the mid-1970s, one classification system has been developed for use in community health nursing. The Omaha System (Martin, 2005; Martin & Scheet, 1992) was developed at the Visiting Nurse Association of Omaha over a span of more than 20 years and is suited for use with individuals, families, groups, and communities.

The Omaha System

The three components of the Omaha System are the Problem Classification Scheme, the Intervention Scheme, and the Problem Rating Scale for Outcomes. The Problem Classification Scheme and the Problem Rating Scale for Outcomes are discussed here in terms for use in a program evaluation. The Intervention Scheme is not discussed because it is not applicable for a program in which the intervention or interventions have been determined in the program plan.

THE PROBLEM CLASSIFICATION SCHEME

The Problem Classification Scheme is a taxonomy of nursing diagnoses useful for identifying, labeling, and organizing concerns of public/community health nursing practice. The scheme is a framework of client-focused problems that are addressed with nursing interventions. Problems are similar to nursing diagnoses but are more common to the practice of public/community health nursing. The Omaha System includes problems about individuals, families, and communities.

The scheme consists of four domains: environmental, psychosocial, physiological, and health-related behaviors. Each domain is organized into four levels: domain, problem, modifier, and sign/symptom. The ordering of this system is from the general to the specific. An example of one problem in the environmental domain is: "Problem 04: Neighborhood/ workplace safety. Freedom from injury or loss as it relates to the community/place of employment." Level 03 and 04 for this problem are: Modifier 03: Deficit. Signs/Symptoms 02: high pollution level (Martin & Scheet, 1992, p. 68).

The Omaha System is useful as the organizing framework for a record system for individuals, families, and communities. A consistent approach for organizing data used by all staff provides a valuable resource for the program evaluator as well as a base for additional program planning. If all nursing staff use the same problem list, compilations of problems for reporting purposes are completed more easily. Also, the consistency of how problems are stated provides a better picture of the health status of the program population.

In addition to stating problems consistently, the Problem Classification Scheme may be used to help identify appropriate programs for individuals, families, and communities. For example, an intervention designed for a specific set of life circumstances is more appropriately applied only to those individuals who possess the specific life circumstances. Others may be included, but the program will not necessarily be effective with people who possess other characteristics.

PROBLEM RATING SCALE FOR OUTCOMES

Another component of the Omaha System, the Problem Rating Scale for Outcomes, can provide structured data that are useful for program evaluation. This scale measures client progress related to specific client problems. For example, the concept of *knowledge* is defined as the ability of the client to remember and interpret information. A Likert scale of 1 = no knowledge to 5 = superior knowledge can be used by the nurse to record progress in reaching the care outcome each time the client is seen or is part of a group session. Behavior and status are also rated on Likert scales of 1 to 5, with each number having a specific definition (Martin, 2005; Martin & Scheet, 1992).

If all staff uses the same scales and the same definitions, ratings on the scales can be summarized to measure a group's progress toward meeting program objectives. An example is a program standard that 80% of participants will increase their knowledge about the benefits of regular exercise. If the knowledge gain of each participant was measured on the 1-to-5 scale, the proportion of the group that increased their knowledge could be readily calculated. Calculations of average achievement of each participant and the total group could be determined as well as the range of scores and other statistics.

In a similar fashion, the achievement of different groups in a program can be compared. If statistically significant differences in achievement levels are observed from group to group, additional evaluation can be performed to detect reasons for these differences.

■ SUMMARY

Program evaluation using an approach to examine effectiveness was presented in this chapter. Program effectiveness focuses on evaluating the extent to which the program met its goals and objectives.

Many instruments and measures of program effectiveness exist in the literature, on the Internet, and in various studies done by master's and doctoral students. The evaluator is encouraged to seek out already developed and tested instruments to save time and resources. If no appropriate instruments are available, the advanced practice public/community health nurse will need to develop and test one or more instruments following the steps identified in this chapter. Assistance from a consultant may be needed for instrument design and analyses of the data collected during the testing phase.

QA/QI can be part of the process for program evaluation by providing data about the actions taken to keep the program structure and process on track. Making changes in the intervention is discouraged because this will confound the ability of the evaluator to determine the extent to which the intervention was related to or caused the outcomes.

Nursing classification systems are useful for program purposes and also help with data collection for program evaluation. The Omaha System developed at the Visiting Nurse Association of Omaha is especially useful for communities because diagnoses related to problems in the community are listed. The system also allows for categorization of outcomes for communities (Martin, 2005; Martin & Scheet, 1992).

The next chapter presents the essential ingredients needed to conduct a program evaluation. Aspects of program effectiveness presented in this chapter are illustrated in practice in Chapter 20.

■ SUGGESTED CLINICAL OR PRACTICUM ACTIVITIES

1. Using the community of your clinical placement, compare and contrast measures of community-wide program outcomes based on the three conceptualizations of community discussed in this text: community-as-client, community-as-relational-experience, and community-as-resource.
2. Review program evaluations designed by a local health department or a non-profit agency to determine what, if any, community-level program outcomes measures were used.
3. Interview an advanced public/community health nurse about the types of classification systems that are used in her or his organization. What suggestions might you offer about the value of classifications systems using resources discussed in this chapter?

REFERENCES

Abdoo, Y. M. (2000). Nurse staffing and scheduling. In L. M. Simms, S. A. Price, & N. E. Ervin (Eds.), *The professional practice of nursing administration* (3rd ed., pp. 459–480). Albany, NY: Delmar.

Carpenito, L. J. (1995). *Nursing diagnosis: Application to clinical practice* (6th ed.). Philadelphia, PA: Lippincott.

Centers for Disease Control and Prevention. (2016). CDCWONDER, Multiple causes of death 1999–2015. Retrieved from https://wonder.cdc.gov/wonder/help/mcd.html

Centers for Disease Control and Prevention. (2017). Lack of health insurance coverage and type of coverage. Retrieved from https://www.cdc.gov/nchs/data/nhis/earlyrelease/earlyrelease201702_01.pdf

Chen, H. T. (2015). *Practical program evaluation: Theory-driven evaluation and the integrated evaluation perspective* (2nd ed.). Los Angeles, CA: Sage.

DeVellis, R. F. (1991). *Scale development: Theory and applications*. Newbury Park, CA: Sage.

Donabedian, A. (1966). Evaluating the quality of medical care. *Milbank Memorial Fund Quarterly, 4,* 166–206.

Donabedian, A. (1969). *A guide to medical care administration, Vol. 2. Medical care appraisal: Quality and utilization*. New York, NY: American Public Health Association.

Fink, A. (1993). *Evaluation fundamentals: Guiding health programs, research, and policy*. Newbury Park, CA: Sage.

Grove, S. K., Burns, N., & Gray, J. (2013). *The practice of nursing research: Appraisal, synthesis and generation of evidence* (7th ed.). Philadelphia, PA: Saunders.

Herdman, T. H., & Kamitsuru, S. (Eds.). (2014). *NANDA international nursing diagnoses 2015–17: Definitions and classifications* (10th ed.). Oxford, UK: Wiley-Blackwell.

Johnson, M., & Maas, M. (Eds.). (1997). *Nursing outcomes classification (NOC)*. St. Louis, MO: Mosby-Year Book.

Johnson, M., Bulechek, G., Dochterman, J. M., Maas, M., & Moorhead, S. (Eds.). (2001). *Nursing diagnoses, outcomes, and interventions: NANDA, NOC, and NIC linkages*. St. Louis, MO: Mosby.

Ludwig-Beymer, P., Ryan, C. J., Johnson, N. J., Hennessy, K. A., Gattuso, M. C., Epsom, R., & Czurylo, K. T. (1993). Using patient perceptions to improve quality care. *Journal of Nursing Care Quality, 7*(2), 42–51.

Mahon, P. Y. (1996). An analysis of the concept "patient satisfaction" as it relates to contemporary nursing care. *Journal of Advanced Nursing, 24,* 1241–1248.

Mandzuk, L. L., & Mcmillan, D. E. (2005). A concept analysis of quality of life. *Journal of Orthopaedic Nursing, 9*(1), 12–18. doi:10.1016/j.joon.2004.11.001

Martin, K. S. (2005). *The Omaha System: A key to practice, documentation, and information management* (2nd ed.). Omaha, NE: Health Connections Press.

Martin, K. S., & Scheet, N. J. (1992). *The Omaha system: Applications for community health nursing*. Philadelphia, PA: Saunders.

McCloskey, J. C., & Bulechek, G. M. (Eds.). (1996). *Nursing interventions classification (NIC)* (2nd ed.). St. Louis, MO: Mosby.

McGlynn, E. A. (1997). Six challenges in measuring the quality of health care. *Health Affairs, 16*(3), 7–21.

McKnight, J. L., & Kretzmann, J. P. (2012). Mapping community capacity. In M. Minkler (Ed.), *Community organizing and community building for health* (pp. 171–186). New Brunswick, NJ: Rutgers University Press.

Meleis, A. I. (2012). *Theoretical nursing: Development and progress* (5th ed.). Philadelphia, PA: Wolters Kluwer.

National Research Council and Institute of Medicine, Panel on Understanding Cross-National Health Differences Among High-Income Countries. (2013). *U.S. Health in international perspective: Shorter lives, poorer health*. Washington, DC: National Academies Press.

Nunnally, J. C., & Bernstein, I. H. (1994). *Psychometric theory* (3rd ed.). New York, NY: McGraw-Hill.

Patient Protection Affordable Care Act (ACA), Public Law 111–148. (2010). 111th United States Congress. Washington, D.C.: United States Government Printing Office. Retrieved from http://www.gpo.gov/fdsys/pkg/PLAW-111publ148/pdf/PLAW-111publ148.pdf

Prochaska, J. O., & DiClemente, C. C. (1985). Common processes of self-change in smoking, weight control and psychological distress. In S. Shiffman & T. Wills (Eds.), *Coping and substance use* (pp. 345–364). Orlando, FL: Academic Press.

Saba, V. K. (1992). The classification of home health care nursing: Diagnoses and interventions. *Caring, 11,* 50–57.

Spector, P. E. (1992). *Summated rating scale construction: An introduction*. Newbury Park, CA: Sage.

Steiner, D. L., & Norman, G. R. (2008). *Health measurement scales: A practical guide to their development and use* (4th ed.). New York, NY: Oxford University Press.

Waltz, C. F., & Bausell, R. B. (1981). *Nursing research: Design, statistics, and computer analysis*. Philadelphia, PA: Davis.

Waltz, C. F., Strickland, O. L., & Lenz, E. R. (2017). *Measurement in nursing and health research* (5th ed.). New York, NY: Springer Publishing.

World Health Organization. (2017). *Classifications. Classification of diseases (ICD). International classification for nursing practice (ICNP)*. Retrieved from http://www.who.int/classifications/icd/adaptations/icnp/en

CHAPTER 19

Conducting a Program Evaluation

Sue Ellen Bell

■ STUDY EXERCISES

1. What sources of data are used for program evaluation?
2. What are the advantages and disadvantages of each type of data source?
3. How do you determine appropriate baseline indicators?
4. What is the relationship between goals and objectives and data analysis?
5. How does one choose the best method for analysis?
6. What is the role of the evaluator in screening and interpreting data?
7. How do you present the evaluation report in written and oral formats?

Program evaluation is an ongoing task that involves determining what variables to measure and how to measure them as well as collecting, analyzing, and interpreting data on the effectiveness and efficiency of programs affecting the individual, family, and community. Evaluation serves many purposes. The most common purposes are to determine the usefulness of ongoing programs and to suggest ways to improve them.

In the past, evaluation often focused on defining the processes of a program. How many educational sessions were provided? How many participants attended? These were common questions that could be answered with relatively little effort. However, in today's marketplace, which focuses on cost and quality, there is increased emphasis on evaluating programs in terms of measurable outcomes of both effect and cost-effectiveness. The strategies used for program evaluation must be rigorous, and the advanced practice public/community health nurse who participates in program evaluation needs a strong foundation in theory and application.

The success of the evaluation is tightly linked to the conceptualization and design phase of the program. Decisions made during program development have a crucial influence on program evaluation. Completing a meaningful evaluation of a program that has been poorly conceptualized is a frustrating, if not impossible, experience.

■ THE ROLE OF THE EVALUATOR

Evaluation does not occur in a vacuum. The advanced practice public/community health nurse who is called on to complete an evaluation may experience role conflict when conducting an evaluation for stakeholders who hold different values. Program administrators may be most interested in documenting the efficiency and cost-effectiveness of a program, whereas program recipients may be most interested in whether the program is reaching most of the intended audience. The successful evaluator must consider the priorities of all stakeholders and complete the evaluation in a manner that demonstrates a commitment to the integrity of the evaluation data.

Advanced practice nurses are familiar with standards of practices that guide the profession. The American Nurses Association, American Public Health Association, and other professional organizations have developed and disseminated standards to guide practitioners. These standards are benchmarks that can be used to evaluate performance. Similarly, the American Evaluation Association (AEA, 2004) has developed guiding principles for evaluators. These guidelines, in revision for review at the 2018 annual conference, provide a framework for the evaluator. Adoption of these principles by the evaluator will contribute to an ethical evaluation process and an evaluation report that is of high quality. A summary of the principles follows, along with discussion of application by the advanced practice public/community health nurse.

Systematic Inquiry

"Evaluators conduct systematic, data-based inquiries" (AEA, 2004, para. 11). Whether advanced practice public/community health nurses use qualitative methods, quantitative methods, or both when conducting an evaluation, they must be well versed in the methodology. At the beginning of the evaluation, evaluators should discuss the strengths and weaknesses of different types of methodologies with the stakeholders in the project. Evaluators should explain in clear terms what the assumptions, strengths, and limitations are of different approaches to evaluation. This type of discussion needs to occur at the beginning of the evaluation, periodically throughout the evaluation, and when compiling the final evaluation report (AEA, 2004). Failing to include stakeholders in evaluation planning and process can result in misunderstanding and conflict between the evaluator and the recipients of the evaluation report.

Competence

"Evaluators provide competent performance to stakeholders" (AEA, 2004, para. 14). It is often difficult for the advanced practice public/community health nurse to possess all the skills of a good evaluator, particularly if this is a new role. When the evaluator lacks a critical skill, a team approach should be used (AEA, 2004). For example, if the recipient of the evaluation wants to conduct a survey of potential clients and the evaluator has had no training in survey design, arrangements need to be made to obtain the necessary expertise. A limited contract or consultation with a survey design team can help the evaluator ensure that the survey is conducted using appropriate survey-design methods.

When the evaluator does not have the requisite skills and there is no way to obtain them, he or she should decline the request to be the evaluator (AEA, 2004). Gaining expertise in the role of an evaluator is an ongoing process, and those who aspire to this role must engage in continuing education and formal course work to upgrade their skills. With the advent of computer technology, the evaluator needs to have a combination of skills that includes both "people skills" and technical skills related to the use of information technology. As evaluators expand their skills, they can complete evaluations of programs with greater complexity.

Integrity and Honesty

"Evaluators display honesty and integrity in their own behavior, and attempt to ensure the honesty and integrity of the entire evaluation process" (AEA, 2004, para. 18). Evaluators need to be honest about the costs of the evaluation as well as the scope and use of the evaluation report. It is the evaluator's responsibility to clarify these issues before the evaluation begins. A written contract should include the fee, expected outcome, and a timetable with due dates for components of the report and the final report. If changes are made in the proposed plan during the evaluation, they should be documented in writing and approved by both evaluator and client.

In some cases, an evaluator may have a potential conflict of interest that must be disclosed to the client (AEA, 2004). For example, if the advanced practice nurse is asked to complete an evaluation on a health department program and a relative or friend is the head of the program, this information needs to be disclosed to the person who commissions the evaluation study. An open discussion and a formal decision are needed about whether the evaluator can complete an unbiased evaluation.

If an evaluator has concerns that the evaluation data are being misinterpreted or misused by certain stakeholders, a plan must be made to deal with this issue. Discussing the concern with other advanced practice nurses or experienced evaluators and the relevant stakeholders can assist in resolving the dilemma (AEA, 2004). If the evaluator continues to have serious reservations about how the data are being interpreted or used, it may be necessary to appeal to a higher authority, attach a dissenting cover memo to the evaluation report, or refuse to sign the final report (AEA, 2004).

Respect for People

"Evaluators respect the security, dignity, and self-worth of the respondents, program participants, clients, and other stakeholders" (AEA, 2004, para. 25). When completing an evaluation study, the evaluator must be sensitive to differences in culture, religion, gender, disability, age, sexual orientation, and ethnicity of potential stakeholders. The dignity and worth of all groups should be respected. If the report reflects negatively on a group, the findings must be handled tactfully in a professional manner. It is important to be honest without overstating the results and to provide a thoughtful, balanced interpretation (AEA, 2004).

Advanced practice public/community health nurses must abide by ethical standards of the profession and principles related to informed consent and the protection of human subjects. As noted earlier, the line between evaluation and research is sometimes fuzzy. If the evaluator plans to publish the results of the report or present the findings at professional meetings, serious consideration must be given to the need to follow federal guidelines related to the protection of human subjects and to seek approval from an appropriate institutional review board.

The advanced practice nurse is also bound by standards of the profession when completing an evaluation. If the commissioner of the evaluation study asks the nurse to complete activities in conflict with the American Nurses Association code of ethics or the state nurse practice act, these activities should be declined.

At times, the evaluator may realize that the evaluation data will cause harm to all or some of the stakeholders in the project. If the evaluation shows that a program did not have the intended effect or had a negative effect, the evaluator may be providing the justification to eliminate the program. This situation needs to be handled carefully. It is important to explore limitations of the report and consider the timing of the report. Will the report do more harm than good? Evaluators must preserve the integrity of the data while minimizing any unexpected harm to the stakeholders or the programs (AEA, 2004).

Responsibilities for General and Public Welfare

"Evaluators articulate and take into account the diversity of interests and values that may be related to the general and public welfare" (AEA, 2004, para. 31). The evaluator needs to be mindful of the broader context in which the evaluation is completed. A democratic society is based on freedom of information, and, unless there are compelling reasons for withholding information, evaluators should share pertinent information with all stakeholders. In addition, evaluators need to balance their relationship with the client who is funding the evaluation with the greater good of society. For example, an evaluator might find that a product or service causes harm to certain individuals. Publication of the evaluation report might have a negative effect on the client, but the evaluator needs to consider the greater good of society. Conversely, when benefits to the client conflict with the principles of integrity, social equity, and nondiscrimination, evaluators must discuss the conflict with stakeholders, and, if the conflict cannot be resolved, a decision needs to be made about continued involvement in the evaluation (AEA, 2004).

The next sections provide the advanced practice public/community health nurse with more tools and knowledge to use in conducting evaluations in a variety of situations for a variety of programs and services.

■ SOURCES OF DATA FOR PROGRAM EVALUATION

Evaluation begins with a thorough community assessment that documents baseline data. Content about community assessment, sources of data collection, and methods for data collection are presented in other chapters of this book. In this chapter, the primary focus is on organizing and analyzing the data so that they can be used in an evaluation report. The quality of the evaluation is largely determined by the quality of the assessment and data-collection methods. For example, before a program for diabetes follow-up in the community is established and later evaluated, many questions must be investigated in the assessment phase. How many people in the community have diabetes? How old are they? What is their education level? What resources are already available to them? What is the level of need? Are they experiencing complications or are they managing their condition? Answers to these questions are critical to establish a baseline for the evaluation. Beginning a new program without baseline data is like starting a trip across the country without a road map. You might eventually get there by luck, but there is no way of knowing if there was a faster way to travel or if your route was better than the many other roads that could have been taken.

Existing Data Sources

A description of existing national and state data sources is provided in Chapter 5. Using these sources as a part of an evaluation may be possible if there is a good match between the existing data source and the project.

CENSUS DATA

The census data of the U.S. population is considered reliable. The Census Bureau has made this information readily available at its website (www.census.gov.), and the evaluator can search for specific baseline data related to a specific project. However, census data need to be interpreted with caution for groups that are traditionally underrepresented in the census, such as the homeless or transient populations. For example, census data collected several years ago may have little relevance in evaluating a program targeted for migrant farmworkers.

DATA ON NATALITY

Local health departments and state governments collect data related to natality, morbidity, and mortality. Data on birth statistics vary from state to state but generally contain information related to birth weight, maternal age, and marital status. Some states collect data related to prenatal care, pregnancy, birth complications, and maternal habits. Interpretation of some of the latter data must be approached with caution because they are frequently gathered from maternal interviews, and there may be some discrepancy between what the mother reports and other objective measures.

When these data are forwarded to the Center for Health Statistics, they are compiled into comparative tables that can be valuable for the evaluator. For example, if the advanced practice nurse is evaluating a program related to infant mortality, the Linked Birth and Infant Death Data set can provide baseline data on national infant mortality patterns (Centers for Disease Control and Prevention [CDC], 2015). The linked files include information from the birth certificate such as age, race, and Hispanic origin of the parents; birth weight; period of gestation; plurality; prenatal care usage; maternal education; live birth order; marital status; and maternal smoking. This information is linked to death certificate information such as age at death and underlying cause of death. These data can provide a baseline for the evaluation plan.

DATA ON MORBIDITY

Clinics, doctors' offices, and emergency departments collect morbidity data. Certain infectious diseases are reported to the CDC for compilation. Although it is better than no data at all, the validity of this information is frequently questioned, especially in relation to some of the less socially acceptable diseases. Therefore, some existing morbidity data related to communicable diseases may be underreported and need to be validated with other sources collected at the community level.

Morbidity data are also gathered through ongoing surveys coordinated by the National Center for Health Statistics (NCHS). For example, the National Health Interview Survey has been conducted since 1957 and provides data to monitor trends in illness and disability and to track progress in achieving the national health goals. Data are collected through personal household interviews conducted by interviewers employed by the U.S. Bureau of the Census. The survey includes specific core questions asked at each interview that can be used to track morbidity data over time. In addition, specialty surveys for adults and children are administered to gain more in-depth information about specific conditions of national interest. Data from this survey can be helpful to the evaluator in comparing a program to national and state benchmarks.

DATA ON MORTALITY

Mortality data are gathered from death certificates. Most states collect data on primary cause of death and contributing factors. Some providers may be reluctant to list certain conditions or health problems on death certificates for reasons of stigma or to prevent problems for the survivors in collecting life insurance benefits. For example, if the patient had life insurance that excluded payment for preexisting conditions, family members may have a long process of substantiating when a chronic condition was diagnosed. It is much simpler to not list it. How frequently this occurs is unknown. Death certificate information, though not perfect, is the best information available about mortality.

In 1997, the *Atlas of United States Mortality* was released to the public (CDC, 2018). This atlas was the first to show all leading causes of death by race and gender for small U.S. geographic areas referred to as Health Service Areas (HSAs). According to the NCHS, the top 10 causes of death included in this atlas (coronary heart disease, cancer, chronic lower respiratory disease, accidents, stroke, Alzheimer's disease, diabetes, influenza or pneumonia, kidney disease, and suicide) accounted for 73.6% of all deaths in the United States from 2010 through 2014, the most recent reporting period. Charts that compare rates for individual HSAs to national rates are available.

ADVANTAGES AND DISADVANTAGES OF EXISTING DATA

The major advantage of ongoing data sets that are compiled at the national and state levels is that they allow for the comparison of local statistics to other regions. These data may provide convincing evidence in the evaluation report that the program being evaluated is having an effect and changes in rates of illness or mortality are not spurious. For example, if the advanced practice nurse is evaluating a program to reduce infant mortality through home visits to high-risk prenatal clients, she can use the national linked birth and infant death data set to document that the program targeted an area with a higher infant mortality rate than other regions of the country.

At the end of the program, the advanced practice public/community health nurse can compare the current infant mortality rate with the baseline as well as comparing the program data to national trends. It may be that for the period in question, the advanced practice public/community health nurse can demonstrate that rates in the targeted region declined while national rates were rising. Alternatively, the evaluator may find that the intervention resulted in no change in infant mortality. At face value, it may seem that the program was not successful. However, if national and state rates were rising while rates in the targeted area remained stable, then the evaluator might argue that indeed the program was a success. Comparative data such as these are crucial in preparing the evaluation report.

The major disadvantage of existing data sets is that they are often not specific enough or do not contain enough data to evaluate the full effect of a program. There is always some lag time before data are available, and the evaluator may have difficulty matching the time frame for the baseline data to the time frame needed for the project. There are always some concerns when any national data set is used. It is impossible for such a broad instrument to capture the nuances that are unique to a targeted area. Therefore, the advanced practice public/community health nurse must consider other sources of data to use in establishing baseline data for the evaluation.

Other Sources of Baseline Data

Other sources of baseline data include key informants, records, and survey results. The methods for collecting data from these sources are discussed in Chapter 6. The focus of this chapter is how to use the data from these sources after they are collected.

DATA FROM KEY INFORMANTS

Often the easiest and most economical source of baseline data is information from key informants. Two problems that must be addressed with this source are (a) identifying valid key informants for the project and (b) quantifying the input in a manner that makes it usable for the evaluation (Pact, 2014).

Key informants are often prestigious community leaders or persons who have administered or interacted with programs such as the one under evaluation. Unless the interviewer has a reliable and valid instrument for collecting data from the key informant, the data may be of little value in evaluating the project. For example, suppose the advanced practice public/community health nurse interviews several county commissioners to determine the magnitude of sexually transmitted diseases (STDs) or sexually transmitted infections in the community. Unless the nurse uses a systematic framework for the interviews, she or he may not get the same information from each commissioner. Furthermore, the commissioners' perceptions may be clouded by bias related to their own experiences rather than hard data. For this input to be valuable in the evaluation phase, the interviewer needs to determine whether the commissioners' comments represent the actual incidence of STDs or perceptions of the incidence of STDs. There may or may not be a close relationship between the actual and perceived incidence.

Although data obtained from key informants tend to be subjective, they can be very useful in helping to identify factors that contribute to the success or failure of a program. Often, key informants have pearls of wisdom that can alert the evaluator to problems that were not identified in more objective forms of evaluation. For example, if the input from key informants suggests that most key informants do not recognize that STDs are a problem, then the evaluation should address the need to develop a method for monitoring and evaluating the perceived incidence of STDs in the community. Particularly in a politically charged area, such as STDs, the perceived incidence will have an effect on reducing the actual incidence. However, if the information is not quantified during the initial interview, it may not be possible to evaluate the change in perception by key community leaders at the end of the project.

DATA FROM PATIENT RECORDS, AGENCY RECORDS, AND PATIENT REGISTRIES

Patient records, agency records, and patient registries are other sources of baseline indicators. These sources can vary widely in terms of reliability and validity (Gliklich, Dreyer, & Leavy, 2014; Waltz, Strickland, & Lenz, 2017). When the evaluator uses records as a basis for program evaluation, a judgment needs to be made about not only the quantity of the data but also the quality. Has there been an ongoing quality-assurance program to track the data for accuracy? Are data-collection instruments standardized in a manner that matches the goals of the project? How have staff been trained in the use of data-collection tools? Answers to these questions and others are critical if records are to serve as a basis for program evaluation. For example, if the goal of a program is to improve the follow-up of women who receive positive pregnancy tests, a record audit of well-kept records may provide useful information. The evaluator should be able to establish the baseline rate of follow-up at the beginning of the project and use this in the evaluation.

However, if the goal of a program is to reduce the abortion rate among teenagers in the county, an analysis of local clinic records may not be reliable. Many teens may choose to go out of their local area to have abortions, so an audit of the county agency record system will not capture the actual rate. In this case, the evaluator may need to have access to other healthcare facilities in the region to evaluate the actual rate of abortions among teenagers in the county.

DATA FROM FOCUS GROUPS AND SURVEYS

Finally, when data are not otherwise available, the evaluator may have to establish baseline indicators from focus groups or survey results. Surveys usually involve a considerable amount of effort, skill, and resources. Chapter 6 provides information about how to develop a reliable and valid survey instrument. When using survey information, the evaluator needs to be concerned with the reliability and validity of the instrument as well as the sampling procedures for administering a survey. Unless there is a good match between the sampling framework for the survey and the targeted population for the project, usefulness of the survey data will be limited.

Many communities regularly complete an extensive community survey that can serve as baseline data for several projects. In fact, as indicated in previous chapters, tax-exempt hospitals are required under the Patient Protection and Affordable Care Act (ACA) to conduct a Community Health Needs Assessment (CHNA) every 3 years (Association of State and Territorial Health Officials [ASTHO], 2017). The purpose of the assessments is to identify needs of the population served by the hospital and to determine ways that the hospital can partner with the community for better overall health outcomes.

Focus groups and key informant interviews provide input for the CHNAs. Focus groups require a skillful facilitator, and, as with key informant data, the input may be difficult to quantify. If the focus group is videotaped or audiotaped and transcribed, meaningful themes might be extracted that can provide important information to consider in the evaluation phase of the project. A program in Canada to promote awareness, knowledge, and uptake of cancer screening used focus groups to explore the experiences of women who served as lay community peer leaders (Ahmad, Ferrari, Moravac, Lofters, & Dunn, 2017). The focus groups provided important information related to the meaning of being peer leaders and perceived barriers of this role in relation to increasing breast and cervical cancer screening among immigrant women. These data were helpful in program planning as well as program evaluation. The focus groups helped to identify additional indicators of program outcomes.

The Youth Risk Behavior Surveillance System (YRBSS) uses a survey format and has been conducted biennially since 1991. Data are collected on six areas of youth risk behavior (CDC, 2016). The six priority areas are "behaviors that contribute to unintentional injuries and violence; sexual behaviors that contribute to human immunodeficiency virus (HIV), other sexually transmitted diseases, and unintended pregnancy; tobacco use, alcohol and other drug use; unhealthy dietary behaviors; and physical inactivity" (CDC, 2016, p. 1).

There is no one perfect method of establishing baseline indicators for program evaluation (DC Healthy Communities Collaborative, 2016). One frequently used procedure is to conduct a needs assessment in two phases: exploration using focus groups and key informants and a quantitative assessment to give some reliable estimates of the extent of the need or problem. The key point is that evaluation begins at assessment, and a good assessment leads to a higher probability of a good evaluation.

■ THE RELATIONSHIP BETWEEN GOALS AND OBJECTIVES AND DATA-ANALYSIS METHODS

Well-written, clear, measurable objectives make evaluation much easier. The planning of a program, discussed in Chapter 12, and development of the evaluation plan go hand in hand.

Goals and objectives help define evaluation data needs. If the program targets specific diseases or conditions, baseline incidence and prevalence data are needed. If the goal of a program is to reduce the incidence of hypertension in a community, then knowing the baseline level of hypertension in the community as well as for subgroups in the community, is crucial.

If programs are preventive in nature, the population at risk must be defined carefully and with as much specificity as possible. For example, if a program seeks to improve immunization rates of 2-year-olds in a community, then an accurate count of 2-year-olds must be determined. Will the project target all 2-year-olds? Are there specific high-risk groups that have different rates from the general population? How will 2-year-olds who migrate in and out of the region during the intervention be counted? Clear and measurable objectives make the evaluation easier and influence the type of analyses chosen.

◼ SELECTING ANALYSIS METHODS

The evaluator uses a variety of techniques to analyze data during and after the program. These range from simple descriptive statistics to multivariate analysis. The type of analysis is dependent on the type of data available and the purpose of the evaluation.

During process evaluation, the evaluator tries to determine the extent to which a program is reaching the intended population, providing services, and expending resources. As presented in Chapter 16, the purpose of process evaluation is to monitor implementation of the program plan and use of the results for continuous quality improvement (Community Interventions for Health, 2017). The target population, coverage of the target group, and monitoring delivery of services are major concerns in process evaluation (Newcomer, Hatry, & Wholey, 2015).

Monitoring participation by the target population involves tracking participants and their continued contact with the program. Types of activities in which participants take part are usually delineated. If participation involves various activities, such as screening, education classes, and counseling, each activity is separately identified.

Code sheets and a framework for data collection are essential. These need to be developed in the planning phase of the project. Each participant needs to be assigned a unique identifier so that cumulative data for that participant can be collected systematically. The coding sheet will ease interpretation for data that can be classified into discrete categories. Simple mistakes in designing a coding sheet can lead to confusion later. For example, if the coding sheet categorizes income as $15,000 to $20,000 and $20,000 to $30,000, where does one code the individual who makes exactly $20,000? If the evaluator is developing the coding sheets, it is important that several people review the codes for clarity and to ensure that categories are discrete and logical.

In most cases, it is better to enter data in the most detailed form possible. It is always possible to recode and collapse data into broader categories, but it is not possible to create data that have never been entered. For example, suppose that one of the components of the program is to administer a questionnaire that measures the quality of life of participants. A summative score of this instrument can be determined. Even though the evaluator is probably most interested in the summative score, it would be more prudent to enter the values for all items on the scale. By doing this, the evaluator can later recode values into subscales or examine individual items. Without the detail of the individual item data, the evaluation will be limited, and questions that emerge throughout the project may not be able to be addressed.

As a part of the process evaluation, statistical calculations will be made to give a clearer picture of the data. Certain statistical tests have assumptions about the level of measurement and the distribution of data that must be met if interpretation is to be accurate. Other statistics have less restrictive assumptions but may be less powerful in drawing inferences. A thorough review of data-analysis methods can be found in most advanced research texts. In this section, the most common statistics found in evaluation reports are discussed.

Descriptive Statistics

Descriptive statistics are used in both process and outcome program evaluations. In a process evaluation, the evaluator will rely on descriptive statistics to quantify the characteristics of the participants and the types of interventions. Descriptive data are more meaningful when represented as percentages or rates rather than raw numbers or counts. For example, the statement "65% of the participants were Hispanic females" is clearer and easier to interpret than the statement "there were 435 Hispanic females in the sample." Similarly, "there were 375 deaths from cardiovascular disease in Jones County last year" is less clear than "the cardiovascular death rate in Jones County was 375/100,000." By using percentages and rates, changes in the targeted group can be compared to national, state, or regional rates.

MEASURES OF CENTRAL TENDENCY

Two categories of descriptive statistics often used in an evaluation report are central tendency and dispersion or variation. Measures of central tendency include the mean, mode, and median (Polit & Beck, 2017).

To illustrate how the mean, mode, and median demonstrate different patterns, consider the following example. In a community-based clinic, the evaluator reported that the mean age of participants in a support group was 41 years. The actual ages of the participants were 25, 30, 40, and 85. In this example, the mode is 25 and the median is 30, whereas the mean is 41. Depending on the question that is being asked in the evaluation, the evaluator may need to consider all these measures. Although all three values are different, it suggests to the evaluator that the data points are not symmetrical and further exploration might be warranted.

MEASURES OF VARIANCE OR DISPERSION

In addition to measures of central tendency, the evaluator often reports two values that reflect the amount of variance in the data. The standard deviation reflects the distance of the scores from the mean. The standard deviation helps the evaluator understand how spread out the data points are, and it is often reported with the mean. The larger the standard deviation, the more variability is in the data.

Another measure of dispersion is the range. The range includes the smallest and the largest value for an indicator. The range identifies the extreme values in the distribution and is very sensitive to changes in even a single value (Polit & Beck, 2017).

MEASURES OF PROGRAM COVERAGE

Coverage of the target population refers to the extent to which the program reached its target population (Newcomer et al., 2015). Objectives for the program usually define what level of participation is desired in the target population. Few programs ever achieve total participation, so it is very important to have an accurate picture of who is participating. Bias can occur if certain groups within the target population participate and others do not. This bias can affect the total effectiveness of the program. As noted in the example earlier, if there is a discrepancy between the proposed target and the actual participants, the objective may be only partially met.

Although a process evaluation focuses on describing who is in the program and what services are being provided, it is also important in many cases to determine who is not in the program. Sometimes, individuals who are a part of the target group never hear about the program; and in other cases, they may make an initial contact with the program but never follow through. The evaluator often needs to quantify these data so that a determination can be made on whether the program is reaching the target group or whether the group represented in the sample is different from the target group in key aspects. For example, suppose that the goal of a program is to increase immunization rates of 2-year-old children in a county. The morbidity data for the county suggested that 30% of the African American 2-year-olds in the county were not properly immunized by their second birthday in comparison to 20% of the Caucasian population. When the program was examined after 6 months, the evaluator found that 80% of the participants were African American, and although the rate for African Americans had increased, the rate for Caucasians had declined. The evaluator needs to look beyond the participants in the program to determine why it is reaching only a portion of the targeted population. To do this analysis, the evaluator needs to determine the degree of coverage.

It is generally expected that the larger the proportion of the target population that is served, the better for the program. However, both undercoverage and overcoverage can be problematic. Overcoverage may mean that potential participants are not adequately screened before entry. This overcoverage can drain resources. If a program calls for 50 participants in a specific category and 100 are enrolled, it may mean that there will not be adequate resources to serve clients in another category. On the other hand, undercoverage of a group suggests that there are perhaps problems in the selection criteria or the recruiting strategies.

Rossi, Lipsey, and Freeman (2004) suggested the following formula for measuring the efficiency of coverage:

$$\text{Coverage efficiency} = 100 \times \frac{\text{Number in need served}}{\text{Total number in need}} - \frac{\text{Number not in need served}}{\text{Total number served}}$$

Values between +100 and −100 indicate the efficiency of coverage. A major difficulty in determining coverage is the inability to delineate accurately the number of people in the target group. Some of the data sets already discussed, such as morbidity data, program records, surveys of participants, and community assessments, can be helpful in determining the level of coverage.

Community surveys, though generally expensive to perform, may be the best method to determine participation levels in a defined population. This method may be the only way to obtain information from nonparticipants and perhaps determine some reasons for the nonparticipation. Often, it is more important to know who is not receiving services than to know who is receiving them. Useful data for program managers compare those who use the program, those who came but left the programs, and those who do not participate. This information helps to judge the worth of the program effort and can help define program modifications to attract and retain a larger proportion of the target population.

Even if an accurate determination of coverage cannot be made, the evaluator will want to track participants who enter a program but do not complete the intervention. To do this, it is important to get information about key variables at the first contact. Descriptive data, such as age, marital status, occupation, living arrangements, education, and income, can help the evaluator compare those who complete the program with those who do not complete the program. Data should be collected early because it is often extremely difficult to track individuals who drop out of a program. Examining differences in completers and noncompleters can help the evaluator reach an understanding of factors that enhanced or hindered participation in the program.

Inferential Statistics

As a project progresses and the evaluation moves to assessing outcomes, inferential statistics and a comparison of outcomes to costs and resource utilization are used. Commonly used inferential statistics include the Chi-square test, *t*-test, analysis of variance (ANOVA), and correlation coefficients (Polit & Beck, 2017). The focus in this discussion is on relating the statistical test to the evaluation question. The reader should consult a statistics text for additional information about the underlying assumptions and logic behind the calculation of these statistics.

COMPARING FREQUENCIES

Chi-square is a statistical technique used to compare frequencies in various categories. The categories do not have to be hierarchical, but they do need to be mutually exclusive. Data can be measured at the nominal level. Suppose the evaluator asks, "Is there a difference in attendance of sessions by gender?" The evaluator can construct a two-by-two table as seen in Table 19.1 and use a Chi-square test to determine whether there is a difference.

COMPARING MEAN SCORES

If the evaluator wants to know whether there is a difference in mean scores between two measures on the same individual or a single measure on two different groups, the t-test may be an appropriate statistic. In the first case, suppose the evaluator has completed an educational intervention for a group and wants to compare the mean score of the participants before and after the intervention. The paired t-test would allow for such a comparison. This test compares mean scores when there are two values of the same variable for each case.

On the other hand, the evaluator may want to compare mean scores between two groups that are not the same. Suppose the question is: "Do men and women have different mean scores on the knowledge questionnaire at the beginning of the program?" In this case, the evaluator would use an independent or group t-test to compare the mean scores for these two different groups. Polit and Beck (2017) cautioned that both tests assume that the variable is normally distributed and that the groups have approximately the same standard deviation. When these assumptions are not satisfied, especially if the sample is small or the groups are unequal, the resulting t value may be inaccurate and inappropriate to report.

If the evaluator wants to compare mean scores for many groups or for many variables, then the ANOVA procedure can be used. ANOVA tests for a difference in means among several groups. A post hoc test can then be used to locate the specific difference between any two groups within the sample. There are many forms of ANOVA, from simple one-way analysis, in which the mean for several groups in relation to one variable is examined, to more complex computations that allow for the introduction of covariates or repeated measures on the same subject. These techniques are discussed in statistics textbooks.

Correlation coefficients allow for comparison of two variables measured at the interval level. Although the previous statistics asked the question, "Is there a difference?" This statistic asks, "Is there a relationship?" The Pearson product–moment correlation is often used to see whether two variables seem to vary in the same pattern. For example, the evaluator

TABLE 19.1 Two-by-Two Table

Men attending all sessions	Women attending all sessions
Men not attending all sessions	Women not attending all sessions

might be interested in knowing whether mean scores increase as a person ages. Performing a correlation between age and the mean score demonstrates a positive correlation of 0.50 ($p = .001$), suggesting that scores do increase as a person ages. As with all the statistical tests, a p value or test of significance generally accompanies the statistic.

The evaluator needs to assess the use of these statistics and others carefully in relation to the assumptions that must be met and the quality of data available. Consultation with a statistician can help the evaluator to use the appropriate statistic and to interpret the findings correctly.

MATCHING STATISTICAL METHODS WITH OUTCOME MEASURES AND DESIGN

One of the most crucial questions the evaluator must answer is what outcome measure is to be used in the evaluation. For example, for a public health program aimed at teaching new mothers about healthful diets, many different types of measures could be used. Testing knowledge "before and after" educational sessions is one option. Testing knowledge of persons who received sessions versus persons who did not is another option. Or one could conduct weekly recalls of dietary intake and compare whether the information had been put into practice. Clearly, there is a difference between acquiring knowledge and behavior. It is crucial to determine evaluation criteria on the basis of the initial goals of the program. In addition, the type of program design will affect the type of outcomes that can be evaluated.

The best design for evaluating the effect of a program is the randomized controlled trial (RCT), in which subjects are randomly assigned to a treatment or intervention and a nonintervention group. This model reduces bias and the results are more generalizable. Subjects are randomly assigned to an intervention or a nonintervention group and self-selection is eliminated. However, RCT designs are rare in the practice of the advanced public/community health nurse. They are expensive studies and often require external funding and the services of a multidisciplinary team affiliated with a major university or research organization.

A more common scenario for the advanced practice public/community health nurse is the evaluation of a program using a quasi-experimental design in which participants are compared within the group or a comparison is made between participants and nonparticipants. The evaluator must be cognizant of threats to internal and external validity that occur when using these less rigorous designs. These concepts are reviewed in Chapter 17. The evaluator must strive for the best design possible within the realistic constraints of the program.

To evaluate the outcomes of a program, inferential statistics coupled with tests of statistical significance are often used. However, McKenzie, Neiger, and Thackeray (2016) cautioned the evaluator to carefully distinguish between program significance and statistical significance. It is possible, particularly when a large number of people are included in the project, to achieve statistical significance that is not significant from a programmatic standpoint. For example, in a large intervention to reduce blood pressure in community-based elders, the evaluator found that the clients in the treatment group had a statistically significant lowering of their diastolic blood pressure when compared to the nonintervention group. However, careful examination of the data found that the actual mean difference in the two groups was 2 mmHg. The intervention group had a mean diastolic level of 84, and the nonintervention group had a mean diastolic of 86. Although the results were statistically significant, it is left to the advanced practice nurse to determine the clinical significance of the difference.

Cost Analysis

In addition to statistical analyses that compare differences or relationships among participants in the program, there is increased emphasis in program evaluation on determining the cost–benefit and cost-effectiveness of programs.

Cost–benefit and cost-effectiveness analyses provide a financial frame of reference for evaluating a project. However, cost–benefit and cost-effectiveness analyses are frequently treated with a fair amount of skepticism. Difficulties with measuring costs and benefits include identifying and measuring every program cost and benefit and expressing each of these costs and benefits in monetary terms. Because the outcomes of many programs are social or preventive in nature, it is often difficult to make an exact determination of benefits and costs. Take, for example, the evaluation of a home-visit prenatal program targeted at lowering the incidence of low-birth-weight infants. Hospital and medical costs that are saved can be calculated easily. However, the mental and emotional costs to a family do not have a readily available dollar value. Nevertheless, the emphasis on estimating the cost–benefit and cost-effectiveness of programs is likely to continue.

Kleinpell (2013) defined cost–benefit analysis as a measure of the cost of an intervention relative to the benefits it yields. The measure is usually expressed as a ratio of dollars saved for every dollar spent on the program. *Cost-effectiveness* is defined as a measure of the cost of an intervention relative to its effect, usually expressed in dollars per unit of effect. Indicators of cost-effectiveness include number of years of life saved, number of pounds lost, or number of people who quit smoking.

Although these definitions of cost–benefit and cost-effectiveness are similar, the basic difference lies in the need to assign a monetary value to the desirable consequences when performing a cost–benefit analysis. Cost-effectiveness analyses are different from cost–benefit analyses in that effectiveness outcomes are expressed in terms of health, such as the number of lives saved. Cost–benefit analyses convert outcomes into dollars.

McKenzie et al. (2016) stressed the importance of clearly defining the problem and specifying the objectives when doing cost-effectiveness analyses. Depending on the scope of the problem, the results of the analysis might vary considerably. For example, if a cardiovascular risk-reduction program has the objective of reducing health insurance costs of the employer, then the cost analysis needs to use monetary costs and benefits that relate to the employer. Calculating hours of work lost, insurance costs, labor costs, and other similar indicators would be appropriate. However, if the objective of the program is to reduce costs for the employees, then a different set of indicators is warranted. The evaluator might use costs of insurance premiums, transportation, doctor visits, and prescriptions.

One of the major objectives of any cost analysis is to compare alternative interventions to addressing a health concern. Therefore, it is imperative that the intervention alternatives use the same framework to calculate costs. Each alternative should be treated in a similar manner.

MODEL FOR ASSESSING COSTS AND EFFECTIVENESS

Russell (2015) proposed a framework for assessing the societal costs and effectiveness of disease and injury prevention programs. This model suggests that a determination of cost should include the direct costs of the program such as personnel, equipment, and space as well as indirect costs, including time for the recipient to attend the program, time lost from work, and time for travel. Similarly, benefits should include direct benefits saved, such as saved healthcare costs, and indirect benefits, such as increased productivity.

Russell (2015) operationalized a cost-effectiveness calculation as:

$$\text{Cost-effectiveness} = \frac{\text{Net cost}}{\text{Adverse outcome averted}}$$

Net cost includes the cost of the program plus the cost of the side effects minus cost of the disease minus indirect cost. Cost of the program includes the costs for management and operation such as space, equipment, materials, personnel time, travel, overhead, follow-up, and treatment, plus the time and expenses of the participants. Cost of the side effects includes the expenses associated with incidental hazards and psychological effects associated with the program. Cost of the disease includes direct costs of care that would have been associated with the disease if it had not been prevented. Indirect costs include the costs from such occurrences as absenteeism or loss of productivity.

MEASURING COST-EFFECTIVENESS THROUGH DISCOUNTING

Discounting is another important concept related to cost-effectiveness analysis of longitudinal programs. *Discounting* refers to program costs and benefits that do not occur entirely in the present. For comparison, all future costs and benefits should be discounted to their present value. Establishing the discount rate is to some extent a value judgment. The main point is that a dollar today is generally worth more to an individual than the promise of having the dollar in the future.

Cost–benefit and cost-effectiveness evaluations require sophisticated analysis, particularly for multiyear, complex projects. However, the concepts of costs and benefits hold much relevance for program evaluation. The advanced practice public/community health nurse will need to consult with the financial officers of the institution to create credible cost-effectiveness models. There is a certain level of subjectivity in determining what to count as costs and what monetary value needs to be put on some benefits. Completing a cost-effectiveness analysis will require that the advanced practice public/community health nurse collaborate with colleagues in business to develop a model that is regarded as valid by a variety of stakeholders.

■ PRESENTING THE EVALUATION REPORT

Organizing evaluation data into a coherent report can be a challenge for the evaluator, but it is essential if the data are to be used to influence future initiatives. The evaluator must give enough detail in the report so that an audience unfamiliar with the program can make meaningful interpretations. At the same time, the report must be organized in a manner so that the important points are summarized clearly and concisely.

Often, the evaluator prepares both a written report and an oral presentation. The written report serves as the official record of the evaluation. The oral report may be presented to the funding agency, the directors of the program, or the larger community.

The Written Report

For projects that span several years, the evaluator may prepare interval reports as well as a final report at the end of the project. Interval reports summarize the results for a specific time frame within a project. For example, if the project is a 3-year intervention to reduce infant mortality, the evaluator will often prepare an interval report after year 1 and year 2. The reports should summarize the progress for each objective, explain any variance from the objective, and make recommendations for the remainder of the project. Most funding agencies require interim reports for multiple-year projects. Many funding agencies will require specific tables and graphs that must be included, especially if the project is part of a larger, multiple-site intervention. Table 19.2 gives an example of a table that might be included in an interim report.

At the end of the project, the evaluator will present an evaluation of the total project. The style of the report needs to be tailored to the audience. For example, if the report goes to a board of directors consisting mainly of community leaders, it will have a different tone than a report that is required for a federally funded program. In the first instance, the tone may be more informal and include anecdotes as well as case studies to illustrate the effect of the project. The evaluator will probably limit technical language and refer the reader to an appendix or to a more detailed report of the project.

On the other hand, a federal agency might require a more detailed report with specific statistical interpretations of the major outcomes. Anecdotal information might be perceived negatively unless it is supported by quantitative data and statistics.

Most evaluation reports include five major areas: an abstract or executive summary, introduction or background, interventions/methods, results, and discussion and recommendations.

The abstract or executive summary gives an overview of the entire project, including the rationale, objectives, major interventions, results, and recommendations. Often, the executive summary is the most important part of the evaluation report because, for many audiences, this may be the first and only part that they read. The length varies from a few paragraphs for a relatively simple project to two or three pages for a more complex project. The evaluator should write this section without using jargon or technical terms. Use clear, understandable words and short, crisp sentences that convey the essence of the project. The executive summary is usually written in the active voice. It is better to use active voice and state, "The project staff accomplished three objectives" rather than "Three objectives were accomplished during the project."

The other sections of the written report provide more detail. The introduction or background provides the rationale for development of the project and lists the major goals and objectives. In this section, the evaluator provides a frame of reference for the following sections of the evaluation report. The evaluator might relate the project to baseline indicators of national, state, or local trends that existed at the initiation of the project. The evaluator might describe the process used to develop the project, including the identification of community leaders who were instrumental. The background information assists the reader to understand the context in which the project was developed.

In the Interventions or Methods section, the evaluator describes exactly what was done. The target population, sampling procedures, and sample characteristics should be specified. Instruments should be described, and the reliability and validity of these instruments

TABLE 19.2 Example of a Table for Interim Report

Year 1 Objective	Evaluation	Recommendation
Enroll 40 high-risk prenatal clients into the program, 25% of whom are from minority ethnic groups	50 high-risk clients were recruited; 10 (20%) were minority	Increase recruitment areas of minority clients, initiate contact through lay advisers and follow-up home visits and phone calls
Maintain an attrition rate of no more than 10% for women enrolled in the program	Of the 50 women recruited into the program, two (4%) have dropped out	Objective met, continue with retention plan, monitor attrition rate

should be reported. The data-collection procedures and the plan for interpreting findings should be outlined.

The Results section of the report describes the findings from the data analysis and answers the evaluation questions. Several charts and tables often accompany a narrative explanation of the findings. Charts and tables need to be clearly labeled and follow an approved format. Tables and graphs need to include the sample size for each analysis and a clear legend that identifies both axes of a graph or all columns of a table. All tables, graphs, and figures should be labeled chronologically. In some cases, the narrative is written without interruption, and supporting materials, such as tables, are placed in an appendix.

Often, the evaluator includes a table that shows how the evaluation relates to the objectives and the intervention. Table 19.3 is an example of a table that may be used to summarize such data.

The last section of the written report provides an interpretation of the results, including a discussion of limitations and recommendations. In this section, the evaluator objectively acknowledges the strengths and weaknesses of the project. Some evaluators try to put a positive spin on the results and emphasize only the positive aspects of the project without acknowledging the limitations. This strategy can backfire and the whole report may be called into question. The role of the evaluator is not to sell the program to future participants or program developers but to provide a realistic interpretation of the results. Acknowledging the problems and offering realistic, pragmatic solutions make the evaluation report more valuable for future programs.

The Oral Report

In addition to the written report, the evaluator is often called on to provide an oral report of the project. Whether the oral report is an opportunity or a dreaded event depends on the preparation and skill of the evaluator as well as the content of the message.

BACKGROUND PREPARATION

When preparing for the oral report, the evaluator needs to do some background work. How large will the audience be? What is their knowledge of the project? Are they likely to be a friendly audience, or is resistance or hostility a possibility? How big is the room? What audiovisual equipment is available? Answers to these questions can help the advanced practice public/community health nurse to prepare an oral report that is well received. In addition, commonsense strategies, such as getting a good night's sleep, eating a small meal, taking a glass of water, and wearing comfortable clothing and shoes, can aid the evaluator in feeling confident, alert, and organized.

TABLE 19.3 Relationship of Objectives and Intervention

Objective	Intervention/Method	Evaluation
Increase to 80% the proportion of 2-year-old children in the county who are up to date on their immunizations (baseline: 60%)	Offer immunizations during WIC appointments and family-planning clinic visits. Use follow-up reminders and postcards for all clients. Complete a home visit within 1 month of delinquent appointments.	At the end of the project, 92% of the participants were up to date on their immunizations; however, the county rate is 75%, indicating there are children not reached by the immunization interventions and need to be immunized.

WIC, Women, Infants and Children Nutrition Program.

REHEARSAL FOR THE ORAL REPORT

Prior to the presentation, it is a good idea to rehearse alone and in front of others. Even the best report will be greeted with a negative response if it is too long and extends beyond the allotted time. It is often more of a challenge to decide what to leave out of the oral report than what to put in it. A rehearsal before a friendly audience who will provide constructive criticism can help the evaluator anticipate problems with the evaluation report.

ESTABLISH RAPPORT WITH AUDIENCE

During the presentation, the presenter will want to establish rapport with the audience. This can occur with a brief introduction or an anecdote. The presenter might disclose information that will help the audience understand the context of the report. Use of humor or a joke can be an icebreaker but needs to be used with caution and not distract from the major objective of conveying the information in the evaluation report. Maintaining eye contact with the audience, speaking instead of reading, and speaking slowly with occasional pauses are examples of good presentation strategies. It is important for the evaluator to not only present the report but also be aware of the audience reaction to the report. Widespread inattention suggests to the presenter that a quick assessment is in order. There may be a need for some impromptu adjustments in the format. Perhaps the presenter needs to interact with the audience by asking questions, or the presenter may need to orient the audience to the components of the report.

CONTENT OF THE ORAL REPORT

Generally, the oral presentation will follow the content of the written report but will probably be given in less detail. The presenter will give background information, outline the key points to be covered, present the evaluation data, summarize the results, and open the floor for discussion. For complex presentations, it is often helpful to provide a handout of the presentation for the audience. If specific tables or graphs are an important part of the presentation, the audience will appreciate a hard copy of these materials.

In this era of technology, most presenters accompany their presentation with visual aids such as slides, videos, computer-generated slides, or handouts. These visual aids can enhance the oral report. In the planning stages of a project, organizers will often budget money for audiovisual materials. A short video or slide show that portrays the staff and participants in the program can convey the real essence of an initiative. The video can be used to introduce the evaluation report or as a summary.

During the presentation, the advanced practice public/community health nurse should use slides or overheads to supplement the material. Using slides helps to keep the presenter on track and can help to minimize the tendency to read rather than communicate the report.

The Dartmouth Biomedical Library (2016) suggested several guidelines for developing effective visuals. These are summarized in Table 19.4.

It is important to keep in mind that visuals are just an adjunct. An enthusiastic voice, a calm interactive style, and an organized demeanor are just as important, if not more important, than professional-looking slides. In fact, slides that have too much information on them or include lots of bells and whistles, such as flying words and audio effects, can distract from the presentation. The advanced practice public/community health nurse needs to strike a balance between communicating with technology and communicating on a personal level.

TABLE 19.4   Guidelines for Effective Visuals

Use Readable, Consistent Typeface

Do not mix more than two typefaces.
Use a font size of at least 20 points.

Use Some Color

Using color can increase attention.
Use color consistently and for emphasis.
Do not vary color too much or the audience will wonder why. For example, use the same background
   consistently unless there is a logical reason to change. No more than five colors per slide are recommended.
Light words on a dark background are easiest to read.

Keep It Simple

Use a few phrases rather than sentences.
Use no more than five phrases and six lines of text to a slide.
Limit the words to those that are key to convey the meaning.
Create slides that present a logical progression of thoughts with each slide building on the previous slide.

Be Consistent in Some Aspect of the Format

Use similar headings for all visuals.
Use parallel structure (e.g., all phrases begin with a verb).

Vary the Look of the Visual

Use pictures or charts when relevant to the message.
Alternate text with charts and graphs.

Supplement the Comments With the Visuals Not the Other Way Around

Do not just read the slides; use them as an outline and fill in details.
Match the content to the audience type and knowledge of the material.
Maintain eye contact with the audience rather than the visual.

▪ SUMMARY

This chapter has provided an overview of how to conduct a program evaluation. The
emphasis has been on analyzing the findings, interpreting data, and presenting the findings to different audiences. The advanced practice public/community health nurse needs
to become adept at all these skills so that effective programs can be replicated and continued. With clear knowledge of the components of the evaluation process, the chance of
continued success is possible.

▪ SUGGESTED CLINICAL OR PRACTICUM ACTIVITIES

1. Review a report of a program evaluation at your assigned agency or another
   nonprofit community agency. Determine what statistical analyses were performed to examine the effectiveness of the program.
2. In the same program evaluation report as in #1, if possible, determine how the
   program outcomes compared with the program goals and objectives. What
   measures were used to determine the program effectiveness?
3. Attend a community or agency presentation of a program evaluation. Compare
   the presentation to the ideas presented in this chapter.

REFERENCES

Ahmad, F., Ferrari, M., Moravac, C., Lofters, A., & Dunn S. (2017). Expanding the meaning of being a peer leader: Qualitative findings from a Canadian community-based cervical and breast cancer screening programme. *Health and Social Care in the Community, 25*(2), 630–640. doi:10.1111/hsc.12352

American Evaluation Association, Task Force on Guiding Principles for Evaluators. (2004). American Evaluation Association guiding principles for evaluators. Retrieved from http://www.eval.org/p/cm/ld/fid=51

Association of State and Territorial Health Officials. (2017). Health systems transformation: Community health needs assessments. Retrieved from http://www.astho.org/Programs/Access/Community-Health-Needs-Assessments/

Centers for Disease Control and Prevention, National Center for Health Statistics. (2015). National vital statistics system. Retrieved from https://www.cdc.gov/nchs/nvss/linked-birth.htm

Centers for Disease Control and Prevention. (2016). Youth Risk Behavior Surveillance System. Retrieved from https://www.cdc.gov/healthyyouth/data/yrbs/

Centers for Disease Prevention and Control. (2018). *Atlas of United States mortality*. Retrieved from https://www.cdc.gov/nchs/products/other/atlas/atlas.htm

Community Interventions for Health. (2017). Evaluation: Process evaluation. Retrieved from http://www.oxha.org/cih_manual/index.php/process-evaluation

The Dartmouth Biomedical Library. (2016). PowerPoint: Guides, tips, and help. Retrieved from http://www.dartmouth.edu/~library/biomed/guides/powerpoint.html?mswitch-redir=classic

DC Healthy Communities Collaborative. (2016). District of Columbia community health needs assessment. Retrieved from http://assets.thehcn.net/content/sites/washingtondc/2016_DC_CHNA_062416_FINAL.pdf

Gliklich, R. E., Dreyer, N. A., & Leavy, M. B. (Eds.). (2014). *Registries for evaluating patient outcomes: A user's guide [Internet]* (3rd ed.). Rockville (MD): Agency for Healthcare Research and Quality. Retrieved from https://www.ncbi.nlm.nih.gov/books/NBK208616/?term=Registries%20for%20evaluating%20patient%20outcomes%20(3rd%20ed.)

Kleinpell, R. M. (2013). *Outcome assessment in advanced practice nursing*. New York, NY: Springer Publishing.

McKenzie, J. F., Neiger, B. L., & Thackeray, R. (2016). *Planning, implementing and evaluating health promotion programs* (7th ed.). London, UK: Pearson.

Newcomer, K. E., Hatry, H. P., & Wholey, J. S. (2015). *Handbook of practical program evaluation* (4th ed.). Hoboken, NJ: John Wiley.

Pact. (2014). Field guide for evaluation. Retrieved from http://www.pactworld.org/documents/field-guide-evaluation

Polit, D. F., & Beck, C. T. (2017). *Nursing research: Generating and assessing evidence for nursing practice* (10th ed.). Philadelphia, PA: Wolters Kluwer.

Rossi, P. H., Lipsey, M. W., & Freeman, H. E. (2004). *Evaluation: A systematic approach* (7th ed.). Thousand Oaks, CA: Sage.

Russell, L. B. (2015). *Population health: Behavioral and social science insights*. Rockville, MD: Agency for Healthcare Research and Quality. Retrieved from https://www.ahrq.gov/professionals/education/curriculum-tools/population-health/russell.html

Waltz, C. F., Strickland, O. L., & Lenz, E. R. (2017). *Measurement in nursing and health research* (5th ed.). New York, NY: Springer Publishing.

CHAPTER 20

Revising Programs

■ **STUDY EXERCISES**

1. Define the term *program revision* within the framework of the program-management model.
2. Describe the steps and issues involved in the process of program revision.
3. Compare and contrast key elements of program revision, process evaluation, quality management, and healthcare redesign.
4. What are the most common sources and types of evaluation data useful for program revision?
5. How is the immediate environment or context of a program important for its long-term viability?
6. Define *sustainability* with respect to a community health program.
7. How do key stakeholders influence the viability of a community program?
8. What political factors may influence the outcome of a community health program?

In this textbook, program evaluation is described in detail from the delineation of purposes and guiding models, to establishing plans and measuring their effectiveness, and, finally, to the actual conduct of the evaluation. The ultimate value of an evaluation depends on how its results are used (Rossi, Lipsey, & Freeman, 2004). The final component of program evaluation, therefore, is decision making about continuation, revision, or termination of a program.

Program revision is not a linear or sequential process, but rather the process requires dynamic responses to day-to-day issues and ongoing data analysis. This chapter summarizes the steps and issues involved in program revision. The discussion about program revision is guided by a program-management model and is illustrated using selected examples of program revision described in the literature. In addition, a case scenario of a community nurse-managed center that began as a grant-funded program is used to highlight salient concepts and principles of the program-evaluation and program-revision processes.

■ **WEIGHING STATISTICAL AND PRACTICAL SIGNIFICANCE**

An increasing number of evaluations of both national and international community health programs are reported in the literature using a longitudinal design. These evaluations address the initial establishment of the program and salient issues, outcomes, rationale, and recommendations for program continuation (Schaffer, Goodhue, Stennes, & Lanigan, 2012; Schwartz et al., 2014; Vaid, Ahmed, May, & Manheim, 2014). However, specific discussions or examples of proposed program modifications or revisions based on program evaluation data, specifically weighing statistical and practical significance of evaluation data, remain limited.

Approaches for Examining Significance

One excellent example described a community approach to asthma management utilizing the PRECEDE–PROCEED model to document the stages of evaluation and resulting program revisions (Fisher, Strunk, Sussman, Sykes, & Walker, 2004). The authors documented unanticipated problems with access to care and subsequently revised the program to emphasize the availability of care through a series of educational and promotional events in the community.

Predominant examples of community health program evaluation and subsequent revision were reported as community research and demonstration studies. Merzel and D'Afflitti (2003) reviewed 32 community health programs from the 1980s and 1990s. These studies included cardiovascular disease-prevention programs, such as the Stanford Five-City Project and Minnesota Heart Health Program, and HIV-prevention studies, such as the Centers for Disease Control and Prevention–sponsored AIDS Community Demonstration Project and the Women and Infants Demonstration Project. Merzel and D'Afflitti found that the majority of these program evaluations revealed modest short-term outcomes, with the exception of the HIV-prevention programs.

PROCESS EVALUATION

Chen (2015) described process evaluation as appraisal of the implementation of a program, including whether problems with implementation were identified in a timely manner and how well the program was implemented. Process evaluation requires assessing, documenting, and analyzing a program's progress. Revision is required when there is an unacceptable divergence between what was observed and what was expected. The purpose of program revision, or corrective action, is to get the program "back on track." This description of process evaluation is consistent with what Rossi et al. (2004) referred to as *program monitoring*. Managers need to continuously monitor information in order to judge the day-to-day operational performance of a program and to make necessary changes in program activities. Three essential areas are addressed when monitoring a program: (a) degree to which a program reaches the target population, (b) consistency of service delivery with the original design criteria, and (c) resource expenditure in the implementation of the program.

QUALITY MANAGEMENT

Quality management, derived from concepts originally developed by W. Edwards Deming, commonly refers to the study of "systems and processes . . . to identify and improve sources of error, waste and redundancy" (Nearpass, 1997, p. 939). Quality management uses input and feedback from key stakeholders to clarify the system problems and potential for improvement. Successful implementation of quality management requires working knowledge of data-driven decision-making methods (Maddox, 1999). Quality management is an anticipatory management approach, which allows program managers to "keep a program on track" through an explicit ongoing process of adjustment, improvement, and revision, as needed.

HEALTHCARE REDESIGN

Porter-O'Grady (1996) has outlined seven basic rules for successful healthcare redesign. These rules evolved from the premise that the healthcare delivery system is in a constant state of flux, and that change, although inevitable, can result in positive and successful outcomes. Although written for large organizations, these rules have equal applicability to smaller programs that are undergoing change. This approach to organizational redesign is grounded on the assumption that extensive and purposeful engagement of all staff is important for the health of an organization or program. This assumption is consistent with the language of program revision, process evaluation, and quality management. These basic rules are useful as operational guidelines for program revision (Box 20.1).

Although change is not always desirable to healthcare professionals, change is inherent in the process of program revision. Therefore, approaches to manage change are essential for success in adjustment or revision of a program. The first rule or guideline is clearly the most significant and sets the stage for success. Change and revision require active participation of stakeholders at every level, both internal and external to the program, and at every stage of the process. The second and third rules acknowledge the importance of leadership and vision for effective redesign or revision of a program. Specifically, leaders must anticipate future challenges and directions and instill in project staff and key stakeholders a coherent understanding of the program aims. The fourth and fifth rules address the distribution of power and decentralization of decision-making authority to the project team in order to facilitate effective action. The sixth and seventh rules focus on the importance of clarity of program goals and objectives as benchmarks for ongoing evaluation.

These seven guidelines are essential directives for success in program revision. Program revision is complex, dynamic, and multidimensional. The process of program revision encompasses formative evaluation, continuous quality management, and the basic principles of healthcare redesign.

THE PROGRAM-MANAGEMENT MODEL

An accurate, objective, and timely program evaluation provides managers with information and knowledge necessary to make judgments about areas that need adjustment if a program is to function at optimal levels and to achieve specified program goals. For revision to be ultimately successful, the overall aims and objectives of the program must

---

BOX 20.1   BASIC OPERATIONAL GUIDELINES FOR PROGRAM REVISION

1. Everyone who is affected by the change must participate and respond.
2. Effective leaders need to "read the signposts" for indications about the direction of change.
3. Leaders promote creation of a vision that articulates the meaning and direction for the work that people do.
4. Leadership builds processes and structures that empower staff closest to the delivery of services to have genuine freedom and authority to make decisions about what is done.
5. Leaders create an organizational structure that supports decentralized decision making.
6. Effective leaders have goals and plans in place that assist staff to move successfully through complexity toward desired outcomes.
7. Leaders make opportunities to focus on evaluation to measure congruence between activities and desired outcomes and goals.

Source: Adapted from Porter-O'Grady, T. (1996). The seven basic rules for successful redesign. *Journal of Nursing Administration,* *26*(1), 46–53. Used with permission.

guide decisions about program adjustment. Such adjustments or program revisions imply the need for change in existing program structures, processes, or other aspects of the program, for example, outreach to the target population.

The purpose of program evaluation is to improve the planning, implementation, and effectiveness of a program (Chen, 2015). Timely information and consideration of the objectives of a program are essential when making decisions about program improvement, continuation, or termination. Program revision, as in every other step in the development and management of programs, is grounded in data that provide the information necessary for sound decision making (Glick, Thompson, & Ridge, 1999). Program revision can be conceptualized using a cyclic model of program evaluation and management, as illustrated in Figure 20.1.

Practical Significance. The model shown in Figure 20.1 illustrates the use of evaluation data as a program-management tool. Evaluation data serve as the basis for decision making within the continuous, cyclic process of program planning and evaluation. Initial assessment data reveal patterns of health needs and resource utilization within the designated population. This information serves as the foundation for the development and implementation of initial program structure, policy, and process. Subsequent information about program structure and process provides guidance for specific dimensions of program implementation such as staffing, budgeting, and service utilization. This feedback provides the direction and focus for ongoing management decisions.

The final type of information, outcome data, is the critical substance of evaluation. Outcome data are used to make judgments about the future of the program. Outcome data include measures of program outcomes such as client health status, program costs, measures of cost-effectiveness, and client satisfaction. Outcome measures are combined with updated assessment of community health status and resources to provide a comprehensive evaluation of program status and community need.

This program-management model is data driven and focuses on the continuous, cyclic processes of planning and evaluation. The model was originally developed for use in

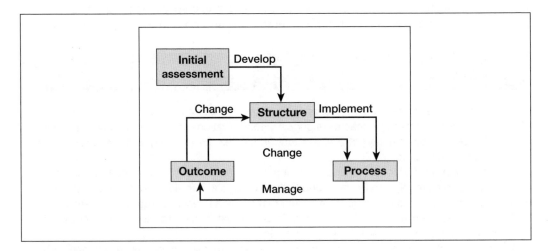

FIGURE 20.1 The role of data in program evaluation.

Source: © Glick, D. F., Thompson, K. M., & Ridge, R. A. (1999). Population-based research: The foundation for development, management, and evaluation of a community nursing center. *Family & Community Health*, *21*(4), 41–50. Retrieved from http://journals.lww.com/familyandcommunityhealth/Abstract/1999/01000/Population_Based_Research__The_Foundation_for.6.aspx

management and evaluation of a community nursing center. The immediate environment or context of a program is equally important for its long-term viability and success. The environment includes cultural, economic, political, and social forces with the potential to influence the processes of program development, implementation, management, and change.

Lancaster (1999) characterized planned change as "intentional and thought-out, occurs over time, and includes mutual goal setting, and equal power distribution, and deliberation" (p. 151). Planned change is a complex process involving many people and issues. Creative ideas must be communicated and are either accepted or rejected. The classic theories about change, developed by Lewin (1951), Rogers (1962), and Lippitt (1973), tend to focus on the behavior, motivators, and responses of individuals within organizations (Lancaster, 1999). Although individual behavior is not the focus of this chapter, it must be noted that program revision involves individuals, and, therefore, the success of program change is inevitably tied to the level of acceptance and resistance among participants.

The results of change within an organization may include improved flexibility and ability to respond, enhanced ability to meet existing needs, and increased consistency between the organizational mission and program capacity and accomplishments. It is not unusual, however, for plans for revision to produce distress, resistance, and a sense of loss among participants who are affected by the proposed change (Sebastian, 1999).

■ SUSTAINABILITY

Issues of sustainability or institutionalization of the program, terms often used interchangeably, are inherent in program revision. The concept of sustainability is multidimensional. It is a dynamic continuation process that encompasses diverse forms (Cramm, Phaff, & Nieboer, 2013).

One of the most perplexing issues that program directors inevitably face is sustainability and viability of the program beyond its initial funding period. Unfortunately, it is common for community-oriented health programs to be discontinued after the initial funding cycle ends. Therefore, attention to long-term viability is a focal point for funding agencies and policy makers when allocating scarce resources (Cramm et al., 2013). Long-term viability of a program is an intended outcome of the process of program management and a specific aim of program revision.

Community-based primary care programs that serve low-income populations face formidable challenges to achieving sustainability, and for those programs that are nurse managed, the obstacles are compounded. Many of the nursing services provided in such settings are not reimbursable through conventional payment mechanisms, and most low-income clients have marginal health insurance coverage. Potential financial problems in such settings may include loss of patients to managed care organizations that contract with state Medicaid agencies, difficulty in attracting patients with better reimbursement potential, frequent staff turnover, and an inability to break even financially (Ervin, Chang, & White, 1998).

Program Adjustment

Decisions about the next phase of the program are made on the basis of program evaluation data, including program outcomes, updated needs assessment of the target population, and availability of funding and resources. A decision may be made to close the program, to continue a program as it is, or to make changes in the structure and/or process of the organizational system to function more efficiently or effectively. The basis for program change can be conceptualized on a continuum from program discontinuation to continuation, as illustrated in Figure 20.2.

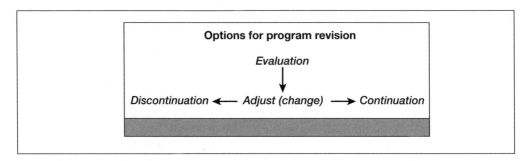

FIGURE 20.2 Program-revision model.

As depicted in Figure 20.2, continuation may vary from essentially "no change" or institutionalization of all or part of an original program structure, through levels of adjustment, and finally to total discontinuation of the program. Adjustments or revisions may also take varied forms in which an external recipient group or stakeholders outside the original organizational structure may adopt the essence of the program mission and goals. Therefore, sustainability implies a dynamic form of institutionalization or integration of a program into supporting structures, which allows the program to survive through change and adaptation to its immediate environment.

Actions to Take With Ineffective Programs

The concept of sustainability includes three explicit perspectives for consideration in the process of program revision: (a) the health benefit or outcomes of the program as originally designed, (b) continuation of the organizational structure of a program, and (c) the responsiveness and capacity of the recipient community. For program revision to achieve optimal outcomes, management decisions must take into consideration data and information about each of these perspectives analyzed in relation to the overall program mission and goals.

Programs judged to be ineffective, on the basis of timely evaluation data, must be carefully re-examined from the perspective of these three key considerations. A series of questions is useful in analyzing data and determining the appropriate course of action:

1. Was the original demand or need for the health benefit or health outcome based on valid assessment data?
2. Is the original information outdated?
3. Has the context or immediate environment of the program changed, such as the cultural, economic, political, and social environments?
4. Are changes in the program context or environment sufficient to alter the need for the program and/or the structure of the community health program?
5. Is the lack of success or sustainability of the program due in part to changes in the responsiveness or capacity of the target community to participate in the program?
6. Have the key stakeholders changed?
7. Have the resources and priorities of the key stakeholders changed markedly?

On the basis of a comprehensive assessment of the successes and failures of a community health program, decisions can be made to institute major program revisions to get the program "back on track" or perhaps to discontinue the program and assess other avenues for starting over.

■ INVOLVING THE COMMUNITY IN THE REVISION PHASE

It could be argued that every member of a community has a stake in the efficiency and effectiveness of programs to improve social conditions. In reality, stakeholders are those who have a direct and visible interest in the program, each having a different interpretation of the meaning and implications of the evaluation findings (Rossi et al., 2004). Such stakeholders include program staff, clients served, the sponsoring organization, funding sources, policy makers, competitive organizations, and the overall community. Involvement of stakeholder community organizations and grassroots members of the community in the planning, evaluation, and revision of a program fosters ongoing community acceptance, client participation, and organizational support for the program.

For community programs to be successful, collaborative partnerships with agencies and organizations that have a stake in the operation or outcome of the program should be established early in the development of a program and should continue through evaluation and program revision. These working relationships among community organizations require consensus about program goals and resources and about respective roles and domains.

The Health Resources and Services Administration (HRSA) led two successful public–private partnerships directed toward the goal of ensuring that vulnerable and underserved populations have access to quality healthcare and to advance education and practice of primary care (Gordon, Kavanagh, Crump, Heppel, & Fiori, 1998). One strategy toward accomplishing this goal was to foster and study the issues and outcomes of public–private partnerships. The lessons learned from this strategy that are relevant for the development and sustenance of community health partnerships include the need to address (a) effective integration of perspectives and resources among participating organizations; (b) development of effective communication to intended groups; (c) dealing with issues relating to leadership, problem solving, and decision-making skills among participating organizations; and (d) aligning respective organizational goals in order to provide an appropriate mix of services to the community. Communication and consensus among participating parties are essential for effective collaboration. The challenges of working together are justified by the outcomes, that is, organizations working together can accomplish what neither can do alone.

Another component that is crucial to successful program revision is grassroots participation by the beneficiaries of the program. These are the community members whose acceptance and participation are essential to the success of the day-to-day operation of the program. Although these community members are the population who has the largest stake in the program's outcome, they are usually the least able to make their voices heard. These beneficiaries of the program tend to be unorganized, geographically scattered, and frequently undereducated and unable to communicate politically.

When such beneficiaries are not likely to be heard during discussions about program development or revision, organizations that represent their interests may speak on their behalf. For example, although homeless people are rarely heard in discussions about programs, the National Coalition for the Homeless frequently serves as their spokesperson (Rossi et al., 2004). (See www.nationalhomeless.org to access the website for the National Coalition for the Homeless.)

■ POLITICAL AND ORGANIZATIONAL ENVIRONMENTS FOR PROGRAM CHANGES

Changes in existing program structures or processes must be grounded in the overall goals and objectives of the project and be consistent with the mission of the larger organization to be successful. The immediate environment of a program is equally important for its long-term viability and success. The environment includes cultural, economic, political, and social forces with the potential to influence the processes of program development, implementation, management, and change.

Berk and Rossi (1999) advised that the substantive roots of program evaluation and revision rest in political concerns and issues that comprise the current "policy space." *Policy space* refers to the immediate contextual environment of a program; it is not static or fixed. Policy space adjusts over time and varies across political jurisdictions. The policy space of a community health program is defined by current political concerns and issues, which may arise at the local, regional, or national level.

The processes of program evaluation and revision are saturated with the political concerns of individuals, groups, and agencies that have an interest in the outcome of the program. These stakeholders may be the actual consumers of the service, groups representing the target or beneficiary population, healthcare providers, policy makers at the state or national level, or agency officials. Ultimately, stakeholders may have different views of important program outcomes: (a) whether the program achieved its purposes and objectives, (b) consistency of service delivery with the original plan, and (c) appropriate resource expenditure for the desired result. Different perspectives and goals among stakeholders may result in different interpretations of the meaning and significance of evaluation data.

Decisions about the outcome of a program evaluation may be influenced by the social worth of a program, the cost-effectiveness of that program, and availability and distribution of resources. Small changes have greater significance when the social worth of the change is great. For example, a program that increased immunization rates among a target group of preschool children by 5% may not be considered worthy, whereas a program of equal cost that decreased the teenage death rate from automobile crashes by 1% may be considered very worthwhile.

The outcome of a program evaluation, therefore, is a process that may be grounded in objective evaluation data but driven by a political process of negotiating and balancing different perspectives and interests. The goal of social programs is to make optimal use of existing resources without creating additional inequities. Decision makers may have to weigh competing arguments and values in making judgments about whether to continue, revise, or discontinue a program.

■ THE CASE OF A PRIMARY CARE COMMUNITY NURSING CENTER

In 1991, the University of Virginia School of Nursing began to explore the feasibility of developing a nurse-managed center to address the unmet health needs of an underserved population of low-income residents of public housing.

Initial Assessment

As part of this initial decision-making phase, community health assessment data were gathered that focused on the health status of the target population and on availability and accessibility of resources in the community to meet those needs (Glick, Hale, Kulbok, & Shettig, 1996). Specific factors that emerged during the assessment included (a) lack of transportation as a major barrier to health service utilization, (b) overuse of the emergency room for primary care, (c) high prevalence of chronic diseases, and (d) child health and parenting concerns. This assessment provided data for decisions about initial development of the program. Later in the cycle of program management, project relevance was evaluated by comparing assessment data with actual demand for clinic services (Glick et al., 1996). The initial assessment data served as baseline data for the evaluation of the relevance of the program.

Development of Structure and Process

In 1992 and 1993, small grants and gifts were obtained to support the program. In the fall of 1993, a major federal grant was obtained to support the program for 6 years. Two clinics were established in public housing with three overriding goals: (a) service—providing primary care services for underserved, low-income residents of the community; (2) education—creating a clinical setting to educate nursing students in the provision of primary care for vulnerable residents of the community; and (3) research—serving as a setting for faculty and student research. One clinic was in a high-rise for elderly and disabled residents, and the other served families composed of predominantly single mothers and their children. The local housing authority provided clinic space, and each clinic was staffed by a School of Nursing faculty member and by a receptionist/secretary. At one of the clinics, the secretary also served as a nursing-care aide. Over time, this structure and process became institutionalized into the existing organizational structures of the School of Nursing, the Housing Authority, and various collaborating agencies within the community.

Outcomes Evaluation and Change

Formative program evaluation is a continuous process of data gathering and weighing statistical and practical significance to measure progress toward program goals. For example, outcomes of the 1998 data related to program goals are as follows: (a) service—the two clinics provided 3,900 patient visits for community residents; (b) education—40 school of nursing undergraduate students had a full semester of clinical experience at the clinics, and five graduate students worked with the program; and (c) research and scholarship—five manuscripts were published or accepted for publication, and there were three presentations at national meetings by nursing center faculty and/or graduate students.

Clinic services were adjusted on an ongoing basis to meet the changing needs of the population. As a case in point, since 1993 the demographic profile and health needs of the residents at the high-rise for the elderly and disabled had changed. Formerly, most of the residents were elderly people, with a small number of younger persons who had physical disabilities. Over time, more of the new residents of the facility were younger people with psychiatric disabilities. This created a new set of health needs and nursing challenges. When the nurse faculty who served that clinic resigned, a decision was made to replace her with a psychiatric clinical nurse specialist who had extensive experience working with the elderly. This program adjustment was based on assessment data about the changed composition of residents and was implemented to ensure that the program remained relevant for the population.

An essential component of the success of a program is community involvement. As an example, at one time some community residents and school of nursing faculty questioned whether the hours that the clinic operated were the best times to meet the needs of community members. The Public Housing Residents Association took the initiative to develop a survey of residents about clinic services. They collaborated with School of Nursing faculty in developing survey items. A question that addressed residents' needs and expectations about optimal clinic operating hours was included. The Residents Association implemented the survey. Responses to the survey indicated that clients were satisfied with current clinic hours, and, as a result, a decision was made not to alter the clinic operating hours. As this example illustrates, in some circumstances, data may be gathered for purposes of program revision; however, the statistical and practical implications of the data may support a decision not to make program alterations.

The political environment has a profound effect on program revisions and changes. This is especially true in regard to program sustainability. The political arena where nursing centers, as all other health programs, must compete for finite resources is complex. The challenge to compete for limited resources became evident early in the program. As services were implemented and became established at the high-rise for the elderly and disabled, it became apparent that there was an overlap in services provided at the nursing clinic and by home healthcare agencies. Moreover, the clinic nurse was involved with most of these ill patients on a day-to-day basis over a long period and was knowledgeable about the needs and problems of each patient. Home health nurses, who frequently did not know the patients, came to the clinic nurse for background information, consultation, and collaboration. At the same time, program administrators were seeking ways to create program income to sustain the program.

A plan was developed and implemented to set up contracts with two local home health agencies for the clinic nurse to provide home health services when prescribed for public housing residents and for the nursing center to be reimbursed by the home health agencies for these services. For several years after the contracts were signed, this arrangement worked well and the nursing center realized some income to support future sustainability. Political realities and economic constraints, however, gradually undermined this arrangement. When home health referrals from local hospitals decreased, the home health agencies needed work for existing staff and stopped referring public housing residents to the clinic nurse for home health services. Hence, the nursing center no longer received this income. This is just one example of how the political and economic environments can impede progress toward meeting program goals and force undesired program alterations.

The future of the nursing center on the continuum of program revision (Figure 20.2) was contingent on issues related to program sustainability. A multitiered approach was used to address sustainability. Strategies included developing a billing system for third-party payment, seeking additional grant funding, seeking contracts for selected services, and developing a collaborative arrangement for city and university support. Complex political, economic, social, and/or regulatory obstacles influenced each of these approaches. The obstacles included state and federal regulatory complexities that impeded reimbursement for nursing services, resistance by physicians to billing for nursing services, competition among agencies for finite local resources, and a dearth of available grant funding to sustain existing programs. Such challenges to sustainability are common among academic nursing centers (Mackey & McNiel, 1997; Schwartz et al., 2014).

For over 6 years, the nursing center fulfilled its fundamental goals of service, education, and research. There was strong grassroots support from the community for continuation of the program, and the School of Nursing was committed to this goal. However, with the inability to garner adequate funding and/or reimbursement for nursing services, program adjustment was inevitable. The nursing center has continued in two public housing locations with modified service levels. Support of the school of nursing, a local community hospital, a regional Area Agency on Aging, and public/community health nurse volunteers have contributed to revised, yet sustained clinic services.

■ SUMMARY

In this chapter, models and issues of program revision as the final step in the process of program evaluation were examined. Some examples of program revision were discussed. Program revision consists of adjusting program structure or process on the basis of a dynamic and ongoing process of data-driven decision making. The purpose of program revision is to take some corrective action to keep the program progressing toward its goals and overall purpose. Options for program revision lie on a continuum from the decision to discontinue a program to various degrees of adjustments, or the decision to continue with minimal or no change. The ultimate program revision issue that must be addressed by established programs is that of sustainability. At every stage in the process, community and staff participation in documenting issues and in decision making is critical for successful program revision.

■ SUGGESTED CLINICAL OR PRACTICUM ACTIVITIES

1. Identify two long-standing community-based health programs in your region (e.g., free clinic, parish nursing, community medication disposal program). Interview the program director and an advanced public/community health nurse about major issues related to sustainability of the program and/or steps required for program revision.
2. With data collected related to activity #1, describe factors that may influence a decision to adjust a program versus a decision to discontinue, start the program over, or design a new program.

REFERENCES

Berk, R. A., & Rossi, P. H. (1999). *Thinking about program evaluation* (2nd ed.). Thousand Oaks, CA: Sage.
Chen, H. T. (2015). *Practical program evaluation: Theory-driven evaluation and the integrated evaluation perspective* (2nd ed.). Los Angeles, CA: Sage.
Cramm, J. M., Phaff, S., & Nieboer, A. P. (2013). The role of partnership functioning and synergy in achieving sustainability of innovative programmes in community care. *Health and Social Care in the Community, 21*(2), 209–215. doi:10.1111/hsc.12008
Ervin, N. E., Chang, W. Y., & White, J. (1998). A cost analysis of a nursing center's services. *Nursing Economic$, 16*(6), 307–312.
Fisher, E. B., Strunk, R. C., Sussman, L. K., Sykes, R. K., & Walker, M. S. (2004). Community organization to reduce the need for acute care for asthma among African American children in low-income neighborhoods: The Neighborhood Asthma Coalition. *Pediatrics, 114*(1), 116–123.
Glick, D. F., Hale, P. J., Kulbok, P. A., & Shettig, J. (1996). Community development theory: Planning a community nursing center. *Journal of Nursing Administration, 26*(7-8), 1–7.
Glick, D. F., Thompson, K. M., & Ridge, R. A. (1999). Population-based research: The foundation for development, management, and evaluation of a community nursing center. *Family & Community Health, 21*(4), 41–50. Retrieved from http://journals.lww.com/familyandcommunityhealth/Abstract/1999/01000/Population_Based_Research__The_Foundation_for.6.aspx
Gordon, L. V., Kavanagh, L. D., Crump, R., Heppel, D., & Fiori, F. (1998). Learning to broaden the impact of health resources through public-private partnerships. *Journal of Health Education, 29*(5 Suppl.), S34–S39.
Lancaster, J. (Ed.). (1999). *Nursing issues in leading and managing change.* St. Louis, MO: Mosby.
Lewin, K. (1951). *Field theory in social science.* New York, NY: Harper & Row.
Lippitt, G. L. (1973). *Visualizing change: Model building and the change process.* La Jolla, CA: University Associates.
Mackey, T. A., & McNiel, N. O. (1997). Success stories: Negotiating private sector partnerships with academic nursing centers. *Nursing Economic$, 15*(1), 52–55.
Maddox, P. J. (1999). Quality management in nursing practice. In J. Lancaster (Ed.), *Nursing issues in leading and managing change.* St. Louis, MO: Mosby.
Merzel, C., & D'Afflitti, J. (2003). Reconsidering community-based health promotion: Promise, performance, and potential. *American Journal of Public Health, 93*(4), 557–574.
Nearpass, M. M. (1997). "Managed competition 101" syllabus. In M. D. Harris (Ed.), *Handbook of home health care administration* (2nd ed.). Gaithersburg, MD: Aspen.

Porter-O'Grady, T. (1996). The seven basic rules for successful redesign. *Journal of Nursing Administration,* *26*(1), 46–53.

Rogers, E. M. (1962). *Diffusion of innovations.* New York, NY: Free Press of Glencoe.

Rossi, P. H., Lipsey, M. W., & Freeman, H. E. (2004). *Evaluation: A systematic approach* (7th ed.). Newbury Park, CA: Sage.

Schaffer, M. A., Goodhue, A., Stennes, K., & Lanigan, C. (2012). Evaluation of a public health nurse visiting program for pregnant and parenting teens. *Public Health Nursing, 29*(3), 218–231. doi:10.1111/j.1525-1446.2011.01005.x

Schwartz, S. M., Mason, S. T., Wang, C., Pomana, L., Hyde-Nolan, M. E., & Carter, E. W. (2014). Sustained economic value of a wellness and disease prevention program: An 8-year longitudinal evaluation. *Population Health Management, 17*(2), 90–99. doi:10.1089/pop.2013.0042

Sebastian, J. G. (1999). Organizational theory and the change process. In J. Lancaster (Ed.), *Nursing issues in leading and managing change.* St. Louis, MO: Mosby.

Vaid, I., Ahmed, K., May, D., & Manheim, D. (2014). The WISEWOMAN program: Smoking prevalence and key approaches to smoking cessation among participants, July 2008–June 2013. *Journal of Women's Health, 23*(4), 288–295. doi:10.1089/jwh.2013.4712

SECTION VI

Future Directions for
Specialty Practice

CHAPTER 21

The Practice Environment

■ STUDY EXERCISES

1. What are the major components of graduate preparation for advanced practice in public/community health nursing?
2. What types of practice venues are projected for practice in the future?
3. Why is a professional practice environment important for public/community health nursing services?
4. What barriers exist for developing a professional practice environment?
5. What factors serve to facilitate the use of research in practice?
6. What activities might the advanced practice public/community health nurse conduct to increase research utilization in policy formulation?

The practice environment for public/community health nurses varies with many factors such as the location of the practice, the focus of the service and programs, leadership for the practice, and autonomy for developing policies that direct practice. A professional practice environment provides the foundation for effective, quality, evidence-based care.

■ GRADUATE PREPARATION FOR PRACTICE

Educational preparation for practice in public/community health nursing has undergone changes over the years since the first edition of this book was published. Several graduate programs have been closed and others have been changed to doctor of nursing practice (DNP) programs. The need for graduate preparation in public/community health nursing is more relevant nowadays than ever, but the interest in such programs has been replaced by increased student interest in nurse practitioner and clinical nurse specialist (CNS) programs with focus on care of the individual.

As a first choice for graduate preparation for public/community health nursing practice, the potential student should enroll in a master's or DNP public health/community health nursing program. These programs provide the breadth and depth of knowledge and skills needed for graduates to practice the full scope of specialty practice in advanced practice in public/community health nursing. The content of such graduate programs is outlined in Chapter 1. Several strong programs are found around the United States.

A second choice would be for the student to enroll in a graduate nursing program that could be augmented by course work in public health, either online or in person. A master's or doctoral program with a focus on primary care would be useful for job flexibility as well as allow the student to incorporate in practice the public health foundational knowledge, for example, advocacy, community assessment, community outreach, health equity, and interprofessional practice. As population health management evolves in the changing healthcare system, many healthcare practices are enhancing their services by recognizing the need for prevention of disease and injury to the community at large while providing primary care to those who come to the clinic for service.

A third pattern for obtaining graduate preparation for nurses interested in graduate preparation in public/community health nursing practice is enrollment in a nursing administration program augmented with public health courses such as epidemiology, community assessment, program planning and evaluation, and environmental health. Clinical experiences should be obtained in health departments or nonprofit organizations that deal with aggregates or populations located in communities.

There are several other options to obtain knowledge and competency in the advanced practice of public/community health nursing. Dual master of science in nursing [MSN]/ master of public health (MPH) and DNP/MPH programs are available in some parts of the country, but are not prevalent. The advantage of these programs is the potential for graduates to be certified in both public health nursing and public health. Although the curriculums of dual-degree programs provide firm foundations in both nursing and public health, the programs are often longer than some doctoral programs.

Master's and doctoral programs for CNS preparation are usually focused on care of ill individuals as well as systems. These programs may be appropriate if the flexibility is available to allow the student to have clinical placements in health departments and other community organizations. The added benefit of these programs is that the graduate may qualify for certification as a CNS and bill for services in a practice setting.

Finally, many accredited DNP programs across the United States include content relevant to the advanced practice of public/community health nursing. Common courses and content, based on *The Essentials of Doctoral Education for Advanced Nursing Practice* (American Association of Colleges of Nursing [AACN], 2006), frequently included in a DNP program and an advanced public/community health program are epidemiology, finance and resource management, global public health, health policy, health promotion and disease prevention, health services administration, information technology, population health management, and program planning and evaluation. This course work could be augmented with clinical practice and scholarly projects that focus on populations and public health problems.

■ LOCATIONS FOR PRACTICE IN THE FUTURE

Although several locations for advanced public/community health nursing have been presented in previous chapters, some additional locations are briefly discussed in this section.

Global Practice Locations

Many opportunities exist for public/community health nurses to provide care in countries outside the United States. Preparation for such assignments should include learning the dominant language of the country, becoming familiar with the culture and norms of the society, gaining a working knowledge of the governmental and healthcare structures, and orienting one's self to the pertinent nurse practice laws.

Several organizations sponsor healthcare professionals to serve in countries across the globe. A search for the right fit for an international placement or employment should start with identifying your objectives and comfort level with aspects of a potential location. The length and terms of an employment site will be important to consider, such as a short-term stint of 2 weeks to 3 months or a 1-year contract. Some placements include travel expenses to return home after 6 months or so. Consider whether the position requires the skills that you possess or do you need to augment the knowledge and skills acquired in a graduate program and in your practice experience.

Nonprofit organizations offer short-term opportunities to explore work in the United States or in other countries. The American Red Cross and other organizations periodically issue calls for assistance after natural disasters, such as hurricanes, earthquakes, and floods. A short-term volunteer experience may provide you with knowledge about how you might adjust to a longer term employment placement.

Walk-In Urgent Care Clinics

Walk-in urgent care clinics, not usually thought of as locations for primary prevention and health promotion, hold great promise for promoting many aspects of public health if approached with programs that match the needs of the populations who use the facilities. One position for an advanced public/community health nurse would be the manager of the clinic. This position would allow the nurse to develop programs and services to promote continuity of care; provide health education, anticipatory guidance, and counseling to prevent illnesses and injury; follow-up with primary care providers; and provide referrals for other social and healthcare services.

Assisted Living Facilities

Most residents of assisted living facilities are people considered elderly. However, many are in relatively good health and able to care for themselves. The potential roles for an advanced practice public/community health nurse are varied. Activities to maintain mobility and cognitive skills may not be present in all assisted living facilities. Programs developed to maintain and enhance balance, flexibility, strength, and cardiovascular health would benefit most residents in such facilities. Other programs to help residents maintain cognitive ability would benefit both residents and staff in keeping residents more independent and safer. In addition, the advanced public/community health nurse can support informal family caregivers who are dealing with challenges of looking after their family members with Alzheimer's disease and related dementia in home- or community-based settings.

The barrier to most of these types of programs is funding. Advanced practice public/community health nurses have the skills to write grant proposals to fund programs and prove the cost-effectiveness of such programs.

Public Housing Associations

In most communities, public housing is rental housing, for example, single-dwelling homes, apartments, or high-rises, which are well kept and safe. It is provided for eligible individuals or families who are in the low-income category, elderly, or disabled. The health needs of these individuals and families are often substantial. Advanced public/community health nurses may have an opportunity to work in a primary care or nursing clinic that delivers basic health services, including primary prevention, health education, health maintenance, case management, and referral. In addition, advanced public/community health nurses may write grants to deliver nursing services in public housing. (Refer to Chapter 20 for an example of a grant-funded primary care nursing clinic.)

The challenge for these primary care or nursing clinics in public housing, which are often grant funded, is sustainability. Despite the clear need for services to these vulnerable populations, there are often issues with provider reimbursement and other practice barriers. Some of these clinics may be operated with volunteer nursing services, or they may use a model such as parish nursing. Volunteers are often the mainstay of these clinics. These types of settings provide opportunity for retired public/community health nurses to continue to serve their communities.

Elected Official and Officials' Offices

Running for elected office is not a usual pattern for public health nurses, but as an elected official, an advanced public/community health nurse could have a great influence on the health of communities. In general, people who run for elected office have been active in their local political party and start by running for local offices such as county commissioner, school board member, or mayor. In addition, many individuals serve on appointed boards and committees such as boards of health.

Professional Nursing and Public Health Associations

An expectation of advanced nursing practice is membership and active involvement in professional nursing organizations such as the American Nurses Association (ANA) or Sigma Theta Tau International (STTI). In addition, advanced public/community health nurses most often join the American Public Health Association (APHA), Public Health Nursing Section, and state and regional affiliate organizations. (For more information, see the organization's website www.APHA.org.) Working at the regional level is an excellent way to build confidence and skills in a leadership role, first as a committee member and then as chair to pave the way for greater involvement at the state or national level. Another important organization for advanced public/committee health nurses who desire a professional career in academia is the Association of Community Health Nursing Educators (ACHNE; see the association's website www.ACHNE.org).

▪ CREATING A PROFESSIONAL PRACTICE ENVIRONMENT

In general, *environment* refers to the conditions and characteristics of an organization. In this instance, the practice environment means the conditions and characteristics of the nursing service, both tangible (e.g., equipment, staff, and the physical facilities) and intangible (e.g., communication patterns, philosophy of the nursing service, and values; Simms, Price, & Ervin, 2000).

Characteristics of a professional practice environment include the following:

- Autonomy of the nursing staff to make patient care decisions
- Accountability of the nursing staff for decisions made and outcomes of care
- Adherence to the professional ethical code of practice
- Flexibility to incorporate new knowledge into practice and pursue effective and efficient patterns of meeting client needs

Creating a Professional Practice Foundation

Elements necessary for a professional practice foundation include use of theory; employment of baccalaureate-, master's-, and doctoral-prepared nurses; maintenance of a quality-assessment and improvement system; and the direction of a qualified nursing administrator. The environment for professional practice includes components such as effective communication patterns, philosophy of the agency, values, and supportive leadership styles (Simms et al., 2000).

As part of the internal environment, *climate* is "the psychological atmosphere that results from and surrounds the operation of the structure; consequently, it is both a result of and a determinant of the behavior of individuals and groups within the structure" (Jones, 1981, p. 160). The climate of an organization is important because it serves as a link between such factors as policies and organizational structure and end results such as satisfaction and turnover (McMahon, Ivancevich, & Matteson, 1977).

Building Blocks for Creating a Professional Practice Environment

The development of a professional practice environment takes time. Success is more likely if building blocks are put into place and are functioning well as the foundation of a professional practice environment. The specific building blocks for a professional practice environment will vary somewhat from institution to institution but have some commonalities. Three broad building blocks are staff involvement in policy and procedure decisions, a quality-assessment and improvement system, and access to research literature.

STAFF INVOLVEMENT

The involvement of staff in decisions about policy, procedures, and other aspects of the practice environment is crucial for the development of skills to be involved in implementing a professional nursing practice. The skills required for committee work, effective communication, leadership, persuasion, and analysis, as well as clinical expertise, will be needed for the work.

One key ingredient of professional practice is use of knowledge. Use of knowledge may be examined within the diffusion of innovations model developed by Rogers (1995). Diffusion is "the process by which an *innovation* is *communicated* through certain *channels* over *time* among the members of a *social system*" (p. 10). The use of knowledge requires the convictions that using the knowledge will be helpful and that the individual can use the knowledge.

QUALITY-ASSESSMENT AND QUALITY-IMPROVEMENT SYSTEM

The processes involved in assessing and improving the quality of nursing care are related to those used in research utilization. Furthermore, the use of research in improving nursing care is included in most quality-assessment and quality-improvement systems. The use of research is usually most prominent when the action to correct a deficiency is addressed. For example, if it is found that patients being discharged from home care are unable to name their medications and state the times they are to be taken, a program to correct this situation may be based on what the research tells us will work.

ACCESS TO LITERATURE

Being able to access literature is crucial because research results in the literature are used to develop research-based protocols. Some community agencies have their own libraries, but this is less the case in small agencies where maintaining a library of current journals is expensive and requires funding beyond the scope of most small agencies' budgets.

However, no longer is it the case that the literature needs to be present in an agency for staff to benefit. Access to literature via the Internet is a cost-effective avenue for increasing the availability of some literature. Connection to the Internet allows searches to be completed at the agency. Following the identification of appropriate references, copies of some articles can be obtained via the Internet, whereas others can be obtained at university, hospital, medical center, and community college libraries.

To facilitate access to university libraries, library privileges should be requested when staff are given adjunct faculty appointments. Another method for increasing access to literature is to appoint nursing faculty to agency committees. Faculty usually have resources to locate and copy articles. At times, students may be asked to share information they have received in their programs.

Assessing the Practice Environment and Climate

The advanced practice public/community health nurse may need to consult with the director of the agency or institution before beginning activities to determine a plan for research-based practice. Sharing the vision for where nursing can be more effective and seeking suggestions from the nurse's superior are often productive ways to engage the individual and get support for the endeavor. At times, a formal proposal may be prepared and presented so that the details of the agreement are documented.

An assessment of the practice environment provides information needed by the advanced practice public/community health nurse to develop the plan and strategies for implementing a research-based nursing service. A survey of the staff will provide a great deal of information about the practice environment and attitudes toward research-based practice. Box 21.1 contains suggestions about areas to include in a survey of staff. A review of the barriers and facilitators discussed in the literature will provide other ideas about questions to include in a survey.

Other surveys may be conducted to obtain information about readiness of the organization for research-based nursing practice. One such survey that may be useful is one of the other disciplines with which nursing works most closely. Any change in nursing practice will no doubt create the need for some change in other disciplines. For example, if nursing changes the time of day for doing a specific procedure in home care, therapists may need to adjust their schedules to accommodate the nursing change.

Although these changes may seem minor on first examination, resentments or conflicts may arise over such seemingly arbitrary changes on the part of nursing. In some situations, it may be advantageous to develop an interprofessional, research-based service rather than nursing attempting to accomplish this alone. For example, in home healthcare services, several disciplines work together frequently to provide care to the same individual or family. A plan to include all or most disciplines in these types of situations will, perhaps, have more chance for success than nursing alone. Another approach is to report on the activities at interprofessional administrative meetings to keep the other discipline heads informed.

In circumstances where nursing is the dominant service (e.g., public health nursing services), or the only service (e.g., community nursing center), the advanced practice public/community health nurse may proceed with a nursing-only approach with some comfort. However, never is it entirely safe to assume that changes in nursing practice in one agency will not have effects within and/or outside the agency.

Surveying Staff About Skills and Knowledge

To obtain information efficiently, a survey of the staff about the practice environment can be combined with questions about their skills and knowledge of research. Standardized survey instruments may be used such as the one used in the Conduct and Utilization of

BOX 21.1   SUGGESTIONS FOR A SURVEY OF STAFF ABOUT THE PRACTICE ENVIRONMENT

Support in the Organization for Making Changes in Practice

How much new practice information is introduced by the nurse manager?

Are staff encouraged to attend continuing-education programs?

Is funding provided for staff to participate in learning activities?

Are staff given time to go to the library or to read professional literature?

Do physicians and other professionals look to nursing for the latest in care techniques and interventions?

Attitudes of the Staff Toward Research-Based Practice

Do staff like to attend research activities, for example, presentations, journal club meetings, conferences?

To what extent do staff think that research is an ivory-tower activity that does not have practical application?

To what extent do staff think that using research provides challenges?

To what extent do staff think that anything not directly related to patient care is a waste of time?

To what extent is staffing not adequate to allow time for involvement in research activities?

Staff Morale and Feelings About the Organization

To what extent do staff like working at the agency?

How much do staff work together?

To what extent are supervisors supportive of staff?

In what ways do supervisors support staff?

Research in Nursing (CURN) study (Horsley, Crane, Crabtree, & Wood, 1983), or an instrument may be constructed. Examples of questions to be used in such a survey are presented in Box 21.2.

Another approach to use to obtain a great deal of information in a short period of time is to conduct focus-group studies involving a cross-section of the staff or with representatives of various categories of staff (e.g., advanced practice nurses, staff nurses, ancillary staff). Having the focus groups conducted by an outside person may also provide an atmosphere for staff to be open about their ideas and opinions. An overview of focus groups can be found in Chapter 6.

The information about attitudes, skills, and knowledge provides the advanced practice public/community health nurse with the starting point for a plan. For example, if the staff have positive attitudes about using research, a plan could begin with developing skills and knowledge to use research in practice. This may entail holding in-service programs for some staff, whereas others may need to take graduate research courses to become experts in specific areas (e.g., critiquing research studies, interpreting statistics).

BOX 21.2   SUGGESTIONS FOR A SURVEY ABOUT STAFF SKILLS AND KNOWLEDGE

Educational Background of Staff

Highest degree earned in nursing; year completed

Highest degree earned; year completed

Currently in school; level; area of study

Demographic Background of Staff

Age

Years worked in nursing

Positions held other than at the staff level

Professional Organization Activities

Membership in organizations

Membership on committees

Elected and appointed offices held

Community Activities

Participation in community activities

Offices held

Volunteer activities

Participation in Scholarly Activities

Presentations

Publications

Research involvement

Development of continuing-education programs

Quality-Assessment and Quality-Improvement Activities

Committee involvement

Leadership positions held

Certifications

If outside consultants are engaged to assist with some aspects of research utilization, the staff will feel more comfortable asking questions and participating if they have the skills and knowledge to be involved at a greater depth than basic nursing knowledge allows. Agency staff are in a better position than outside consultants to provide ideas about what may work best in their own agency.

Making Contacts With University Nursing Faculty

Although the preference is to have nursing faculty involved, not all universities have nursing programs. At times, a faculty member in another discipline will be appropriate and willing to help with the process of research utilization. Expertise in conducting research in health services, public health, health economics, education, psychology, and several other areas would be valuable to the endeavors of the nursing service. It is important that the advanced practice public/community health nurse has in mind exactly what is needed from the consultant because someone outside nursing may not be versed enough to guide the efforts.

A consultant knowledgable about statistics, research design, sample size, effect size, and other technical aspects of studies may provide the assistance needed for staff to determine how to use the research findings in practice. However, assistance of nursing faculty may still be needed for the translation of the research into practice protocols, if the research is not clear about the intervention. Often, research findings are more general than prescriptive, so the nursing staff must develop interventions on the basis of the research and will not always find the exact intervention protocols spelled out in journal articles (Grove, Burns, & Gray, 2013). For example, many studies have demonstrated the relationship of social support to health outcomes (Uchino, Bowen, Carlisle, & Birmingham, 2012). The exact intervention using social support may not be clearly explained in the literature or may not be appropriate for the population targeted by the nursing program. Thus, the nursing staff are left with the task of developing the details of the intervention on the basis of what the research has reported as being effective in similar situations.

Developing the Structure for Implementing Evidence-Based Practice

With the results of assessments of the nursing staff and the organization, the advanced practice public/community health nurse is ready to begin the development of the structure for implementing evidence-based practice. At this point, it is advisable to have more involvement of the other advanced practice nurses as well as nurse managers. Some of the senior staff should have been involved from the beginning, but the development stage is even more crucial for greater involvement. As with any change, the more involved staff are, often the more committed they will be to make the changes.

The following steps are suggested for the development endeavor:

1. Identify the areas of greatest discrepancy between current status and where the nursing service needs to be (e.g., more negative than positive attitudes toward research utilization).
2. Form task forces to recommend strategies for addressing the areas of discrepancy.
3. Implement strategies to correct the discrepancies.
4. Evaluate the success of correcting the discrepancies.
5. Secure the services of faculty to assist with the process of literature review and critique of research.
6. Implement the steps of the research utilization process as listed earlier in this chapter (Grove et al., 2013; Simms et al., 2000).

Evaluation of how the whole process is proceeding is important for corrections to be made early and often, if difficulties are encountered. In some situations, the process may need to be slowed down because of turnover in key positions. Strong resistance from the staff may also require slowing the process. If the number or type of nursing staff is inadequate (e.g., no master's-prepared nurses), implementation may need to be delayed until someone can be hired.

Often, the advanced practice public/community health nurse is the only master's-prepared nursing staff member in an agency. Implementation may be possible with this situation, but the burden on the public/community health nurse may be too great coupled with other job responsibilities. In these instances, consultation from nursing faculty is necessary for success of the project. If funds can be made available, a part-time faculty member may also be hired to coordinate the planning and implementation of the evidence-based practice project.

■ RESEARCH UTILIZATION FOR POLICY FORMULATION

Although not usually thought of in research utilization, policy formulation requires the use of research to be more successful in solving the problems of the country. For example, laws that require children to have immunizations before entering school have been made on the basis of the research that demonstrates that specific immunizations are effective against specific diseases. Legislation not based on research is often costly without the benefits hoped to be achieved. For example, the state of Illinois required that all people applying for marriage licenses have a test for HIV. The test was very costly at the time of the legislation, and no recommendations from the scientific community had ever intended that testing at that time be used on the general population. After a review of the results of testing, the law was repealed because the yield of positive tests was small compared with cost.

Legislation may be the result of processes other than logic, but the opportunity always exists that logic and research results will be used to write good legislation. The advanced practice public/community health nurse, with an understanding of the research utilization process, has an opportunity to influence the policy-formulation process to improve the health of communities.

The different areas of knowledge for the advanced practice public/community health nurse to acquire are the formal and informal systems of policy formulation, the points at which certain strategies may be more successful, names and positions of people who influence policy formulation and adoption, and the names of organizations that have more influence in the policy-formulation arena. Specific knowledge about these areas should be aimed at the level of policy formulation that the nurse wants to influence, that is, local, state, or federal. Legislative governmental bodies are the obvious targets for policy influence, but there are other groups that could benefit from influence on policy (Institute of Medicine, 1995; Mason, Leavitt, & Chaffee, 2014; Milio, 1981, 1996). For example, health departments may develop policies that are deterrents to access to care (e.g., only daytime, weekday hours). If low-income working families want to access health department services, they often must miss work. This is not possible without loss of pay, so services are often underutilized by the very people who they have been targeted to reach. Numerous such examples abound in the healthcare sector.

Systems of Policy Formulation

Policy formulation is the challenging process of clarifying problems with "good data and evidence about what works" in order to develop a course of action that will achieve a desired solution (Mason et al., 2014, p. 52). The plans may cover a small arena (e.g., employees in a specific business) or have far-reaching effects on every person in the United States (e.g., the tax code). The advanced practice public/community health nurse can influence policy at many different levels.

Policy is formulated both formally and informally. To have an influence on the process, the nurse must have knowledge of both the formal and informal systems of policy formulation. Basic knowledge of how governments are structured, how they function, and how bills become laws is part of preparation for nursing practice. To build on that basic knowledge, the advanced practice public/community health nurse will need to become involved in observing the process in action by activities such as attending governmental meetings, preparing and presenting testimony on proposed legislation, serving on nursing organizations' legislative committees, and volunteering to work in political campaigns.

Strategies to Influence Policy

Being a true expert in planning strategies to influence the formulation of health policy requires more than an interest in the topic and goes well beyond what can be offered in a few paragraphs in a textbook. Nonetheless, there are valuable lessons to be learned by reading, observing, and becoming involved in activities about policy.

Some nurses have completed policy internships at the national or state level. Others have been fellows in programs such as the Primary Care Health Policy Fellowship Program at the Public Health Service, which elects fellows every year from various health professions. Many nurses work as lobbyists for state nurses' associations or other organizations.

Timing is an important aspect of strategies for influencing policy. The political, social, and economic climates are key factors in determining what legislation is appropriate to introduce. Popular support for an issue is often important for politicians to pass a piece of legislation.

People Who Influence Policy Formulation

Successful influence on policy also requires knowing the officials and staff who are responsible for writing the legislation. Contacting them regularly contributes to the nurse's credibility as well as indicates interest in legislation. A technique for regular contact is to form a nurses' advisory committee with an elected official at the federal, state, or local level. Although the offer to form an advisory committee may not always be accepted, elected officials are reluctant to refuse help from voters.

Special interest groups and lobbyists form a large section of society that influences policy formulation. These groups are powerful usually because they contribute large amounts of money to election campaigns (Shi, 2014). Although nursing does contribute to campaign funds, the amount of money is so small as to be insignificant compared with the special interest groups. Knowing the names of special interest groups, lobbyists, and other players who influence policy will assist the advanced practice public/community health nurse to better plan strategies for working with officials.

■ SUMMARY

The use of research in nursing practice is an important aspect of the role of the advanced practice public/community health nurse. A practice environment that supports research utilization provides a beginning foundation for ongoing evidence-based practice. The advanced practice public/community health nurse has the knowledge and skills to lead efforts to accomplish the goal of evidence-based practice, which results in better care with more effective programs and desired outcomes.

Professional practice is characterized by autonomy, accountability, adherence to an ethical code, and flexibility to incorporate new knowledge into practice. As a foundation for professional practice, four elements needed are use of theory; baccalaureate-, master's-, and doctoral-prepared nurses; a quality-assessment and quality-improvement system; and a qualified and supportive nursing administrator.

Building blocks for a research utilization environment include a professional practice environment and at least staff involvement in policy and procedure decisions, a functioning quality-assessment and quality-improvement system, and access to research literature. Rogers's (1995) diffusion of innovations model is useful when planning for research utilization in the practice setting.

The seven-step research utilization process was discussed in application to care of the community, family, and individual. Guidelines for using research were listed. Barriers and facilitators for use of research were summarized from the literature, but each agency needs to explore its own factors to be more successful in developing an evidence-based nursing practice.

■ SUGGESTED CLINICAL OR PRACTICUM ACTIVITIES

1. Interview a registered nurse who holds an elected or appointed governmental position in your county or state.
2. Attend a public hearing of a proposed regulation or law to observe how the hearing is conducted and examine how an advanced public/community health nurse may be able to contribute to the process through testimony or other means of advocacy.
3. Meet with an advanced public/community health nurse to discuss how local ordinances or state laws affect the quality of life of a community.

REFERENCES

American Association of Colleges of Nursing. (2006). *The essentials of doctoral education for advanced nursing practice*. Washington, DC: Author. Retrieved from http://www.aacnnursing.org/DNP/DNP-Essentials

Grove, S. K., Burns, N., & Gray, J. (2013). *The practice of nursing research: Appraisal, synthesis and generation of evidence* (7th ed.). Philadelphia, PA: Saunders.

Horsley, J. A., Crane, J., Crabtree, M. K., & Wood, D. J. (1983). *Using research to improve nursing practice: A guide*. New York, NY: Grune & Stratton.

Institute of Medicine. (1995). *Nursing, health, & the environment*. Washington, DC: National Academies Press.

Jones, J. E. (1981). The organizational universe. In J. E. Jones & J. W. Pfeiffer (Eds.), *The 1981 annual handbook for group facilitators*. San Diego, CA: University Associates.

Mason, D. J., Leavitt, J. K., & Chaffee, M. K. (2014). *Policy and politics in nursing and health care*. St. Louis, MO: Elsevier, Saunders.

McMahon, J. T., Ivancevich, J. M., & Matteson, M. T. (1977). A comparative analysis of the relationship between organizational climate and job satisfaction of medical technologists. *American Journal of Medical Technology, 43*(1), 15–19.

Milio, N. (1981). *Promoting health through public policy*. Philadelphia, PA: F. A. Davis.

Milio, N. (1996). *Engines of empowerment*. Chicago, IL: Health Administration Press.

Rogers, E. M. (1995). *Diffusion of innovations* (4th ed.). New York, NY: Free Press.

Shi, L. (2014). *Introduction to health policy*. Chicago, IL: Health Administration Press.

Simms, L. M., Price, S. A., & Ervin, N. E. (2000). *The professional practice of nursing administration* (3rd ed.). Albany, NY: Delmar.

Uchino, B. N., Bowen, K., Carlisle, M., & Birmingham W. (2012). Psychological pathways linking social support to health outcomes: A visit with the "ghosts" of research past, present, and future. *Social Science & Medicine, 74*(7), 949–957.

Index